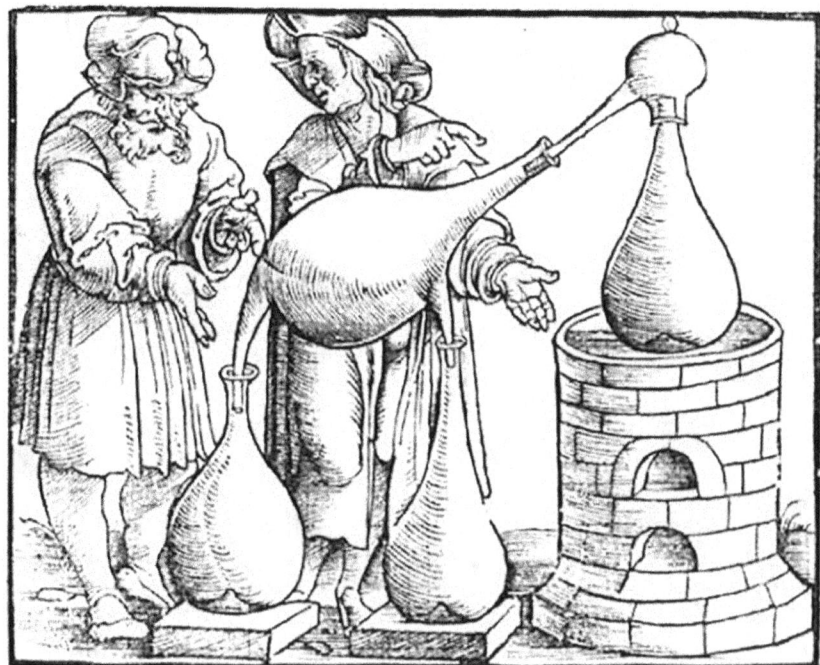

Poetry in the Clinic

This book explores previously unexamined overlaps between the poetic imagination and the medical mind. It shows how appreciation of poetry can help us to engage with medicine in more intense ways based on 'de-familiarising' old habits and bringing poetic forms of 'close reading' to the clinic.

Bleakley and Neilson carry out an extensive critical examination of the well-established practices of narrative medicine to show that non-narrative, lyrical poetry does different kind of work, previously unexamined, such as place eclipsing time. They articulate a groundbreaking 'lyrical medicine' that promotes aesthetic, ethical and political practices as well as noting the often-concealed metaphor cache of biomedicine. Demonstrating that ambiguity is a key resource in both poetry and medicine, the authors anatomise poetic and medical practices as forms of extended and situated cognition, grounded in close readings of singular contexts. They illustrate structural correspondences between poetic diction and clinical thinking, such as use of sound and metaphor.

This provocative examination of the meaningful overlap between poetic and clinical work is an essential read for researchers and practitioners interested in extending the reach of medical and health humanities, narrative medicine, medical education and English literature.

Alan Bleakley is Life Emeritus Professor of Medical Education and Medical Humanities at Plymouth Peninsula School of Medicine, UK. He is a widely published poet, psychologist, and psychotherapist, and has written many academic books, most recently *Medical Education, Politics and Social Justice: The Contradiction Cure* (Routledge 2021).

Shane Neilson is a poet and medical doctor who practises in Guelph, Ontario, Canada. He has written several books of poetry and poetry criticism. In 2022, he will publish *You May Not Take the Sad and Angry Consolations* and *Saving*.

Routledge Advances in the Medical Humanities

Storytelling Encounters as Medical Education
Crafting Relational Identity
Sally Warmington

Educating Doctors' Senses Through the Medical Humanities
"How Do I Look?"
Alan Bleakley

Medical Humanities, Sociology and the Suffering Self
Surviving Health
Wendy Lowe

A Whole Person Approach to Wellbeing
Building Sense of Safety
Johanna Lynch

Rethinking Pain in Person-Centred Health Care
Around Recovery
Stephen Buetow

Medical Education, Politics and Social Justice
The Contradiction Cure
Alan Bleakley

Poetry in the Clinic
Towards a Lyrical Medicine
Alan Bleakley and Shane Neilson

For more information about this series visit:
www.routledge.com/Routledge-Advances-in-the-Medical-Humanities/
book-series/RAMH

Poetry in the Clinic

Towards a Lyrical Medicine

Alan Bleakley and Shane Neilson

Routledge
Taylor & Francis Group

LONDON AND NEW YORK

First published 2022
by Routledge
2 Park Square, Milton Park, Abingdon, Oxon OX14 4RN

and by Routledge
605 Third Avenue, New York, NY 10158

Routledge is an imprint of the Taylor & Francis Group, an informa business

British Library Cataloguing-in-Publication Data
A catalogue record for this book is available from the British Library

Library of Congress Cataloging-in-Publication Data
A catalog record has been requested for this book

ISBN: 978-1-032-04724-9 (hbk)
ISBN: 978-1-032-19594-0 (pbk)
ISBN: 978-1-003-19440-8 (ebk)

DOI: 10.4324/9781003194408

Typeset in Bembo
by codeMantra

Shane Neilson:
For Poetry, as Poetry.

Alan Bleakley:
To my loving wife Sue and family – constant sources of inspiration and amazement

Contents

Figures

Preface

Our credo

Let's put our cards on the table. We're not sure that poetry can do anything *for* medicine. Further, hoping that poetry might act *as* medicine – or therapeutically – seems to us to be misjudged, where much poetry, like all good art, unsettles, disturbs, and even poisons received opinion. We understand the claims for poetry as therapeutic or cathartic (Shapiro 2009). But such claims are surely compromised where the poetry concerned is often mediocre or plain bad, and would not pass muster in dedicated poetry circles. If poetry acts as pharmaceutical (Sieghart 2017, 2019), then we must ask that the poetry is of good quality, tried and tested.

Our view also is that poetry is best not used instrumentally, in a means-end setting, such as aiming to *improve* medicine or medical education. Again, poems that set out to complicate, complexify, or "make strange" habitual frames of mind or activities are not really about "improvement". Rather, they question, compromise, and disturb settled definitions of "improvement". So, what is poetry *for* in medicine? Instead of addressing, or even asking, this question, we will make a statement that will act as our credo.

Our starting point is that medicine *is* poetry.

Our task is to illustrate and illuminate this claim. We even think that biomedicine, much maligned for its (necessarily) reductive linearity and informational stance, is poetry. Here's a definition of atrial fibrillation taken from an online glossary of medical diagnoses:

> Atrial fibrillation (AF or Afib) is the most common type of irregular heartbeat. It increases with age. If you have AF, the impulse does not travel in an orderly fashion through the atria. Instead, many impulses begin simultaneously and spread through the atria and compete for a chance to travel through the atrioventricular (AV) node.

Pretty dull, standard biomedical fare, no? The purely informational content is freighted in stark technical terms further reduced to initialisation (AF, Afib, AV). There are also the plain descriptive sentences: "the most common type",

"It increases with age". Yet the passage is not purely informational because, inevitably, metaphor and imaginative content creeps in: "the impulse does not travel in an orderly fashion" could have been used to dryly describe the beginning of a love affair, especially as the impulse is located in the heart; and then "many impulses ... compete for a chance to travel" suggests that our affections are scrambled as metaphor emerges and engages. Furthermore, the phrase "compete for a chance to travel" brings the imagination to bear, so that you see and feel these itchy "impulses" getting more impulsive. No matter how buttoned-down language seems, there is poetry straining against the seams, it seems (where poetry lurks, puns – good, bad, and indifferent – will be close by).

Metaphors are common in clinical medicine. For example, when an occluded artery becomes "furred up", or a heart attack becomes "central, crushing chest pain" we shift register from information to metaphor. Resemblances or likenesses of this kind are particularly common in clinical diagnostic work (Bleakley 2017). Gwinyai Masukume (Masukume and Zumla 2012), an obstetrician and public health researcher, collects and curates medical metaphors (https://foodmedicaleponyms.blogspot.com/), lovingly describing some cherry-picked likenesses such as "cauliflower warts" and "chocolate cysts". As we move into areas of medicine such as global public health, we find high rates of metaphor frequency. In a recent article on vaccine hesitancy across African nations, Danielle Ofri (2021) notes "an unsettling aspect of global health" illustrated by "The Nigerian vaccine boycott":

> ... even the most strenuously wrought achievements—ones that required years of painstaking logistical, financial, and diplomatic effort—could be gutted by the mere puff of rumor. The local strain of polio ultimately spread to twenty countries, as far afield as Yemen, Saudi Arabia, and Indonesia. Fifteen hundred children were paralyzed; it cost a half-billion dollars to contain the outbreak. The lesson ... was that global vaccination efforts would never succeed without a detailed understanding of rumor and a rigorous process for creating trust.

Here, a doctor (also an accomplished writer) commenting on a public health issue draws heavily on tried and tested metaphors ("vaccine boycott", "unsettling aspect", "strenuously wrought", "painstaking effort", "gutted", "local strain", "as far afield", "contain the outbreak", "the lesson", "detailed understanding", "rigorous process"), perhaps to create a sense of trust in us. The language used thus far is familiar, easily intelligible. But then Ofri coins a new metaphor in which the delicate and ephemeral are made material: "the mere puff of a rumour". Lovely.

As in the examples above, biomedicine cannot help itself. It stretches past the purely informational and finds its most effective (which also means beautiful) expression as metaphor. This is our ideal for a clinical imagination.

To return to our starting point, imagine that medicine does not need poetry to nourish and enrich it, but that we need a poetic imagination to spot and exploit the poetry that is already in medicine. Our work is archaeological and geological, digging where we stand. Our starting point again is Medicine = Poetry, a deceptively complex equation that describes the general case and not necessarily the specific instant, where, sometimes, Medicine ≠ Poetry. The more reductive medicine becomes, the less the poetry shows (although the explanatory power can increase). But, of course, poetry itself (or the poetic imagination) helps in recognising and expanding poetry in medicine, and this hinges again on the creation of expansive metaphors. Clinicians gaining a poetic imagination as a key aspect of their overall practice helps all of this.

Our organising principles

This book is a work in progress. We say that not just because it breaks new ground, and so hopefully will attract critical response leading to reformation, but primarily because you, the reader, will reform (or reformulate) the work according to your reading of it. The book has emerged as a "complex conversation" between two people, Alan Bleakley and Shane Neilson, who are passionate about poetry and want to place it in their fields of practice with some consequence: Bleakley in medical education, psychology and psychotherapy, and Neilson in medicine. More, we are both academics who want to renovate ideas and who share a common background in formal education in sciences. We recognise and cherish the aesthetic in science.

Complex conversation

William Pinar (2019) coined the phrase "complicated conversation" to describe the then-emerging field of curriculum reconceptualisation that took "curriculum" as an object of study within pedagogy. Curriculum was revisioned as process rather than content, the latter better described as "syllabus". While "complicated conversation" is an attractive term aesthetically, having a balanced metrical rhythm (Pinar himself properly puts aesthetics at the heart of pedagogy), it has been superseded by complexity theory. What was deemed "complicated" described a linear problem that can be solved rationally (sending a person to the Moon), where the "complex" describes a nonlinear, open system (weather patterns, human encounters) where relationships of parts to the whole are key, and instability is commonplace. Medicine and poetry display high levels of ambiguity and instability excepting the level of form, where biomedicine is governed by linear aspects of science, and poetry by formal rules. The complicated and the complex can then run concurrently. William Doll (2012), a colleague of Pinar and also an educationalist, is a student of complexity theory. Doll prefers the term "complex conversation" over Pinar's "complicated conversation" to more accurately describe pedagogical theory generally and curriculum development specifically. We follow his lead here.

"Complex conversation" in our case refers to many hours of patiently re-working each other's primary texts to achieve a truly collaborative product that is the book before you. Scoping the field, preparing ground, digging in, and digging over (and over), we have attempted to bring poetry into fruitful conversation with medicine to illustrate our assumption that medical thinking and the poetic imagination at their best are meaningfully equivalent (i.e. they don't just randomly coincide). Both of us have long-standing interest in narrative medicine (Bleakley 2005; Neilson 2009), but we were both wary early on that narrativism had become a dominant discourse in the medical and health humanities, where a sense of imperialism emerged, and in the process non-narrative poetry was crowded out. We needed to clear the ground first before invoking our complex conversation in a stern effort to offer a critique of narrative medicine's over-reach.

We approach medicine as a cultural object in need of appreciation before explanation, nested in layers of meaning and historically determined. By bringing medicine into a complex conversation with poetry, we developed a complex conversation between ourselves in how best to present that exchange. We did not particularly set out to find poetry examples that fitted our case. These largely fell into place serendipitously. An organic conversation led by metaphors and a critical imagination emerged and we followed its trails, prompts, and provocations.

The general case and the specific application

Our primary method is that of tempering abstraction with illustration and example. Quite in tune with classical narrative workshop advice in this respect, we share a frustration with texts that tell, but do not show. As far as possible, we illustrate our points through examples drawn from clinical work: medical, psychiatric, and psychotherapeutic. Our product is necessarily like a woven carpet – we have made a pattern to our liking, but turn the carpet over and there are loose threads everywhere. We invite our readers not to replicate our carpet's design, but rather to follow those threads and re-weave new fabric. And hooray to the loose thread that unravels our non-schema such that a new carpet can be woven.

We have a running theme about the tension between the general case and the specific application. This mirrors the infamous divide between evidence gained from population studies and large-scale trials (general principles) and the specific patient (application). But this also applies to ideas and their concrete instances: where the general case is an abstraction, but the specific illustration is a concrete example.

The primacy of the aesthetic object

We see poems as "objects" whose primary work is to turn events into experiences, or deepen us in some way. This is often a beautifying, but sometimes an entry into the sublime. The work of poetry is primarily aesthetic – to educate the senses, to bring us closer to the qualities of things in noticing, to tap into feeling states and explore their qualities, and to encourage appreciation prior to explanation. But poetry too is by turns ethical and political – about values and power.

By "objects" above we don't mean solid "things", but a cosmos of language in its various forms (spoken, written, performed), including semiotics (signs and symbols) that brings us into relationship with phenomena (events) in such a way, again, that they are transformed as experiences. A poem is both a product and a producer of imagination. It acts to cause change and in the process is itself changed (through close reading and through interpretation), as it changes the reader or listener. It is less a catalyst (here, it would remain unchanged in any reaction), or intermediary (a translator, a messenger, or an instrumental means to an end, although poems are often used this way, for example for therapeutic purposes), but rather a mediator that causes expansion of activities, while it expands too.

Poetry can be seen as akin to Nietzsche's (1889/1997) "philosophising with a hammer", or doing away with false idolatry as challenging unproductive habits and conventions. But there is a double meaning here, where Nietzsche points to the value of thinking that actually changes things rather than remaining purely speculative. Nietzsche's project to bring on the "twilight of the idols" is a process of engaging with the qualities of the world, creating new forms, and creating humans in forms that realise their worth or value. Yet an ethical dimension must temper the aesthetic project of poetry (beautifying, enlarging sensibility) as rules of conduct. In order to achieve this, we must agree to democratic habits or forms of collaboration (as politics).

Oddly, the history of medicine is one that privileges a practical *phronesis* (wisdom in action) without due regard to aesthetic and political dimensions. Only recently has medicine formalised a deeper awareness of ethical responsibilities, now packaged as "professionalism". In this way, medicine evolved beyond a duty of cure to a more complex duty. Because one of us (Bleakley 2021) recently published a book about medicine and politics, we thought it was time to turn to the relationship between medicine and aesthetics. As poets we have focussed this relationship squarely on poetry and medicine.

Our disorganising principles

We follow Aristotle's (Poetics: Chapters 24–25) guidance to concentrate not simply on the poem, but on the wider poetic imagination that can be applied to any context. Our connection between poetry and medicine can be widened to the poetic imagination and medicine, following Aristotle below.

First principle

From Aristotle (ibid.): "One ought to choose likely impossibilities in preference to unconvincing possibilities".

Second principle

From Aristotle (ibid.): "And if a poet has represented impossible things then he has missed the mark, but that is the right thing to do if he thereby hits the mark that is the end of the poetic art itself, that is, if in that way he makes that or some other part more wondrous".

Third principle

From Aristotle (*De Anima II*, 6): Aristotle describes three kinds of perception that will be familiar to all poets and doctors.

The first is surface perception, where the eye sees, the ear hears, and the tongue tastes. Such direct perception is not deceptive: "We must speak first of the objects of sense in relation to each sense. ... I call special-object what cannot be perceived by another sense, and about which it is impossible to be deceived, e.g. sight has colour, hearing sound, and taste flavour, while touch has many varieties of object".

Second and more complex, several senses operate together: "... while those that are spoken of as common are movement, rest, number, figure, magnitude, for such as these are not special to any, but common to all". Thus, a crudely drawn circle can be "seen" and "felt" as a circle because imagination completes the gestalt.

The third, and final one, is the attribution of sensibility to objects that is the labour of imagination, where "[A]n object of perception is spoken of as incidental" (ibid.). I interact with another person, object, or phenomenon and intimately describe a character, filling in the gaps through an active, intelligent, and affective imagination. This draws in qualities such as forgiveness, love, and despair – the poetic imagination at work.

Our fourth and final disorganising principle is to apply the poetic imagination democratically, without prejudice.

An apology to readers and a lifeline

Like us, you will be constantly frustrated by not having full poems, or decent segments, quoted on the page as we discuss these works. We are severely hampered by copyright protocols that only allow a few lines in quote to be excerpted from most modern poems before payment from publishers who hold the copyrights is legally incurred. The exceptions are modern poets whose work is now in the public domain, such as Wallace Stevens, and the contemporary Canadian poets who have given permission for their work to be used. You should ask why we are unwilling to pay copyright. After all, the poets deserve this. Of course, they do. But, first, the payments would have to be made by us, the authors, as the publishers do not take on that responsibility, and we cannot afford to do this much as we wish to support poetry. Second, we would be paying publishers mainly and the authors would not receive their just rewards. Many of the modern authors we quote are in copyright, but dead, so royalties go entirely to their publishing houses. Thus, to make the connection between the few lines quoted and the whole poem, we ask you to follow the online links to where poems are housed (mainly *The Poetry Foundation*). (See also Appendix 1: Links to poems.) Routledge has provided a link to this book's listings of poems we draw on, and, in turn, you can link to the relevant website that houses the poem. Please read the poems in full!

References

Aristotle. De Anima. *Line by Line Commentary on Aristotle's De Anima Books I and II, ET Gendlin.* Chicago: IL: University of Chicago. Retrieved from https://focusing.org/sites/default/files/legacy/aristotle/Ae_Bk_1-2.pdf

Aristotle. 2013. *Poetics.* Oxford: OUP.

Bleakley A. Stories as Data, Data as Stories: Making Sense of Narrative Inquiry in Clinical Education. *Medical Education.* 2005; 39: 534–40.

Bleakley A. 2017. *Thinking with Metaphors in Medicine: The State of the Art.* Abingdon: Routledge.

Bleakley A. 2021. *Medicine, Politics and Social Justice: The Contradiction Cure.* Abingdon: Routledge.

Doll WC, Fleener MJ, Trueit D, St Julien J (eds.) 2012. *Chaos, Complexity, Curriculum, and Culture: A Conversation.* New York: Peter Lang.

Masukume G, Zumla A. Analogies and Metaphors in Clinical Medicine. *Clinical Medicine* (London). 2012; 12: 55–56.

Neilson S. Caring Masked as Narrative Medicine. *Canadian Medical Association Journal.* 2009; 181: E93–E94.

Nietzsche F. (Trans. R Polt). 1889/1997. *Twilight of the Idols, or, How to Philosophize with the Hammer.* Indianapolis, IN: Hackett Publishing Co.

Ofri D. 2021. Heidi Larson, Vaccine Anthropologist. *The New Yorker.* June 12. Retrieved from https://www.newyorker.com/science/annals-of-medicine/heidi-larson-vaccine-anthropologist

Pinar W. 2019. *What is Curriculum Theory?* 3rd ed. London: Routledge.

Shapiro J. 2009. *The Inner World of Medical Students: Listening to Their Voices in Poetry.* Oxford: Radcliffe Publishing.

Sieghart W. 2017. *The Poetry Pharmacy: Tried-and-True Prescriptions for the Heart, Mind and Soul.* London: Particular Books.

Sieghart W. 2019. *The Poetry Pharmacy Returns: More Prescriptions for Courage, Healing and Hope.* London: Particular Books.

Acknowledgements

The authors would like to thank all those colleagues, friends, and co-writers who have made this project possible, particularly those poets who have generously contributed their work to this book. Without their words and those of fellow poets, the world would be a much bleaker place.

Shane Neilson would like to thank Dr Miranda Hickman.

In particular, we would like to thank Grace McInnes (publisher, Health and Social Care) and Evie Lonsdale (editorial assistant, Routledge Health and Social Care) at Taylor & Francis for their continuing support and decidedly "hands-off" approach.

This book has been an inspiring and intense transatlantic collaboration between Shane Neilson and Alan Bleakley (during a global pandemic) for the sake of poetry and what it can do for the human spirit and beyond. We have been pressed into service by forces and presences known and unknown to restore poetry to its rightful place in conversation with medicine.

Part I

Setting out to alter the narrative

1 In difference (and not deference) to narrative medicine

Prolegomena

Later, we engage critically with narrative medicine as represented in the influential work of Rita Charon and associates at Columbia University in New York (Charon 2006; Charon and Wyer 2008; Charon et al. 2016). We show how non-narrative poetry has not simply been overshadowed, but rather eaten whole, by narrativist approaches. There is time enough for this. But for now, we want to start our book with the evergreen reason for why we're writing it. So let us tell you a story.

During the rise of the narrative medicine movement in the noughties, the California-based medical educator and psychologist Johanna Shapiro (2009) published a book on medical students' poetry and how this can illuminate the nature of their studies and identity formations. But the strange feature of Shapiro's book – given that the students' poetry is its springboard – is that poetry (as we understand the genre and phenomenon) is entirely engulfed by narrativism. For Shapiro (ibid.: 42), all students' poetry is a form of story and is treated as such in her analysis, where further, poetry is explicitly understood to be an art consisting of information: "This book is predicated on the argument that poetry can be understood as a form of qualitative data".

More, Shapiro, a psychologist, proceeds to (predictably?) psychologise her material. By this, we mean placing an emphasis on what happens to the individual person internally, and not focussing on that person's engagement with the world. The developmental psychologist Jean Piaget (Inhelder and Piaget 2006) called the first approach "assimilation" (the world is adapted to the individual's needs) and the second approach "accommodation" (the person adapts to the world). Shapiro's book is appropriately entitled *The Inner World of Medical Students*. In contrast, the celebrated poet Geoffrey Hill (in Phillips 2000) was adamant that poetry is not about personal growth, the poet's ego, or the betterment of individual "wellbeing". Rather, poetry is a gift to culture and an invitation to diversity and inclusivity, where, as Hill says, "genuinely difficult art is truly democratic". Carefully crafted, thoughtful verse adds to the richness of poetry's field independent of its author. If, by inhabiting that field, we feel differently about the world or ourselves so much the better, but poetry may infect us differently.

DOI: 10.4324/9781003194408-2

The first half of our book will explain how Shapiro's (in our view) rather bizarre approach – when surveying the field as a whole – is actually normative. But for now, we ask, with the fervour of poets: how could such a misreading and misapplication have ever come to be?

Taking 576 poems written by 386 medical students (sampled from published examples in medical and medical humanities journals), ranging across all years of study, Shapiro subjected the poems to "content analysis" from which the following themes emerged inductively: the experience of cadaver dissection; becoming a doctor; becoming a patient; doctor-patient relationships; student-patient relationships; language and culture differences; death and dying; issues of inequity and social justice; and students' general reflections on life and love.

These themes are then made sense of by drawing on the narrative framework categories of the medical sociologist Arthur Frank (1995), who identified a typology of four kinds of "illness narratives": chaos, restitution, journey, and witnessing. These were seen as guiding metaphors organising patients' experiences around a theme. Shapiro, in utilising Frank's narrative-based typology, then imposed narrativism on poetry, whether or not the original poetry was written in a narrative or non-narrative style. Poetry was given no room to exert its unique character where it was deformed into narrative, and further reduced to data or information.

More, the overall message of the book is that students write poetry instrumentally – the poetry is put to use. *That* it is put to "use" is one contentious argument; *how* it is put to use is another – in Shapiro's analysis, the point of poetry is to fulfil the requirements of Frank's four illness narrative types where the students' poems supposedly describe: (i) making meaning of chaos; (ii) restitution for something lost; (iii) illness as a journey; or (iv) acts of witnessing. Shapiro (ibid.: 41) sees overlap between these categories, but claims that "[M]ost of the poems that I reviewed made sense within these Frankian-influenced narrative typologies". Thus, the typologies were not inductively drawn out from the data, but the pre-existing typological framework was used as a classification and meaning-making device. In the process, all poetry was made to go through the narrative mill. A product of this reduction from raw poems to categorical types is the boiling down of wide metaphor content, where Shapiro (ibid.) says, "[T]wo overarching metaphors dominated my conclusions". To wit, illness described as a "foreign land" and coping with illness as an "heroic journey".

As poets, we find this worrisome. As scholars, we appreciate the work done in classification and yet return, inevitably, to the misframing. Shapiro's work is conducted according to a misapprehension of what non-narrative (primarily lyrical) poetry is and what it does. Was no poet or poem available to tug the robe of this confident narrativist to whisper, *Memento Mori*?

We will see many more examples of poetry being used for instrumental purposes (as Shapiro advertises above) throughout these opening chapters as we gradually lose the poetry itself to data, used to supposedly "improve" our understanding of medical education. But wait, there are bigger blows: Shapiro's data may be untrustworthy for we do not know how representative this sample is of gender and ethnic mix among medical students, and it is obviously North American-centric. Such medical students' poems represent a privileged source. While Shapiro's brief is not to look beyond the poetry, foregrounding this does remind us of the need to highlight minority, suppressed and excluded poetic voices. To merely stuff the students' poems into the Western canon box advertises a missed opportunity.

More, the medical students' poetry is technically suspect (we illustrate this with examples later). The cynical side of us rejoices at this milling of suspect poetry into data: better to have good information than questionable verse. Not all of Shapiro's examples are poorly conceived or crafted, but, as Shapiro (ibid.: 44) herself admits, "[I]t is true that much of this writing is imperfect, unpolished, lacking in formal craftsmanship, and does not appear to pay attention to the formal structural or rhythmic conventions of poetry". In defence of such paucity, Shapiro (ibid.: 45) quotes Gillie Bolton, once a key figure in UK medical humanities circles, who says, "poetry does not have to be great so long as it is useful to the writer and to an appropriate audience". Hmmm – we baulk at the mention of "useful" in this context, and cannot agree that it is a good excuse for potentially poor verse. Indeed, we strenuously disagree. Would we use the same framework and terms to describe a doctor or surgeon's work?

We wince in a familiar fashion when we read Bolton's predictable invocation of "useful": poetry is useful for what? Bolton leaves that question wide open. At least Shapiro brazenly says that poetry has an instrumental use to "improve" the perceptions of medical students. But again, of what use is poetry? Presumably, for those relatively few publishers who make a profit out of selling poetry books, poetry is useful for making that profit, and constitute the rare instances when poetry becomes commodity. Perhaps, for many of the medical student poets that Shapiro or Bolton refer to, poetry is not central to their lives and they could take it or leave it, so poetry serves a decorative function. For Bolton and Shapiro, poetry has therapeutic value. Not one of these justifications appeals to us.

We do recognise that relationships to poetry are multiple and complex. Some will say that poetry saved their lives, where others will say that it ruined theirs. Seamus Perry (2019) writes of the Scottish poet W. S. Graham, who re-located in the far West of Cornwall: "Many poets end up having a hard life but W. S. Graham went out of his way to have one. His dedication to poetry, about which he seems never to have had a second thought, was remorseless". And yet, by his own admission, Graham was slowly drinking himself to death. In a posthumous address to his near neighbour, the painter Peter Lanyon, Graham said of his alcoholism: "The poet or painter steers his life to maim // Himself somehow for the job". Graham couldn't live without writing poetry, but couldn't write poetry without drinking, so poetry did not act as therapy at all, but was complicit in self-harm.

The Indian poet and scholar Meena Alexander says that poetry is the primary art form for "the essentially unsayable", but we do not buy into poetry as unreachable, or even necessarily revelatory. We like the fact that poets are baldly and boldly political, like Linton Kwesi Johnson (from the album "Bass Culture" 1980), the Jamaican dub poet and activist based in London, commenting on police harassment of black people:

> Hours beat, the scene moving right
> When all on a sudden
> Bam, bam, bam, a knocking pon the door
> "Who is dat?", asked Weston, feeling right
> "Open up, it's the police, come on, open up"
> "What address do you want?"
> "Number 66, come on, open up"
> Weston, feeling high, replied, "Yes, this is Street 66, step right in and take some licks".

The poetry, of course, is performed (as a dub song: https://www.youtube.com/watch?v=UnAV1Ec4Z9M) that adds a critical dimension. In the subsequent age of Black Lives Matter, antagonism between black communities and the police, the front line of institutional racism, has been exposed as part of a complex health issue. Since the beginning of the Covid-19 outbreak in the UK, for example, black and ethnic minority groups have lower life expectancy than the white population (The King's Fund 2021). Social deprivation, inequalities, and injustice are major factors in susceptibility to Covid, and lowering of life expectancy. Stop and search by UK police is heavily biased against black communities (Gov.UK 2021).

So poetry, indeed, can have an instrumental function in representing oppression in order to contest or resist oppression. Poetry, of course, can be of use, and can be operationalised. But it must also have the useless valence in play, an optional-applied rule at play at all times. Otherwise it dies. At the level of politics poetry is about the political *relation* and not ideology, or necessarily resistance. Poetry helps one to see and feel, perhaps to understand more, if not perfectly, than to afford a deeper imperfection; and in this affective identification, one creates in oneself the inapplicability of the oppression, the resistance condition. In short, poetry is transformative, but through and by indirection.

Clearing out the interruptions to poetry

It is bad enough that poetry's appearance in terms of scope might be frustrated by certain kinds of privilege. But do committed literary scholars really need to keep frustrating the appearance of poetry in full expression through tactics such as "tired" instrumentalism (poetry serves a purpose other than its full expression as an art form, where its cumulative work is reductive of surprise, complexification, meaning, or defamiliarisation of the familiar), and narrative oppression (poetry is subsumed in narrative). For example, returning to the Program in Narrative Medicine at Columbia University, Rose Bromberg (2008: 63), then resident poet, wrote, "There's a special relationship between poetry and medicine, and great value that physicians, other healthcare professionals, and patients could derive from making better use of this art form". Thus, poetry gains value by putting it to good use in medicine. But what about stand-alone poetry and not poetry as springboard?

Bromberg then suggests what poetry can do, advertising naked instrumentalism: "Poetry can sharpen listening, attentiveness, observation, and analytical skills. It can refine the artistic side of medicine: Poetry allows us to express ourselves, fosters creativity, and accepts ambiguity. It enhances empathy, self-awareness, and introspection". Poetry too is therapeutic, cathartic and is about personal growth, for which Bromberg makes big claims:

> Poetry about illness includes addressing not only the symptoms of illness, but the *experience*, which includes emotions and responses. We use various ways to share and validate our physical, emotional, intellectual, and spiritual perspectives, commonly through written and spoken language. The way we perceive and use poetry devices, for example: diction, tone, voice, organization/arrangement, meter/rhythm; the interactions and physical and emotional spaces/silences between the healthcare professional and patient or between the poem and reader, helps us to define and interpret ourselves and others, and to direct thoughts, feelings, and actions. Communication thus improves. Changing the cadence may influence healing and even outcomes.

And, predictably, poetry is drawn into the maw of story, controlled by the narrative gaze in personal-confessional and identity-constructing mode: "The poetic voice orders thoughts and allows for control, clarity, and reflection. It shapes our past narrative, and how we may construe our future narrative".

If we chip away at this claim by exposing brazen instrumentality and the narrative tic, two of our bugbears, poetry itself is left with nothing. Bromberg offers "an example of a brief poem I wrote to express relief and provide comfort after an unpleasant medical experience":

SERENITY

White
water lilies
float
atop the pond;
a petaled quilt
to keep
me
warm.

We have empathy for Bromberg's unpleasant medical experience, but less for the poem itself, again used as a directed and specific self-therapeutic instrument (means–end writing) rather than for the sake of poetry. The haiku-like feel of the poem takes on none of the challenges of the haiku form, although that is no great offence; we are surely in the presence of the spirit of haiku, an identification that we are pleased to make. There is formal awareness to be found here, uncommon in the land of medical poetry. Yet it is the insistent hard consonant "t" alliteration seems to go against the grain of the poem's title "Serenity". Softer assonance (the "o" of "float", "atop", and "pond") nearly pulls off the poem's objective, and yet something is off here too. The vowel sound itself suggests to us surprise, a mouth gaping. Finally, the lone metaphor feels off. We like the lily quilt but how might it keep one warm, appearing as it does on a surface of water? To us, the poem has an "instapoetry" feel, made to be paired with an image and written in some kind of repellent cursive font. And when poetry requires visual assistance for effect, then it is not well.

Bromberg's poem is metaphor-lite ("petaled quilt"). This does not align with conscious wrangling with metaphors by poets such as William Carlos Williams who, claims Alec Marsh (1992) has "an aversion to metaphors, and especially similes, because he connects their transformative power to that of financial manipulation". In other words, there is a stated rationale behind the form. Williams saw American financial (capitalist) obsessions as harmful to democracy, and he applied this same value system to poetry, where excessive production of metaphor (or overproduction of tired metaphors) was likened to accumulating capital for the sake of it. Williams's great gift, however, was to turn a whole poem into a metaphor.

Bromberg's rather clumsy apposition of "cold" and "warm", and "cover" and "undercover", do not effectively spell out a metaphoric "serenity" to us, but rather a vague and loose comfort, a gentle ease created by the briefest of impression. For us, the poem's brevity is perhaps its success. One cannot grip onto it too much for analysis; there are flowers and there is water: ergo, serenity via those associations. Or the poem can get away with deficiency because it's brief. Within the typical formulaic medicine-poetry formats (instrumental, therapeutic) poetry like Bromberg's above is hard to comprehensively resist because of its brevity and innocuousness. Our bottom line is that the poet seems not to have applied sustained rigour and critical attention to the work.

The same cannot be said of William Carlos Williams. We are both fans of the rigorous yet beautiful lines of Williams, whose autobiography was written between 1948 and 1951 (Williams 1967). Two chapters, in particular, in Williams's unapologetically and uncharacteristically scattergun account – one about poetry ("Projective Verse" Chapter 50) and the other about medicine ("The Practice" Chapter 54) – can be seen as forming one body, where poetry and medicine not only co-exist but actively feed each other. Williams explains that "The poem springs from the half-spoken words of such patients as the physician sees from day to day", and that this comes "… after a lifetime of careful listening" (ibid.: 362). Structurally, "The poem is made of things–on a field" (ibid.: 333). Poetry is then *placed*. It is, of course, ultimately placed in the hands of the reader, or the ears of the listener. But prior to this it finds place on a field of action, as a whole piece, through speaking about things (objects) musically and tonally. Williams describes the scene we have just described, where "An advance of estimable proportions is made by looking at the poems as a field rather than an assembly of more or less ankylosed lines ..." (ibid.329).

Here, poetry and medicine collide in the term "ankylosed". Technically, this means fusion of bones, causing stiffness of a joint for example. Ankylosed lines in Williams's worldview are then stiff from habitual overuse of poetic devices that approach the poem as parts to be built structurally, rather than an expressed whole (the field). Such poems can be arthritic. The field, a gestalt or holistic grasp of the subject/object of the poem, is loose-limbed, *articulated*. The tension between these two approaches to poetry is archaic, grounded in two types of Creation myth: the world built day-by-day, hierarchically, and the world given whole, with equal participation.

Williams quotes from Charles Olson's manifesto "Projective Verse", first published in 1950. Olson suggests that the poem's transfer from writer to reader is one of honouring how the poem appears to want to arrange itself first syllable-by-syllable (from the head by way of the ear), and then line-by-line (from the heart by way of the breath). This is what gestalt psychologists call the emergence of a differentiated foreground from an undifferentiated background. Williams then draws in the metaphor of the house and its furnishings to illustrate this process of (re)construction of the poem (ibid.: 332–34). First, the house has a *topos*, a location, and this location is already invested with a history, sometimes troubled. It is on the site of this historical reference that the house (the poem) is expressed, so that it is already invested with meaning, where, says Williams: "The poem is our objective, the secret at the heart of the matter – as Sheeler's small house, reorganized, is the heart of the gone estate of the Lowes – the effect of a fortune founded on tobacco or chicle or whatever it was". Williams is drawing on a house and a family that he knows, in the Hudson River Valley near New York.

The man and his wife, in Williams's fable, build a "house" of poetry and live in it, furnishing it. This is their vocation, where they "made it a cell ... to give the mind its stay". Further, as the house outlives its inhabitants, so the poem is limited by the lifespan and life experiences of the writer: "The poem ... is the construction in understandable limits of his life". In other words, the poem is what Heidegger would call a temporary Place of Dwelling for language, reflecting this person, in this life with its own peculiar constrictions lived authentically; or bluntly, objectively: "The poem is made of things – on a field". Williams concludes this chapter as, "Nothing can grow unless it taps into the soil". The Place of Dwelling that is poetry's house is a grounding in a field of possibilities. We might represent the latter by replacing one vowel in Williams's line: "Nothing can grow unless it taps into the soul". But do you see what we mean about "rigour" in Williams's conception of the poetic field?

We turn now to Williams's Chapter 54 "The Practice" – on medicine, and we see how this, for Williams, is the other half of poetry's house, free from ankylosing. Just as the poem coalesces as objects arranged in the field, so Williams, when visiting patients, would develop his form: "In a flash the details would begin to formulate themselves into a recognizable outline, the diagnosis would unravel itself, or would refuse to make itself plain, and the hunt was on" (ibid.: 356–57). Then, "… the patient himself would shape up into something that called for attention, his peculiarities, her reticences or candors". Williams continues that medicine was "… the very thing which made it possible for me to write" (ibid.: 362).

Such "House Calls" made by Williams (again locating his medicine in space) are brilliantly glossed by the literary physician Robert Coles and the photographer Thomas Roma (Coles and Roma 2008), where Williams sets out his rationale for seeing patients on their own turf rather than in the clinic. This rubs against the grain of modern medicine, where seeing patients in the clinic rather than the home, argued Michel Foucault (1976), offered the "housing" for both an identity for doctors and for a legitimising of power differential between doctor and patient. The clinic offers the abstract "white space" in which the patient can be displayed for inspection/examination (and then objectified) as if in a gallery. Williams's habit of house-calling resists such objectification.

And so Williams frames our argument. Poetry and medicine once more feed each other, diagnoses springing from the poetic imagination, words springing from encounters with patients. This is the soil from which this book has grown. It encompasses more than Williams speaks of as it embraces the entanglements of clinical diagnostic work, patient encounters and the field of poetic expression, articulating the movement from syllable-driven mind and ear, via line-driven heart and breath to form fields or places of habitation: houses of poetry as clinics, clinics as places where poetry already is.

Importantly, we will put into perspective the science that is the basis for the doctor's diagnostic thinking as it relates to poetics. We also move away from poetry written by physicians to embrace the significance of a range of poems for medicine, making a general case to hopefully illuminate specific and idiosyncratic clinical encounters. As we do this, we are again wary of the instrumental use to which the poetry can be put that strips the work of its original value. And yet poetry needs its optional applied-function too so that it keeps its future open. We suggest one might protect medicine from a purely applied mentality as well, as counter-resistance from the opposite pole. Whatever connections we make between medicine and poetry, we will be careful to maintain their respective original currencies.

Our book is not an apologia for poetry. We don't want to convert doctors to become poets or artists. Again, we want to introduce a poetic imagination into medical work. When Aristotle (384–322 BC) described "Poetics" he did not restrict this to formal written and spoken poetry, but embraced a more ambitious worldview as a *poetic imagination*. We ask you, the reader, to also be constantly vigilant about the issue of instrumentalism, or means-end thinking, in relation to our topic of poetry and medicine. Where does medicine use poetry instrumentally such that medicine benefits but poetry is left unaddressed, failing to develop from the relationship, acting simply as a catalyst for medicine's growth? Poetry is desiccated in this way, expended, an extracted resource. And then, because of this misreading, this misuse, it is also misapprehended, unable to do that which medicine needs. Where does poetry draw on medicine to milk it dry without giving anything back other than sour comment about reductive science, or objectification of patients? We hope that we are charitable to both poetry and medicine while remaining critically alert to the failings of both in their more-than-chance encounters. More than anything else, we want you to recognise our true love for both medicine and poetry. It is not our objective to abuse one in favour of the other.

Where "plot" collapses into field and soil

In the absence of the priest, the doctor and therapist hold privileged positions in society. Patients and clients will open up to them bodily and emotionally in ways that they will not with partners, family members or close friends. In contrast with personal therapies, conventional biomedicine cannot respond to such emotional needs, powerful though biomedicine is as an explanatory tool. Further, biomedicine is grounded in research data gained from population studies that can't embrace individual idiosyncrasies. Focussed on quantities rather than qualities, and fact rather than belief, such medicine is necessarily reductive, impacted. The patient is treated as isolated disease or symptom. We recognise that this critique is as old as when the scientification of medicine was first identified and biomedicine first named as an epistemology over a hundred years ago (Porter 2003). This is not biomedicine's "fault" – no blame is attached, for biomedicine works within its singular epistemology. (Our culture's use of biomedicine is another matter entirely.) Medicine, as we saw from William Carlos Williams's remarks earlier, is wider than its informing science. It is about often complex human encounters and human suffering.

To compensate for the inherent lack in the biomedical approach, doctors are now "trained" (rather than educated) in "communication skills" and "professionalism" – a set of standardised and codified responses that often lack both authenticity and spiritual nourishment. Formulaic, and often learned in vitro under simulation rather than in vivo in patient encounters, such approaches are like flowers plucked from their nourishing soil – they easily wilt. To draw on the poet Wallace Stevens's line from "Certain Phenomena of Sound", this is an equivalent of "Cat's milk is dry in the saucer". Such "training" is readily confounded by surprise and uncertainty, the vagaries of the workplace, the rich experience of full cream. This book is that metaphorical cream, and provides a new critique – where poetry matters in medicine – merely recalling that which was already present in historical practice. Poetry has mattered long before biomedicine was ever dreamed. We will show how poetry matters to medicine today.

Authentic patient contact demands something beyond the exercise of a desiccated biomedical understanding and instrumental communication skills. This deeper element turns the raw into the cooked and cultured. In fact, prior to the anthropologist Claude Lévi-Strauss's (1964) famous coining of these metaphors to describe, respectively, nature and culture, the poet Robert Lowell coined the raw and the cooked metaphors to describe two kinds of poetry – a more sophisticated cooked or cultured brand and a raw "howl" of visceral verse characterised particularly by Allen Ginsberg and Beat poetry (https://poets.org/text/raw-and-cooked-robert-lowell-and-beats). We like both kinds, but we are sceptical of raw poetry that turns its back on technique gained through study and experience. We don't think that poetry flows by just turning on the tap. To elaborate the metaphor, there's plumbing, pipework, and filters. Most of all, there's water sources – where the water is drawn from. We're keen to show how the sources of poetic inspiration and medical inspiration may share much in common; but more, that moving from source to tap requires labour. Recall Williams's reference above to "a lifetime of careful listening" to patients to gain expertise as both doctor and poet.

We detail in the following chapter how narrative medicine has (with partial success) stepped into the role of offering cooked culture to medics where biomedicine delivers raw nature. Narrative is different from a plain prose account that is purely informational, descriptive, or lacking imagination (prosaic), such as a factual doctor's letter or an autopsy report. Narrative too is different from a discursive argument that is primarily rhetorical, such as a philosophical or theoretical analysis. Rather, narrative is a structured spoken or written account of connected events through time. Usually there are characters and a plot. The plot normally has a twist or a crisis point and the story escalates towards this point. There is then a resolution. Where narrative engages medicine, patients' accounts are overlaid with plot. Williams's (and, as we shall see, the poet Charles Olson's) "plot", however, is of another variety and shifts us from story's time sequences to poetry's negotiation of space. Here, the "plot" is the field and garden that is cultivated.

Patients may, indeed, recount their symptoms in terms of temporal plot. However, they may just as readily offer disconnected events as a spatial account (this happened *here*, that happened *there*, right *here* is where I hurt) lacking temporality. Projecting plot onto such events is a way for the doctor to make narrative sense of the patient's account, but it does not necessarily reflect the patient's experience and may even distort it. There are many deviations from this general rule as stated, and narratology has become quite complex over the years; yet the general case – and as you will see, we very much appreciate the general case! – is fairly described here. Certainly it is this general case that has the most pedagogical value to the general physician.

Because narrative collapses and choreographs experience, it follows that narrative medicine too has limits. Again, to pun, we might collapse the desire to impose narrative plot on a patient's account, with turning that account over, as the other kind of plot – that of soil, of land, of defined space. The account may be of a soiling, and a spoiling through symptom the causes of which are as yet undiagnosed. Another approach is needed to practice a non-reductive, humane medicine with awareness that mines the moment deeply; seeks connections of intensity; excels in working with affect; generates the conditions for epiphanies or sudden insights; tolerates ambiguity and open-endedness; is forever open to the creative; and works with space, place, and the moment, rather than obsessing with time.

This describes the work of a poetic, rather than a prosaic, imagination. Non-narrative lyric poetry – which we will fully define in a moment – does different work from story, seeking a particularly intense experience of defamiliarisation, as "thinking otherwise" and "making strange". Largely through metaphor, poetry seeks to grasp and express the soul of a therapeutic encounter, which might be conceived of as wonder and beauty. To accomplish this, poetry explores its objects of attention in intimate detail. We have both previously written at length about metaphor in medicine (Neilson 2016, 2019a, 2019b; Bleakley 2017) and metaphor will appear as friend and guide throughout this book. Sometimes metaphor will let us down or disappoint; over-description of objects through simile is a common error in poetry (as it is in medicine with neophytes, where medical students understandably tend to overdiagnose). We are aware too of Williams's warning – posted earlier – that metaphor production and collection can be a kind of capitalism, a business strategy, or poetic commercial venture (especially where metaphors are cheap and easily gained, tired or overused, such as "medicine as war").

Suffocated, buried alive, even eaten, and certainly largely ignored by narrative medicine, non-narrative poetry must be saved from abuse first, and perhaps neglect thereafter, although we have managed expectations as to the potential impact of our work. Before we can illustrate how poetry operates in the body of medicine, living within medicine's circle of influence, we must first clear the ground, or weed the plot, by critiquing narrative's limits. Only then can we illustrate poetry's power, elegance and beauty. Our critique of narrativism will occupy this and the next four chapters. We will dig over the soil thoroughly, as critique.

We can hear our friends the narrativists clamouring in the background at our claims, wondering if we intend to cleave the work of metaphor from narrative and try to make it exclusive to poetry. *Well, narrative medicine does this work too*, they exclaim. We patiently respond with the words of poet and critic Stephanie Burt (2019: 194), who suggests, "If you want a compact, aurally intricate representation of somebody's interior life, poems might well be the first place you look". Further, poetry offers "a bracing challenge to all storytelling, to all prose sense". Over and over again in this book, we will try to convince you of how transformatively useless poetry is in the general medical encounter – that "general case" again – at the level of improving outcomes.

(Burt [ibid.], in fact, offers a version of this barefaced contradiction as the title to her book: *Don't Read Poetry: A Book About How to Read Poems*. We encourage you to look it up!) And yet it somehow makes all the difference at the same time. We stand by this contradiction and expand on it.

We walk the paradoxical line between saying poetry does nothing yet is everything. We ask you to take our contradiction as a resource. While we walk that line, we notice a mercantile (capitalised to differentiate it as a brand) type of narrative medicine invest in biomedical proof of effectiveness, a full stop to instrumentalism. What we are selling, if we are selling anything at all, is not a workshop or a student livestream, but rather an entirely different way of thinking medically. We are selling you poetry-thought. It's free. But it will cost you. The cost is to imagine medicine (and life) differently, and this is transformative. We gleefully admit that this is a claim also offered by narrativists, yet we arrive at this "outcome" obliquely, as an incidental yet profound consequence – and not as an achievement, learning goal, objective, or competence set in stone.

Wallace Stevens often used birds as symbols of transformation to see the world anew. In "Sunday Morning", he sees the inquiring mind wanting to break free of binding conventions:

> I am content when wakened birds,
> Before they fly, test the reality
> Of misty fields, by their sweet questionings.

(From here on, when we refer to a poem, wherever it is available, we offer an online link to the whole work, and these poems are listed in Appendix 1: https://www.poetryfoundation.org/poetrymagazine/poems/13261/sunday-morning.)

This intense, specific and place-based poetic diction is not the language of the "story", not the gaze of the narrative eye. If the birds are set free, they ultimately settle, somewhat domesticated, to bring further gifts. In the same poem, Stevens describes,

> the green freedom of a cockatoo
> Upon a rug.

This poetic style resists the impulse to impose "plot" on a patient's disconnected and fragmentary account. But it does turn over the soil of the reader's imagination and encourage us to think differently. It defamiliarises, a term we explore in depth in Chapters 3 and 5 in particular. To try to impose narrative plot on Stevens would be comic, and yet poetry gets a small share of such narrative medicine treatment on occasion.

Returning to narrative readings in medicine, of course, "this happened" and then "that happened" to the patient, but the person in front of us now is in the *grip* of a fever, or has *exploded into* a terrible itchy rash; couldn't *staunch* a nosebleed; has just *missed* her period, is 16 and *terrified* that she is pregnant [Williams (1967: 361) describes, "The girl who comes to me breathless, staggering into my office, in her underwear a still breathing infant, asking me to lock her mother out of the room"]; or has a *blinding* headache that won't calm down. Yes, there is a "story" here; there's always a story. But there is also always poetry, in each explosive or nurturing word that, in turn, is metaphoric, signalling transformations of meaning and experience.

Further, how does the patient experience the "story"? As "story"? Is the so-called "co-constructed" story between doctor and patient actually, as in so many cases, even the most narratively sensitive one, dominated by the doctor's capital, invested back into the medical business? Maybe there is something more instant, deeply compressed, emotionally charged and metaphorically loaded going on in both the patient's account and the doctor's response – maybe something poetic?

In the same poem mentioned above ("Sunday Morning") Stevens says, "Death is the mother of beauty". Is this some morbid desire on the part of the poet? Not at all – "death" can be taken here as change, so that transformation becomes the mother of beauty. We are asked to see something in a new light. The metaphor does the heavy lifting as a form of defamiliarisation, met above, also the key role of poetry according to Viktor Shklovsky (1991), one of the Russian Formalists who we will discuss in more depth, especially in Chapter 5. Medical interventions such as a spot-on diagnosis, or a surgical success, can, of course, be wholly transformative, but we must be able to articulate how and why such transformations occur beyond the exercise of bare instrumental practice. Will we put up with blandness, or even kinds of ugliness, in medical exchanges with patients, or will we strive for something far deeper and engaging, not just of beauty but also of compassionate wisdom? One royal road to get here is via the apparently permissive route of "King or Queen Narrative" (sometimes, cheekily, we think of this as "Knave Narrative") – the established model of narrative medicine with which we critically engage over the next few chapters. Yet we will see that such a route brings hazards. Another – the path not taken – is poetry. Welcome to this errant path.

Summary of argument

Medical work and non-narrative lyric poetry are shaped by sets of variable structures or frames that have remarkable similarities, one of which is vulnerability and fragility. Medical work and non-narrative lyric poetry can both be readily denatured. Medicine's potential for applying mundane science imaginatively, to match patients' needs through emotionally charged and creative personal encounters, is frequently frustrated unnecessarily. The informing science is often translated and practiced in mechanical terms, inviting tired, even dead, metaphors such as "the body as machine". For its part, diagnostic work often dehumanises by rendering patient as symptom and illness as disease. Treatment can be reductive, even combative, by metaphorising medicine as conflict and combat.

But medical work can strive for quality beyond the merely efficient, efficiency being what we identify as the chief scourge (and symptom of lack of imagination) of the "training" and "competence" movement (Bleakley, Bligh and Browne 2011). Medical work must not scare away Wallace Stevens's "wakened birds" or be scared off by the appearance of the "cockatoo upon a rug". These are not hallucinations but real – as metaphors, always embodied, often object-oriented, plots of soil ready to be turned and planted out. They point to meanings as yet unrealised. We point to a medicine of potential fuelled by poetry.

By "medical work" above we mean in particular diagnostic reasoning, but also the whole arc of a medical intervention from consultation, examination and testing through diagnosis, prognosis, treatment, follow-up and overall care. By "lyric poetry", we mean collapsed, intensive, non-narrative forms of descriptive poetry that create emotional responses leading us to see the world differently. Sometimes it is useful to say what a thing is not, to rely on a negative definition, which we find a delicious irony in a positive book of this kind. Lyric poetry is, generally speaking, not the following: concrete poetry, conceptual/ experimental poetry, and most especially, epic poetry. To define each of these precisely, and further precisely discuss the exceptions, is beyond the scope of this book. Suffice to say that the most common kind of poetry to be published in the English-speaking world is the kind we intend with our category. It is, again, a general case.

The diagnostic and poetic arcs are tacit in origin. Ask an experienced specialist physician how she makes decisions and she will undoubtedly say that she "just knows" – in other words, she is working from pattern recognition or "clinical gestalt", a result of apprenticeship and then long experience leading to "adaptive expertise" (Kneebone 2020). She is standing in Williams's and Olson's field as syllables form into lines, the mind feeding the ear, the heart feeding the breath, the words (both hers and the patient's) forming whole structures of meaning and delight.

This does not mean, of course, that she, as expert, is guessing. Rather, while the process of pattern recognition is automatic or intuitive, it is shaped by a tacit store of anatomical and biomedical knowledge engaged by a number of cognitive strategies. The latter include key trigger words, a cache of previous cases coded as "illness scripts" that become "general cases", semantic qualifiers ("hard vs soft", "proximal vs distal", "acute vs chronic"), and a range of heuristic devices such as mnemonics, aphorisms, and metaphors (these terms are unpacked throughout, with a particular focus in Chapter 7).

A complex unconscious web of memorised and coded material then informs the surface decision. Further, memory is linked to anticipation in a future-facing cognition that embraces fast-changing and ambiguous contextual cues, where prediction is required and tolerance of ambiguity is fundamental. Medical judgements are never made in isolation because the starting point is a dyadic doctor-patient encounter and this often blooms into a web of healthcare provision with the patient formally at the centre as spider, but sometimes trapped as prey, especially as other factors come into play: such as political influences, management decisions, and healthcare insurance costs. As overall care brings in other healthcare colleagues and associated services, so it is linked to a range of artefacts such as tests and imaging equipment that constellate around the patient.

These are not necessarily sucked into the vortex of narrative, but can represent poetry's engagement with things, which is poetry's forte: bringing the objects of the world into new light by scrutinising them closely (what in poetry is called *ekphrasis* and in medicine close noticing). But this is not just sensate noticing; it is also a witnessing of suffering and of the human condition. Wallace Stevens (1951: 31) said that poetry doesn't reveal things, but instead lurks in material things where the world of poetry is "indistinguishable from the world in which we live". Normally, we don't see the world in the direct and intense way that poetry demands. It's up to poets to master the element of surprise to capture the intrinsic expressions of objects that count as revelations. For poetry, there is a parallel set of heuristics and devices such as verse forms, rhythm, cadence, assonance, consonance, dissonance, musicality and syncopation, intensity, density, alliteration, enjambment, rhyme, and repetition. However, these are consciously enacted, unlike the tacit or implicate order of medical reasoning.

Creativity as medical and poetic devices

You would expect both poetry and medicine to embody creativity, otherwise they would both be pedestrian: flat and dull. Medical melodramas are among the most successful serials on television, but there is an awful lot of flat medicine (and flat poetry) in real life, fed by (often dull) strategies in medical education to augment their biomedical pedagogies by charging a handful of medical students to write raw or undeveloped poetry in the name of the "medical/health humanities". This, of course, is the general case – in specific medical schools there is genuine innovation at work. When the first literary scholars, such as Kathryn Montgomery Hunter (1991) and Anne Hudson Jones (2013), were brought into medical schools, they meant business, despite meeting bewilderment and cynicism from some quarters.

In both medical work and poetry, close description and imaginative conjecture are at work and these can be intensified creatively. We want to pause at this point to think more about what we mean by "being creative", because poetry at its best springs us from the jail of the prosaic and pedestrian to the freedom of permission for the exercise of imagination.

For many, "creativity" is a weasel word, concealing more than it reveals, and, like "narrative", is intent on spreading so thinly that it loses its proper intent, or attempts to outreach its limits, a point we elaborate across these opening chapters. Because "creativity" is not a weasel word for us, but rather one that poetry depends on, we feel it is worth a brief scoping analysis. Multiple types of creativities (Bleakley 2015) are central to the practices of both thoughtful medicine and inventive poetry, and these types invite different qualities of expression.

Danielle Ofri (2013) suggests that much medical school "education" is actually a functional "training" in which creativity is stifled, where "rote recitation inhibits the ability to think beyond diagnostic straightjackets". "Medical school", says Ofri,

> can seem like an industrial line of ongoing exercises of committing lists to memory, the only creativity being the mnemonics for memorizing branches of the facial nerve or diseases with anion gap metabolic acidosis. When students present such cases, there is a sense of roteness. A patient with chest pain, for example, becomes "Rule-out M.I. (myocardial infarction). Get an EKG, serial troponin levels, stress test, cardiology consult …"

Mnemonics, an Art of Memory (Yates 1966) technique, can be included in our first tier of imaginative devices that expand medicine. But Ofri is right to denigrate reductive medical training based on rote exercise, as this extends beyond the necessary limitations that biomedicine refuses to acknowledge, annexing the entire territory of medical practice. In the example she gives, the patient's experience of chest pain is occluded instead of being central to the diagnostic rota. What is the point of finding a problem if the patient herself is never known? Functionality and "listification" flatten the patient's experience, squeezing out any enriching poetic account. The diagnostic steps must be rehearsed within the world of biomedical terminology, but should not be limited to the biomedical frame. Poetry will prevent the patient's experience from being occluded because it cannot abide a dead rhetoric. It paradoxically floods functionality with its uselessness, reclaiming the excess of the human from its partial conceptualisation by biomedicine.

Though biomedicine tries to obscure poetry in the so-called "descriptive" language, no language – even the technical variety – can prevent poetry from rearing its head and stealing the show. For instance, there is some poetry at work in the descriptors of the chest pain case mentioned above: "metabolic acidosis" is easily remembered because of its assonance, a stress on the "a" and "o" vowels. Just thinking this way though, noticing this fact, shifts register from the prosaic to the poetic. It naturally follows that the importance of functional listing is not elevated in the formulation of care, unlike the patient's anxiety mirrored in her heart rate.

Poetic work will encompass the patient's world, entering the rhythm of the heart, the immediate predictive arc of anticipation or what is to come, the anxiety and uncertainty embedded in the situation, a sense of awe and wonder at the body's diction, an efficiency of practiced intervention, and a moving dialogue with the patient that embodies care and instils confidence.

William Carlos Williams (1967: 361–62) cherishes the exchange of words between doctor and patient as necessarily poetic. What else could they be? Otherwise they are brute, senseless:

> We begin to see that the underlying meaning of all they want to tell us and have always failed to communicate is the poem, the poem which their lives are being lived to realize. No one will believe it. And it is the actual words, as we hear them spoken under all circumstances, which contain it.

The medical work, for Williams, is "… to recover underlying meaning as realistically as we recover metal out of ore". The poem is in the patient's words, where the poetic imagination is served by close noticing and witnessing, so that the patient is observed in exquisite detail, while idiosyncrasies are registered – not in objectification but in particularisation. Much of these offered riches are provided by traditional narrative medicine pedagogy. But like so much else in life, it matters how you get there, as the form of extraction and recovery of the precious metal. Poetry goes a different way from narrative. Perhaps it is a way you need. Perhaps it is a way you prefer. And, perhaps it also gets to different places at different times, for a one-size-fits-all method is – distressingly – redolent of the biomedical. In summary, poetry can do things narrative cannot, and with panache, grace, and beauty – sometimes with wisdom too. And sometimes it will upset you or shift your perspective radically. We like the descriptor used by Emily Dickinson, who claims that poetry educates us into looking "slant" at the world.

Getting back to creativity, the founder of the contemporary narrative medicine movement, Rita Charon (in Jones and Tansey 2015: 61) agrees with a remark by Nellie Herman – a novelist colleague of hers – that "creativity is the most important ingredient in how we are to improve healthcare". But, again, precisely what is meant by "creativity"? It is used here as a catch-all, like "narrative", akin to the general case rather than the idiosyncratic person with the atrial flutter. Different kinds of narrative do different work, as do differing kinds of creativity. The work of poetry is primarily granular particularity, so let us approach "creativity" as poets: we can both articulate a typology of creativity as we can exercise invention and imagination at the level of the individual's creative work.

While pre-Homeric lyre-playing poets sang epics that so pleased audiences because they all knew the storylines in advance, what also mattered was their licence for invention or improvisation around themes. This is what gave particular singers character. Thus, "creativity" might be seen in such oral invention prior to the written form. However, "creativity" is actually a modern word, first appearing in a dictionary from 1678 as a synonym of "productive", implying labour. It wasn't until the 19th century that "creativity" appeared as "originality". Scholars of the creative process have made distinctions between creativity as product (the poem and the diagnosis), process (pondering, notes and drafts; and diagnostic reasoning), a creative individual (the poet; and the doctor), and contexts for creativity (the writing programme, criticism, audience reception, or reader response; and the consultation, the clinic, the bedside) (for an overview, see Bleakley 2015: 10–31).

James Hillman (1972) developed a typology of creative acts as differentiation, novelty, ferment, problem solving, eminence, and renewal. Differentiation is "taste" or the ability to distinguish between qualities. Novelty, ferment (effervescence or fizz) and problem solving speak for themselves, as does renewal or regeneration. Eminence is an interesting choice. It means those who are naturally elevated or distinguished by some characteristic or achievement. Bleakley (2015) describes "creativities" – in the plural – that may intermingle: (i) as an ordering process and problem solving (99% perspiration and 1% inspiration); (ii) as rhythm and cycle; (iii) as originality and spontaneity; (iv) as the irrational; (v) as problem stating; (vi) as inspiration or revelation; (vii) as making strange (indirection, thinking otherwise, defamiliarisation and rendering the familiar unfamiliar); (viii) as serendipity; and (ix) as resistance to the mundane. Admixtures of these are to be expected.

We will see how varieties of creativity appear in poems and medical work that take us out of the general case ("creativity") and into particulars (here, creativity is an indirection; or there, a revelation; and here, a product of perspiration or application – the fruit of labour). Throughout, we make statements as if they were true (an old saw in medicine is "if you hear hoofbeats, think horses, not zebras", or go for the most likely scenario in diagnosis); yet time and again, the particular, the odd, the individual patient disproves the general case. Poems are unique in this sense, and yet we will continue to generalise ("lyric poetry") and occasionally spout empty proclamations ("a life well spent"). We'll leave the final word to William Carlos Williams (1967: 343), who says, "The poem is a capsule where we wrap up our punishable secrets". How creative is that? And how this utterance resists being pigeonholed within our typologies of creativities! The poem may express truisms or controversies germane to the public world (the general case), but it is also the individual psyche writ large, necessarily confessional. The poem in the clinic symptomises some of the time. What else would you expect?

References

Bleakley A. 2015. *The Medical Humanities and Medical Education: How the Medical Humanities Can Shape Better Doctors*. Abingdon: Routledge.

Bleakley A. 2017. *Thinking with Metaphors in Medicine: The State of the Art*. Abingdon: Routledge.

Bleakley A, Bligh J, Browne J. 2011. *Medical Education for the Future: Identity, Power and Location*. Dordrecht: Springer.

Bromberg R. Poetry and Medicine. *Medscape Journal of Medicine*. 2008; 10: 63.

Burt S. 2019. *Don't Read Poetry: A Book about How to Read Poems*. New York: Basic Books.

Charon R. 2006. *Narrative Medicine: Honoring the Stories of Illness*. Oxford: Oxford University Press.

Charon R, DasGupta S, Hermann N, et al. 2016. *The Principles and Practices of Narrative Medicine*. Oxford: Oxford University Press.

Charon R, Wyer P. Narrative Evidence Based Medicine. *Lancet*. 2008; 371: 296–97.

Coles R, Roma T. 2008. *House Calls with William Carlos Williams, MD*. Brooklyn, NY: Powerhouse Books.

Foucault M. 1976. *The Birth of the Clinic: An Archaeology of Medical Perception*. London: Routledge.

Frank A. 1995. *The Wounded Storyteller: Body, Illness and Ethics*. Chicago, IL: University of Chicago Press.

Gov.UK. Stop and Search. February 22, 2021. Retrieved from https://www.ethnicity-facts-figures.service.gov.uk/crime-justice-and-the-law/policing/stop-and-search/latest#by-ethnicity

Hillman J. 1972. *The Myth of Analysis: Three Essays in Archetypal Psychology*. New York: Harper & Row.

Hunter KM. 1991. *Doctors' Stories: The Narrative Structure of Medical Knowledge*. Princeton, NJ: Princeton University Press.

Inhelder B, Piaget J. 2006. *The Psychology of the Child*. New York: Basic Books.

Jones AH. Why Teach Literature and Medicine? Answers from Three Decades. *Journal of Medical Humanities*. 2013; 34: 415–28.

Jones EM, Tansey EM. (eds.) 2015. The Development of Narrative Practices in Medicine c.1960–c.2000. *Wellcome Witnesses to Contemporary Medicine*. Vol. 52. London: Queen Mary University of London.

Kneebone R. 2020. *Expert: Understanding the Path to Mastery*. London: Viking.

Lévi-Strauss C. 1964. *The Raw and the Cooked*. Paris: Plon.

Marsh A. Stevens and Williams: The Economics of Metaphor. *William Carlos Williams Review*. Vol. 18, No. 2, A Special Issue on Williams and Stevens (Fall 1992), pp. 37–49. Retrieved from https://www.jstor.org/stable/24565089

Neilson S. Pain as Metaphor: Metaphor and Medicine. *Medical Humanities*. 2016; 42: 3–10.

Neilson S. 2019a. The Practice of Metaphor. In: (A Bleakley (ed.) *The Routledge Companion to the Medical Humanities*. Abingdon: Routledge, 144–54.

Neilson S. Poetry Will Save Your Life. *Canadian Family Physician*. 2019b; 65: 820–22.

Ofri D. 2013. Creativity in Medicine. (First in *New York Times*). Retrieved from https://danielleofri.com/creativity-in-medicine/

Olson C. 1950. "Projective Verse". Retrieved from https://www.poetryfoundation.org/articles/69406/projective-verse

Perry S. What a carry-on. *London Review of Books*. Vol. 41, No. 14, 18 July 2019. Retrieved from https://www.lrb.co.uk/the-paper/v41/n14/seamus-perry/what-a-carry-on

Phillips C. Geoffrey Hill. The Art of Poetry No. 80. *The Paris Review*. Issue 154, Spring 2000. Retrieved from https://www.theparisreview.org/interviews/730/the-art-of-poetry-no-80-geoffrey-hill

Porter R. 2003. *Blood and Guts: A Short History of Medicine*. Harmondsworth: Penguin.

Shapiro J. 2009. *The Inner World of Medical Students: Listening to Their Voices in Poetry*. New York, NY: Radcliffe Publishing.

Shklovsky V. 1991. *Theory of Prose*. London: Dalkey Archive Press.

Stevens W. 1951. *The Necessary Angel*. London: Knopf.

The King's Fund. The health of people from ethnic minority groups in England. 17 September 2021. Retrieved from https://www.kingsfund.org.uk/publications/health-people-ethnic-minority-groups-england

Williams WC. 1967. *The Autobiography of William Carlos Williams*. San Francisco, CA: New Directions Books.

Yates F. 1966. *The Art of Memory*. London: Routledge and Kegan Paul.

2 The imperialism of narrative

Disclaimer

We love story, but we refuse to worship at its shrine. What we don't like is this story: narrativists employing narrative in an imperialistic manner. For example, the highly respected historian Hayden White (1987: 1) says of narrative, "So natural is the impulse to narrate, so inevitable is the form of narrative for any report on the way things really happened, that narrativity could appear problematical only in a culture in which it was absent …".

In other words, narrative ways of thinking are habitual and normative; more, narrating is an "impulse" or a biological necessity. This claim rather complicates White's scenario of imagining "a culture in which it was absent". He cannot have it both ways: either narrativism is a biological imperative and then universal, or it is a cultural imperative and then takes on differing intensities and tones, with a possibility of absence. Further, and paradoxically for a biological impulse, narrative "report" is taken as a measure of veracity ("the way things really happened"). White then not only biologises but also scientises narrative. We thought stories on the whole offered fictions, but White seems to be referring to our everyday recounting of incidents and episodes. In which case, he cannot get away with ironing out rhetoric, inflation, hyperbole, white lies, and the rest.

White does not apply the same logic to poetry. Is non-narrative poetry "natural" and an "impulse", or "inevitable"? Like a lot of narrativists, he conveniently squeezes poetry out, refusing it entry to the house of narrative. Indeed, there is no entry for "poetry" in the index to White's influential text. Poetry has been dodged, a White-out.

Narrativism (and then narrative medicine) has become a dominant discourse, a God-term, or what Jean-François Lyotard (1979) calls a "grand narrative", an overarching theme or method that can become ideological and oppressive. Lyotard too falls under the spell of story, as ideologies or Big Ideas are labelled "narratives", where the "local" or idiosyncratic "story" – such as a person's life history or patient's account of illness – becomes a "little narrative" or *petit récit*. We can add "Narrativism" (necessarily capitalised as a Lyotardian "grand narrative") to Capitalism, Marxism, Religious Orthodoxies,

DOI: 10.4324/9781003194408-3

Consumerism, Existentialism, Humanism, and so forth. As Narrativism is applied to medicine, doctors become interpellated in an ideological apparatus as they internalise a set of values and act according to them. Surely this is no bad thing as either a counter, or a parallel thinking process, to a biomedical scientism that peddles reduction and instrumentality? If everyday narrative is, indeed, moulded by interpellation into grand narratives, then we must again look askance at Hayden White's claim that narrative recounting is total recall: "the way things really happened".

What we see is that narrativism applied to medicine (narrative-based medicine, or narrative medicine) can act as an oppressor of non-narrative poetry. More, this has not been recognised by the narrative medicine community, doubling the power of oppression (see in particular Bahar Orang's essay opening Chapter 14).

We have been irritated enough over the years to wonder why narrative medicine scholars and practitioners indiscriminately lump non-narrative lyric poetry in with all kinds of other writing: narrative prose (the novel, short story, essay, literary biography, autobiography and autoethnography – the latter perhaps the most popular genre right now in the medico-literary canon). We see this as selectively rejecting the very quality that literary scholars demand of their students: discrimination. In fact, again we see lyric poetry as having been swallowed whole by narrative medicine as a kind of colonising, where it usually reappears not as poetry in its own right but as serving an instrumental, therapeutic function. We will illustrate this argument with plenty of examples throughout this book. From the outset, we are forthright that our critique of narrative medicine is a vigorous one, focused on the most popular variety of narrative medicine as developed by Rita Charon (Charon 2001, 2006; Charon and Montello 2002; Charon and Wyer 2008; Charon et al. 2016) and others at Columbia University in New York. We capitalise this latter, more popular, variety as "Narrative Medicine" to be specific, and our critique largely concerns this variety. But before we can offer our critique, we shall neutrally offer a brief history of generic narrative medicine (lower case, to distinguish the general movement from the specific Charonian Narrative Medicine approach) so that our analysis can have a solid referent.

A spotted (potted and spotty, non-chronological – read: poetic) history of generic narrative medicine

Narrative medicine is a branch of narrative studies that spread from wider literary studies in the 1980s as part of the "narrative turn". As biomedicine, grounded in quantitative science and population studies, became the dominant discourse in global medicine, critics of this view wished to recover the qualitative face of medicine with its focus on the care of the individual patient. A resistance movement to perceived biomedical reduction started slowly in the 1970s, gaining considerable traction two decades later. Kathryn Montgomery Hunter (1991) – with an academic background in literature and no clinical experience – and others introduced literary perspectives to better understand the human face of medicine. This could be essentialised as focusing on qualities of language in clinical encounters. In Hunter's (ibid.: 193) case, this was based on the premise that doctors are not pure scientists, but "rational science-using" practitioners whose clinical reasoning is already grounded in a hermeneutic method: close attention to cues and clues as a kind of interpretive "sleuthing". This reflected the way that Conan Doyle (a doctor himself) inscribed the investigative method of the fictional Sherlock Holmes.

Hunter (ibid.; 2005) described how such clues were provided in patients' verbal accounts, and how sleuthing was advertised by doctors' retelling of these accounts within their own registers of medical knowing. She called such knowing "Doctor's Stories" – formally, as the subtitle indicates, "The Narrative Structure of Medical Knowledge" – launching the movement in North America that we now generally recognise as generic narrative medicine. Hunter described this structure of medical knowing aware that doctors themselves do not consciously articulate their reasoning in narrative terms.

The medical doctor and scholar Rita Charon (2001) mirrored and progressed Hunter's model by formalising narrative ways of knowing as a parallel set of knowledge and skills to biomedical work. She termed this "narrative competence" and developed a unique brand that, again, we will distinguish from generic narrative medicine by capitalising as Narrative Medicine. On occasion, we slyly and civilly question elements of Narrative Medicine by branding it as Narrative Medicine[TM]. We take "sly civility", as a form of quiet civil disobedience, from the critiques of imperialism of Homi Bhabha (1994) and Gayatri Chakravorty Spivak (2008) engaging "postcolonial affect", or feelings of displacement as an effect of colonisation. For us, it is poetry that has been displaced, as we indicated in the previous chapter. And it is poetry that feels the hurt as much as poets themselves.

We say this because as poetry is utilised instrumentally (e.g. as a device in medical education to "improve" medical students and doctors as a prelude to "improving" patient care and safety), poetry in its own right is not developed. You might say, *Well surely if medical students or clinicians are writing poetry in the context of their work, then poetry is being developed?* We say, *A good deal of poetry written in such circumstances is written therapeutically or cathartically, without due regard to formal aspects of poetry and without reference to the extant body of published poetry.* Indeed, we have already said so in print a number of years back, writing about an anthology of narrative medicine writing (Neilson 2009: E93):

> And what of the question of aesthetics? The authors suggest that the experience of narrative medicine need not concern itself with the quality of the writing, and emphasize process and content over form. This is perhaps the chief weakness of the narrative medicine trend: good writing is keener observationally and possesses more penetrating insight, than the mere doodlings of amateurs. Narrative writing, as advocated here, is like a kindergarten class where everyone is praised.

If poetry is separated from quality and history, then it does not have the oxygen to survive. Will the majority of medical students' poetry be read by generations to come? Will it be critically received? Most importantly, will it impact in any way on the development of poetics, for example as innovation? Narrativists do not care about such questions, for wouldn't concerns about quality lead to a discouragement of production, a compromise of generative "process", and then a threat to the business model?

To return to our history, in the UK, as part of a global generic narrative medicine sympathetic to both Hunter's and Charon's pioneering work, Trish Greenhalgh and Brian Hurwitz (Greenhalgh and Hurwitz 1998) had coined the term "narrative-based medicine" to also describe an embracing qualitative approach to the individual patient that was seen to complement quantitative biomedicine. This movement is glossed below.

Early narrative medicine spread its wings to embrace bioethics. What had traditionally been taken as a branch of moral philosophy centred on universal principles (paralleling an evidence-based approach) was revised through literary lenses. Where the specifics of the individual "case" had been absorbed into the general principles of beneficence, nonmaleficence, autonomy, and justice, Tod Chambers (1999) in particular took these classic principles-based ethics cases and, drawing on literary theory, analysed them to expose their rhetoric. Chambers provocatively titled his 1999 text *The Fiction of Bioethics*, where he described bioethics cases not as factual accounts, but as inventive narratives written by ethicists. The "fictions of bioethics" are, of course, not first-hand accounts of patients' experiences, but representations of those experiences. A later Hastings Center report, *Narrative Ethics: The Role of Stories in Bioethics*, edited by Martha Montello (2014), offered a roll call of key figures in the field at the time such as Howard Brody, Rita Charon, Arthur Frank, Hilde Lindemann, and Anne Hudson Jones. These distinguished authors focused not only on critical readings of representations of reciprocity and dialogue between patients and caregivers but also advertised the use of literary techniques such as close reading of ethics "cases", as pioneered by Chambers.

A growing body of enthusiasts in medicine and healthcare eagerly took up narrativism's ideas and techniques. This flowering was realised in particular through innovative pedagogies such as viewing the patient-doctor relationship as one of co-construction of identity through an "agreed story" in "crafting relational identity" (Warmington 2020). But academic naivety also permeated the culture, reflected in a lack of self-critique and values clarification. Typical of the way that medicine and medical education have vigorously embraced the narrative wave is advertised in George Zaharias's uncritical (2018: 176) overview:

> Stories are our life's blood. We like to listen to stories, and it is through
> stories that we make sense of the world, that identity is shaped, and that
> we attempt to communicate what matters to us. ... Narrative-based

medicine (NBM) is the application of narrative ideas to the practice of medicine. Like patient-centred care, it came into being in reaction to the inadequacies of the biomedical model.

Note the biological metaphor ("life's blood"), echoing Hayden White's (and others') framing of narrativism as "natural", an "impulse". Rhetorically, this grounds narrative in a bodily knowing, a natural sense of things, already creating an aura: a sense of holiness or untouchability.

In a more genealogical fashion, Jones and Tansey (2015) describe formal interest in narrative in medicine from the early 1960s centred on the UK. Prior to this, psychiatry had long employed story-based practices (psychoanalysis, of course, is dependent on story). By focusing adult patients on memories of childhood, Freud also created temporal frames, forcing his patients into storying their symptoms; this narrativising was doubled in intensity as Freud wrote up his case studies with a narrative focus. In Freud's wake, many post–Second World War British General Practitioners absorbed the seminal work of Michael Balint (1896–1970), a Hungarian psychoanalyst who spent most of his adult working life in England. His legacy is not just the ongoing existence of cathartic "Balint groups", but more so the larger reality sponsoring those groups: that medicine must acknowledge the importance of emotion and that the doctor-patient relationship is not just technical or instrumental but potentially therapeutic on both sides.

Accounts of the history of narrative medicine are dominated by North-American-centric and Eurocentric accounts. Up to now we have largely followed the North American framing. Bates and Hurwitz (2016) provide a more Eurocentric account, emphasising Balint's significant contributions as noted above. The establishment of UK "narrative-based medicine" was headlined by the 2015 decision of *The Lancet* to include narrative-based case reports rather than purely instrumental accounts. We recognise this embrace of narrative as a mixed good, both a tempering of objective cases with story, and a morphing of story towards data-led accounts. Victoria Bates's (medical historian) and Brian Hurwitz's (General Practitioner and medical historian) account of the roots of narrative in modern medicine points to a number of historical precedents to narrative medicine in "the clinical casebooks of the early modern era" (ibid.: 559). Case reports in medicine, originally called "a narrative", can be traced to the 18th century and served two purposes. Individually, they afforded the singularity of illness, but collectively they offered diagnostic opportunity through classifications such as typologies (e.g. "cancer cases", "heart cases", and, later, "studies of hysteria").

Interestingly, perhaps because they are historians first rather than scholars of literature, Bates and Hurwitz "use story and narrative almost interchangeably" (ibid.: 560), preferring the composite "history" (the patient's "history"). They point to etymological roots of both "history" and "story" that suggest commonalities (e.g. French *histoire*), then take a conceptual leap: "We take narrative to be the umbrella term for these *storia* and argue for their continuing valency in both medicine and 'the emergent discipline' of the medical humanities" (ibid.).

It is unclear how the leap from *histoire* to narrative is made, while other scholars, as we have seen, continue to make a distinction between story and narrative, particularly where patients offer stories, while doctors and narrative medicine scholars make narratives out of these stories. Formally, "story" has been defined as the telling "of events unfolding in linear time", where a "narrative" is the formal "artful organization" of the raw materials of story "that may complicate their chronology, suggest their significance, emphasize their affect, or invite their interpretation" (Greene 2012). Through this definition, again patients tell stories while doctors create narratives out of these accounts, the latter artfully arranged within medical frames. Conjoining "story" and "narrative", as Bates and Hurwitz do, conveniently bypasses this distinction of origins and potential issues of colonisation of "story" by the apparently more sophisticated – and certainly more self-assured, even bossy – "narrative".

The first book length accounts of medical narratives that appeared in the second half of the 20th century are characterised as "illness narratives" – thinking here in particular of Arthur Kleinman (1988), who in *The Illness Narratives* called illness a disruption to biography that can prompt sense-making through reflection and writing (diaries being common media). Another important figure is Art Frank (1995), who in *The Wounded Storyteller* concentrates on disruption of identity through illness, and the subsequent difficulties of articulating such an ill and disrupted self through writing. Jumping ahead a little, we recognise Joanna Bourke (2014) who, in *The Story of Pain*, stresses the use of a wide range of artefacts – such as diaries, letters and poems – to articulate experiences of pain.

Thomas Lacquer (1989) claims that illness narratives afforded a new aesthetic genre, different from objective autopsy reports and case histories that introduced fictional and subjective elements, a precursor to contemporary "frontline" medical autobiographies and television soap operas, or "medical fictions" (Moody and Hallam 1998). Such narratives bounce back and forth between voices of patients and doctors. By the 1970s, these narrative forms were joined by ethnographers researching medical contexts, formally in terms of detailed linguistics (Byrne and Long 1976; Mishler 1986), and more informally as "dig where you stand" partial ethnographies sketching broad-brush accounts of medical life, including institutional contexts (Becker et al. 1961).

Erving Goffman (1961) recorded formal "frontstage" and informal "backstage" activity in an asylum, drawn from a year-long fieldwork study at St. Elizabeth's Hospital in Washington, DC, where Ezra Pound had been treated. The institution was famous for its early arts therapy initiatives. Paul Atkinson (1995) researched what he called the "liturgy of the clinic". Medical work and medical talk were analysed using some literary methods such as accounting for the work of rhetoric in medical communication. Building on this, Bates and Hurwitz (2016) introduced an "ethnopoetics", where aesthetic and affective dimensions to clinical work were represented in quasi-literary terms, as a kind of "soft", conversational research.

Such accounts began to follow a classic narrative arc of journey: setting out, meeting obstacles, a turn in events, and a resolution. The arc of arousal and resolution described the process of diagnosis itself, the medical establishment now adopting the patient's story as its capital – as Medical Narrative. Where literature and medicine finally met, as noted medical schools began to employ literature scholars, the inter-discipline of the medical humanities was established with narrative medicine and the history of medicine as its base (now fused in some institutions, such as the medical humanities work at King's College, London being incorporated into the English Literature department and not the medical school or History section). Medical ethics meanwhile, as noted above, having separated out from medicine's interest in history and literature in particular, drifted back into view as narrative fodder.

The formal use of literary techniques such as "close reading" – discussed throughout this book – was a natural consequence of this integration of literary scholars and narratologists into medical schools. By 1994, faculty with expertise in literature were employed in one third of medical schools in North America (Montgomery Hunter, Charon, and Coulehan 1995). In the UK such scholars worked in English and Humanities departments in Universities, and not in medical schools, having little interest in medical education or pedagogy. These literary scholars, working in particular with physicians who write, have created a vibrant culture of narrative medicine that we respect and honour. However, our main question remains: has narrative medicine recognised its limitations? For example, what happened to non-narrative poetry as a consequence of the rise of narrative medicine?

One of the key concerns of contemporary narrative medicine returns us to the distinction often made between the patient's story and the medical narrative. Howard Brody (1994) in North America and John Launer (2018) in the UK were leading figures in making a case for a collaborative co-construction of narrative between patient and doctor. But this agreement on authentic story is complicated by the fact that stories may be initiated in dyads, but they are soon parts of extensive healthcare, carer, family and health insurance networks, supported in turn by artefactual and information webs. More, stories may become detached from patients as distributed content on websites dedicated to disseminating medical information or creating special patient groups as a kind of narrative-based witness culture. Patients may be valorised as spiders at the centre of a web, but there is more likely a scattering of flies caught in the web as prey for the spider who is now the institution of medicine or healthcare, and whose narrative has become that of the occupier or imperialist. Theories, techniques and schools of narrative medicine can occupy the same role of colonist, as we shall see.

With a history of narrative medicine briefly outlined, and with recognition of the positive contributions made by narrative medicine to medical education, pedagogy and scholarship, we shall proceed with our detailed critique of Narrative Medicine as developed by Rita Charon and colleagues.

Whose tale is it? I told you a story but you narrativised it back!

Generally speaking, "narrative" and "story" are used interchangeably in narrative medicine, though, as noted above, there is a tacit rule that "story" refers to what the patient says, where "narrative" refers to how the doctor stitches together reception of the story and its return to the patient with the clinician's gloss. Making formal meaning of the patient's account requires a robust biomedical understanding of the patient's condition and a delicate return of this knowing in supportive terms that, to paraphrase Charon (2006), "honors the story of illness". We applaud this clear and central intention of Narrative Medicine to hand the "story" back to the patient; our problem is with the intervening narrativising moment, when the capital of the patient's story is appropriated by the doctor.

What will be lost to the patient before the story reappears in the "honouring"? Will story capital be fairly re-distributed and how much of it will be appropriated by narrative texts? We sweated blood over how we can represent dedicated poets' work in this book, yet in medical schools' medical/ health humanities courses, we see medical students writing raw untutored poetry and we see such poetry published. A second issue is ownership and rights. We see the value of a Gift economy here; we just don't think that it has been properly acknowledged and scrutinised as an ethical issue. Are we really "honoring the stories of illness" in publishing poor poetry? And is there genuine "narrative reciprocity" (Charon 2006; Charon et al. 2016) where poems are published to expand the CVs of medical educators? It is ironic surely that the publishing mill is no different in kind in the narrative medicine field than in the biomedical fields.

Of course, we recognise that Narrative Medicine's intention is to return the patient's story to her with interest, the addition to the capital being the labour of the doctor who employs the story clinically for the benefit of patient care. Wrapped around this is the narrative medicine academic industry with its research, grants, publications, and conferences. We just do not see this complex unpicked and scrutinised with academic rigour drawing on models such as Marxism (from economics), Gift transactions (from anthropology), or identity constructions (from Psychology and Sociology).

We recognise that Narrative Medicine's hard-earned capital is derived from investment in literary studies, and is not that of initial patients' "stories" – the raw matter from which the "narratives" are mined. Thus, Charon (Charon et al. 2016: 1) defines her version of narrative medicine as: "(a) rigorous intellectual and clinical discipline to fortify healthcare with the capacity to skilfully receive the accounts persons give of themselves – to recognize, absorb, interpret, and be moved to action by the stories of others". Despite the underlying promise of an innovative way of making a tender and caring relationship with a patient, we note that Narrative Medicine is couched in muscular, tough, hardtack talk: "rigorous", "discipline", "fortify", and "capacity". The "discipline" allocates the empathy. Charon means business, both metaphorically and literally. There is then investment in metaphors of Narrative Medicine's making and not from the patient's cache.

Such a "relational" capability for Narrative Medicine, a much-needed extension and corrective to bottom-line biomedical medicine, is specifically set again in what Charon calls "narrative competence" – a formalised set of frameworks and techniques drawn from literary studies that is Narrative Medicine's key labour. This augments "patient-centred", "person-centred", or "humanistic" approaches to medicine; and has become a key feature of the wider movement of introducing the arts and humanities into medicine (as the medical humanities) and healthcare (as the health humanities) (Bleakley 2015).

Charon (2016: 196) recognises the distinction between the patient's story and the doctor's narrative in comments on "voice", relating to perspective or point of view: who is saying what and how might this be received and returned to the source? The early 20th-century Russian Formalists (Vladimir Propp studying the formal structure of folk tales, and Viktor Shklovsky promoting the value of the text for the text's sake, freeing it from ideological purposes and recognising the quality of surprise) distinguished between *fabula* or what is actually described in an account (equivalent to the patient's "story") and *syuzhet,* how that original account is represented in text or talk (such as the "case" history). Shklovsky (1991) first coined these terms. We have more to say, critically, about Russian Formalism in Chapter 5. The mid- to late 20th-century French structuralists mirror this distinction in the terms *histoire* and *récit*, respectively, again a distinction glossed over by Victoria Bates and Brian Hurwitz above, who collapse story and narrative solely into *histoire*.

Charon (2006: 40) defines "the major features of narrative" as, "Some event happens or state of affairs obtains within a temporal sequence and specified setting to and by characters or agents, and the opening state gives way to an altered state". (We note the awkward construction of this sentence and repetition of "state".) Further, a speaker absorbs or represents the events from a particular point of view. The key elements are "time, characters, narrator, plot and the relationships that obtain between teller and listener". Applying this to medicine, Charon (ibid.: 50) claims that plot is the key clinico-narrative intervention: "Clinical practice is consumed with emplotment. Diagnosis itself is the effort to impose a plot onto seemingly disconnected events or states of affairs". "The effort to impose a plot" is clearly a directive even if it is done with understanding as its goal. "Effort" makes it muscular (again). It is not a revelation, an epiphany or sudden insight into the patient's condition but rather an imposing of meaning along with a reconstruction. This doesn't seem to us to be a patient-centred diagnostic move, but (once more) at best a medicine-centred accruing of capital at the worker's (patient's) expense, and at worse a doctor–centred narrative oppression as colonising of experience.

Well, we are wary of the imperialistic reach of Charonian Narrative Medicine in particular, for several reasons. We begin with the oppressive generality with which the tradition of Narrative Medicine approaches its potential clients. The absorption of story into medicine may potentially create an illness – one of mundanity – through the evisceration of quality, surprise, tension and danger. This potential instrumentalising of narrative approaches means again that they are no longer myth-busters, politically empowering, imaginatively dangerous, but simply techniques – as is explicitly apparent in Charon's key term "narrative competence".

Most worrisomely, perhaps, is the lack of self-critique within the Narrative Medicine tradition. Of her system of Narrative Medicine[TM], Charon (2016: 5) says, "All who seek care and all who seek to give care can unite in a clearing of safety, of purpose, of vision, of unconditional commitment to the interests of patients. This is the vision of narrative medicine". We are suspicious of both the piety and idealism of this "vision statement", but there is a bigger problem. Throughout her work, advertised particularly in the single authored *Narrative Medicine: Honoring the Stories of Illness* (2006) and then in the multi-authored set of essays *The Principles and Practice of Narrative Medicine* (2016), there is an absence of reflexive self-critique: no sustained account of the model's limitations (a standard requirement, for example, for research articles in peer reviewed journals). The 2016 text certainly expands the scope of Narrative Medicine from the 2006 text (for example with greater emphasis on social justice and diversity) but it still fails to critically address the epistemological assumptions of narrativism as applied to medicine, and does not acknowledge (and answer) established critiques of narrativism generally, such as that of Galen Strawson (below).

Our next concern rests with the market monopolisation of the pedagogy of Narrative Medicine. Critical of the way that health insurance practices, backed by medicine, led to a dehumanising commodification, Narrative Medicine[TM] is now itself commodified, a business proposition based on the highly successful Masters programme at Columbia University, running since 2009; and in parallel workshops and seminars, now run internationally. This is again why we continue to use the term Narrative Medicine[TM], fully aware that the weak cultural power of poetry prevents us from ever dreaming of such a lucrative product in our own field of interest! As Robert Graves said, "There is no money in poetry, but then there's no poetry in money, either". If there is money in narrative, it's little wonder why Narrative Medicine[TM] has so little time for poetry.

While initially criticising medicine for its commodification as a sell-out to business interests, Charon, in the best North American Protestant-Capitalist tradition, has packaged and marketed her Narrative Medicine methods as effectively as she has established their evidentiary natures. The Narrative Medicine website does not show a bunch of eager students, but rather a stack of Charon et al.'s (2016: 2) text (part of the business's capital – visit the Narrative Medicine website a few times and an advert for the business, using the text as its head, will irritatingly pop up on your screen, uninvited), that is rather hubristically placed on a par with William Osler's historic medical text:

> The goal of narrative medicine from its start has been to improve health-care. This accounts for the title we have chosen for our book, *The Principles and Practice of Narrative Medicine*. Echoing William Osler's 1892 *The Principles and Practice of Medicine* that set the standards for the practice of internal medicine, we believe the work that has emerged in narrative medicine has the potential to help move an impersonal and increasingly revenue-hungry healthcare toward a care that recognizes, that attunes to the singular, and that flows from the interior resources of the participants in encounters of care.

We applaud the drive to challenge impersonality in medicine, but we are cautious about a text that makes general claims for the efficacy of a narrative medicine flowing from "the interior resources of the participants in encounters of care", where the general case of the narrative frame overlays the unique patient's story.

Where "[t]he goal of narrative medicine from its start has been to improve healthcare", surely this is no different from the aims of biomedicine where biomedical insight can lead to a correct diagnosis and treatment? The limits to Narrative Medicine should be self-evident to its followers, but are seemingly too close for critical consideration. Rather than projecting "plot" onto another's plotless experience (is this any different than prescribing a pharmaceutical through biomedical diagnostics?), why not, again, take the given language of this experience (the patient's account) in its own right as a *political* gesture? Consider Beckett's *Waiting for Godot* and how the sense of the thing is possible to plot, but also quite ridiculous. To understand this play, one must untether oneself from time and feel timeless, infinite dread. Yes, the play unfolds in the time of performance; but what time is it in Purgatory, Mr. Wolf? Or, if we want to supplement the patient's account, why not politicise it in favour of that patient, acting as advocate for social justice? This is to take the lyric "I" of romantic poetry and turn it to the lyric "we" of socially aware, democratic poetry.

When Charon (2006: 3) notes that scientific medicine's tendency to objectify patients in a way aligned with the commodification of care – "Patients lament that their doctors don't listen to them or that they seem indifferent to their suffering" – this rhetorical stance tars all doctors with the same brush, another example of overindulging in the general case. But the same is true on the patient end of things. North American applied narrative practices offer little acknowledgement of how cultural differences may affect how "stories" are envisaged, constructed, told and received. For example, Arden Hegele (2017) argues that the dominance of formal narrative approaches has overshadowed the importance of ceremonial healing traditions such as idiosyncratic Native American use of story. Sayantani DasGupta and Edgar Rivera

Colón's (2016) chapters in Charon et al. (2016) edited collection go some way to addressing this lack and we applaud this, but Narrative Medicine is not yet in a position to advertise diversity and inclusion until it considers its North American-centrism (Woods 2011a, 2011b). Further, as we have indicated, narrative medicine, narrative ethics, and narrative-based medicine are rarely treated as differing perspectives, but more often indiscriminately lumped together.

One key, ongoing object of our irkful ire is the refusal of Narrative Medicine to engage with the literature critical of narrative dominance. Rather, it seems intent on blimpish self-celebration. We consider this literature in brief below.

Critiques of narrativism's imperialism

"It's the economy, stupid!" was coined by James Carville in 1992 while working on Bill Clinton's Presidential campaign team against George H. W. Bush. Actually, it's one of three catch phrases that stuck. The unsuccessful other two were "Change vs more of the same" and "Don't forget health care". Any decent rhetorician would have seen the last two as weak in comparison with the memorable first. Of course, it's the "stupid" label that is memorable. In medical education, we might say, "It's the narrative, stupid!" Oh, yes, of course! How stupid of me! The narrative imperative is insistent as we have seen. The psychologist Jerome Bruner (1987) in particular popularised the view of "Life as Narrative", this being the title of his influential 1987 paper. Bruner's title holds open the possibility of other metaphors for life, yet he later argued that life *is* narrative, no longer a metaphor. Bruner concretised Hans Vaihinger's (1924) model of life as enactment of the philosophy of "as if", turning the speculative into the empirical "it is". Of course, "life as narrative" remains a metaphor, but a dead one, as harmful in its hegemony as "the body as machine" and "medicine as war".

Generic narrativism outside medicine – the mother or father of the family of medical narrativisms above – has itself become a hungry monster, or outgrown its limits. This can be seen in Jens Brockmeier's (in Tansey and Jones 2015: 55–56) summary of a second wave of narrative studies termed "post-classical". Here, narrative is widened beyond literature and literary studies to "non-literary" narrative occasions encompassing all face-to-face human encounters, as if every time we meet we also recount or construct stories. This extends to "visual and performative ways in different semiotic environments, not least in digital media platforms". Everyday exchanges embody a narrative "form of life", again scooping up all experience in the narrative pail. Even our unconscious life is narrativised (we shouldn't be surprised, this was Freud's contribution to culture as noted earlier; where Jung in turn mythologises all experience as the grandest of all grand narratives). Patrick McNamara (2015) claims that "empirical data" from studies of thousands of dreams show that: "Most of us experience dreams as stories". Of course, the dream may be re-membered or retrospectively reconstructed as narrative (mirroring narrative reconstructions of patients' disconnected accounts), where the raw experience may not even be story, but rather discrete non-temporal events actively dissolving storylines. Welcome then to the coronation of narrative.

By refusing to engage, narrative imperialism has so far survived external views critical of narrativity such as Seamus O'Mahony's (2013) work in medical education, when he speaks explicitly ""against narrative medicine" and its misreading of patients who don't present with "stories" but with disconnected pieces of information or fluctuating affect". In medical humanities, Angela Woods (2011a, 2011b) cautions against narrativism's overreach that suggests medical humanities enthusiasts haven't had the courage to speak out against a dominant discourse of narrativism for fear of being sidelined. And Abbott (2007) contrasts "standard quantitative inquiry" in sociology "with its 'narratives' of variables as well as those parts of qualitative sociology that take a narrative and explanatory approach to social life" with an innovative "lyrical sociology",

> characterized by an engaged, nonironic stance toward its object of analysis, by specific location of both its subject and its object in social space, and by a momentaneous conception of social time. Lyrical sociology typically uses strong figuration and personification, and aims to communicate its author's emotional stance toward his or her object of study, rather than to 'explain' that object. The analysis considers many examples and draws on literary criticism, the philosophy of time, and the theory of emotion.

Abbott then interestingly identifies quantitative measurement as one kind of story, as well as "explanatory" qualitative descriptive approaches. While he does not explicitly invoke poetry, as one can see from the quote above he favours mobilisation and appreciation of affect, the collapse of time into simultaneity and the spatial (specifically place or location), as well as the lyrical, over the instrumental (with its emphasis on synthetic emotional expression rather than analytic explanation). These expressions do not set out primarily to explain, but rather to expose and explore. In alignment with his efforts to reform sociology to include poetic qualitative methods and not be dogmatic about narrative, we titled our book accordingly, for our goal is the same in the medical context.

Perhaps the most infamous critique of narrative medicine is that of the philosopher Galen Strawson. For example, in a review of Jerome Bruner's (2002) *Making Stories*, Strawson (2004b) sees an ouroboric worm at work, eating its own tail. Those who are already committed narrativists necessarily devour the idea that life and identity are storied; thus, we get

On one side, the narrators: those who are indeed intensely narrative, self-storying, Homeric, in their sense of life and self, whether they look to the past or the future. On the other side, the non-narrators: those who live life in a fundamentally non-storytelling fashion, who may have little sense of, or interest in, their own history, nor any wish to give their life a certain narrative shape. In between lies the great continuum of mixed cases. How did the narrativist orthodoxy arise? I suspect that it is because those who write about it and treat it as a universal truth about the human condition tend, like Bruner, to be profoundly narrative types themselves.

We are not Strawson acolytes. We find his critique of narrative orthodoxy (and then, by association, of narrative-based medicine) can be rejected as far too sweeping, even crude, but it remains sobering nevertheless (Strawson 2004a). As a philosopher, he should recognise that his argument starts from an unproven premise with no confirmatory evidence: that there are "narrativists" and "non-narrativists", implicit personality styles like Liam Hudson's "divergers" and "convergers". Although Strawson recognises that these identities are on a spectrum, such typologies can be dangerous, hiding a range of subtleties and complexities. Strawson's sweeping critique has the paradoxical benefit of being refreshingly blunt however. He likes to poke in the eye: "At one point Bruner talks up the 'program in narrative medicine' recently instituted by Columbia University's College of Physicians and Surgeons, but all it amounts to is the idea that doctors should listen to their patients". Yes. Doctors should, hardly a revolutionary idea. But is story only what we should do with such listening? Again, William Carlos Williams (1967: 362) talks a lot about learning how to listen in "a lifetime of careful listening", but his ear and his breath move within the field of the searing single line and not the narrative plot.

Further, Strawson (2004a) argues that a narrative view of life is neither naturally given (the psychological view) nor naturally good (the ethical view), where not living in time is often seen as a form of madness. He distinguishes between a "diachronic" type who sees the world in narrative terms and assumes this is right and good; and an "episodic" type who does not perceive herself primarily as in a flow of time and does not see narrative perceptions as necessarily right or good, but may, for example, prefer spatial metaphors. Again, Strawson at least admits to "a great continuum of mixed cases", but if these exist then they confound rather than better articulate his typology. He takes Montaigne as an Ur-example of an episodic type who is uninterested in either recollection or what the future may hold, but lives in the moment. We note that in sympathy, Jean-Paul Sartre defines existential angst as the inability to step out from the stream of time and exist in the moment as a spatial existence, or finding place, echoing Buddhism. This further echoes Martin Heidegger's sense of location or Being out of time, as "dwelling" and "indwelling". Poetry, for Heidegger, offered a direct sense of Being in place, rather than being displaced in time.

Strawson's intuitive argument offers no empirical evidence for its claims – they remain as provocations and suppositions. We appreciate this as poets, since poetry as a rebellious art is much the same! Despite claiming a "continuum of mixed cases", Strawson proceeds to set up an opposition between episodic and diachronic types as a rhetorical technique for engaging in conflict rather than conversation. Also, as Matti Hyvärinen (2012) notes, Strawson frames "time" in terms of a life history, but does not engage with the bigger world of time – human history, biological history as evolution, cosmic history as the consequence of the Big Bang. Neither does Strawson draw on what would appear to be an obvious ally in Buddhism, where a life course bookended by birth and death is not seen as a vertical event, but rather a horizontal spreading, a continuity. But Strawson's combative style does engage us with critical thinking and not the seemingly endless strings of plaudits that Narrative Medicine seems to crave, ducking self-critique or recognition of limitations.

With what shall we identify? The problem of false identification

Narrative Medicine invents identification between the doctor's narrative and the patient's story disguised as diagnosis. We say "invents" because the patient does not necessarily identify with the story returned as narrative, and a false identification ensues. There is a surplus to this process of narrativising the patient that may, indeed, promote dis-identification (the patient thinks, "I don't recognise what you just said"). The surplus is doubt and uncertainty. Is there an alternative to this to-ing and fro-ing within the narrative universe?

In anti-narrativism mode again, Strawson finds common ground with the poet Rainer Maria Rilke's remarks on the poetic imagination as a way of opposing "identity narrativism". Rilke says that the horizontally spreading lyric poem (and not the vertical "story") is formed through intentional opposition to identity and ownership. The poet must uncouple from narrative identity, or storying oneself, by allowing the poem its own identity and liberty. It is through the poem that one achieves dissociation from a fixed identity while maintaining a sense of place (in the projected field as Charles Olson would insist). Only by dissolving the notion that the poem arises from "my" memory and is then "my" child do we give the poem the independence to roam and flourish, open to reception across a community of readership. In "Letters to a Young Poet", Rilke (2013) says,

> Depict your sorrows and desires, your passing thoughts and beliefs in some kind of beauty – depict all that with heartfelt, quiet, humble sincerity and use to express yourself the things that surround you, … If your everyday life seems poor to you, do not accuse it; accuse yourself, tell yourself you are not poet enough to summon up its riches.

Here, Rilke expertly undoes subjectivity: know and "express yourself through the things that surround you". Poets closely notice such things, from which a self is sculpted. Perhaps the medicalised narrative overlaying the patient's story does not fit that story, but more, creates a sense of mistaken identity. The patient, despite the best efforts of the narrative medicine-infused doctor, feels that she is "in" the doctor's story and not in hers. This is an old criticism of medical exchange dressed up in newer terms. The patient feels herself to be a misfit. A clear example of this is in patients' resistance to prescriptions, crudely called "noncompliance" or "poor medication adherence" (Kleinsinger 2010).

Ironically – possibly by accident – Jerome Bruner (1986: 3) takes a similar stance to Rilke in the opening pages to *Actual Minds, Possible Worlds* where he quotes the poet Czeslaw Milosz, who follows Rilke's sentiments. Milosz admits to being "in the power of a daimonion, and how the poems dictated by him came into being I do not quite understand". The poem must be set free, says Milosz, not only from ownership by the poet but also from overwhelming literary analyses of poetry that can strangle or swamp the poem. But there is a trap here too – poetry is not just inspiration but also craft. If we tell medical students interested in writing poetry to hang around until the muse appears, they will soon abandon us. Show them technique and they will soon embrace it. Duck the technique part and we will have a cache of poor poetry, a condition bemoaned in Chapter 1.

If, for example, we are stuck with deadening metaphors in medical work, such as "poor medication adherence" that has the overlay of biomedical thinking, and if Narrative Medicine does not really address this metaphor lack, because it too has a sackful of dead or heavy metaphors of the muscular variety as we have seen (rigour, effort, discipline, fortify), then we should look elsewhere for our metaphor cache. Of course, the patient may already be describing her symptoms and life in rich metaphorical terms and we missed it, too busy thinking ahead to our narrativist overlays and interventions. Poetry might help here, offering radar, attunement.

Our reading of Milosz (1982) from *The Witness of Poetry* is that setting poetic thought and scientific thought in opposition is more a complaint – that science so easily becomes reductive through paucity of metaphor, or continued use of tired metaphors. Science should be constantly reinventing its metaphoric cache. We can make the same complaint about contemporary medicine: where has the continually inventive metaphoric imagination gone? The most disheartening metaphoric move for Milosz is science's insistence on physical causation – or the "concrete" event. This refuses the imagination – Ariel in Shakespeare's *The Tempest* imprisoned in a tree (literalism) by Sycorax and released by Prospero (gaining the life of metaphor and the soaring spirit).

Milosz described poetry as "the passionate pursuit of the Real" – capitalised because the Real is the Imagination, and the spirit of inquiry. Milosz's (1968) "Ars Poetica" asks, "what is the point of poetry itself?" The poet bemoans the limits to both narrative and poetry: "I have always aspired to a more spacious form / that would be free from the claims of poetry or prose", a form that is "something indecent … which we didn't know we had in us", "… as if a tiger had sprung out, / and stood in the light, lashing its tail", for "we are other than how we see ourselves in our ravings". Milosz then recognises the boundaries of both narrative and poetry, neither of which is capable of capturing an animal howl, a present danger.

There is a danger in making too clean a break between narrative and non-narrative poetry, where both descriptors hide a mass of ambiguities. Also, we are still in the territory of the general case here, for there are many types of "narratives". If we adopt Strawson's rhetoric, from the point of view of narrativists (in general!), any utterance or text is morphed into a story. In turn, Hyvärinen (2012: 9) accuses Strawson of reducing "narrative" almost to a parody of the conventional story, where "narratives of the self are plural, often fragmentary, and much more changeable and volatile than narratives in Strawson's model". (For more challenge to Strawson, see Arca 2018.)

If Strawson's critique is the most abrasive, it is the critique by Angela Woods (2011a, 2011b) that strikes us as the most trenchant. She writes with scepticism towards narrative medicine and its overreach, where "This has led to a neglect of other modes of reflecting upon and representing experience, such as poetry, phenomenological philosophy, or photography", although Woods does not progress the case for these media. However, Woods does provocatively ask if the search for meaning is a meta-narrative that we have every right to resist in the guise of narrative sceptics. She quotes the philosopher Crispin Sartwell (2000), who says that in extremes, in ecstasy, in writhing pain, and, of course, in death, does narrative matter?

"Narratively speaking", suggests Sartwell, we are "not getting anywhere" in most of our trivial everyday activities. Yet in breathing, eating, watching television, walking around, and, of course, in sleeping, imagining, and dreaming, narrative time can be severely disrupted. Sartwell asks why we fail to take the trivial non-narrative seriously. He asks also if we can take comfort in insignificance. Of course, as Woods points out, this is a message of discomfort that can also be taken as an inspiration. Is this not the point of an author such as Samuel Beckett who points to the absurdity of narrativity? We think it tyrannical and spiritually denaturing to live in a world that insists on linearity and meaning. Much meaning can be derived from grand narratives, but what comfort comes from them? Comfort is taken in small things, in accumulations of instants.

Rita Charon (Charon et al. 2016: 116) promises that learning "narrative competence" will help us to distinguish between "reading Elizabethan drama" and "a Beckett play". Let us then leave the last word in this chapter to a hero of ours, Samuel Beckett (*Endgame*: 83), who signals the end of story, upsetting the applecart. Beckett is a narrative sceptic. *Endgame* depicts the time-allergic act of becoming clogged, miring us in the certainty of uncertainty and the trivial instant:

Moments for nothing, now as always, time was never and time is over, reckoning closed and story ended.

In the following chapter, we continue our critique of Narrative Medicine by suggesting that, far from offering a parallel track to biomedicine and a critique of its limitations, Narrative Medicine can become biomedicine's bedmate.

References

Abbott A. Against Narrative: A Preface to Lyrical Sociology. *Sociological Theory.* 2007; 25: 67–99.

Arca KC. Opaque Selves: A Ricoeurian Response to Galen Strawson's Anti-Narrative Arguments. *Ricoeur Studies.* 2018; 9(1). Retrieved from https://ricoeur.pitt.edu/ojs/index.php/ricoeur/article/view/387

Atkinson P. 1995. *Medical Talk and Medical Work: The Liturgy of the Clinic.* London: Sage.

Bates VL, Hurwitz B. 2016. The Roots and Ramifications of Narrative in Modern Medicine. In: A Whitehead, A Woods (eds.) *The Edinburgh Companion to the Critical Medical Humanities.* Edinburgh: Edinburgh University Press, 559–76. Retrieved from https://www.ncbi.nlm.nih.gov/books/NBK379256

Becker HS, Hughes EC, Geer B, Strauss AL. 1961. *Boys in White: Student Culture in Medical School.* Chicago, IL: University of Chicago Press.

Beckett S. 1957. Endgame. Retrieved from https://edisciplinas.usp.br/pluginfile.php/3346220/mod_resource/content/1/ENDGAME%20BY%20SAMUEL%20BECKETT.pdf

Bhabha H. 1994. *The Location of Culture.* London: Routledge. Retrieved from http://www2.tf.jcu.cz/~klapetek/bha.pdf

Bleakley A. 2015. *Medical Humanities and Medical Education: How the Medical Humanities Can Shape Better Doctors.* Abingdon: Routledge.

Bourke J. 2014. *The Story of Pain: From Prayer to Painkillers.* Oxford: OUP.

Brody H. "My Story Is Broken; Can You Help Me Fix It?": Medical Ethics and the Joint Construction of Narrative. *Literature and Medicine.* 1994; 13: 79–92.

Bruner J. 1986. *Actual Minds, Possible Worlds.* Cambridge, MA: Harvard University Press.

Bruner J. 2002. *Making Stories: Law, Literature, Life.* Cambridge, MA: Harvard University Press.

Bruner J. Reflections on the Self. *Social Research.* 1987; 54: 11–32.

Byrne P, Long B. 1976. *Doctors Talking to Patients.* London: HMSO.

Chambers T. 1999. *The Fiction of Bioethics.* Abingdon: Routledge.

Charon R. Narrative Medicine: A Model for Empathy, Reflection, Profession, and Trust. *Journal of the American Medical Association.* 2001; 286: 1897–1902.

Charon R. 2006. *Narrative Medicine: Honoring the Stories of Illness.* Oxford: Oxford University Press.

Charon R, DasGupta S, Hermann N, et al. 2016. *The Principles and Practices of Narrative Medicine.* Oxford: Oxford University Press.

Charon R, Montello M (eds.) 2002. *Stories Matter: The Role of Narrative in Medical Ethics.* London: Routledge.

Charon R, Wyer P. Narrative Evidence Based Medicine. *Lancet.* 2008; 26: 296–97.

Frank A. 1995. *The Wounded Storyteller: Body, Illness and Ethics.* Chicago, IL: University of Chicago Press.

Goffman E. 1961. *Asylums.* New York: Anchor Books.

Greene R (ed.) 2012. *The Princeton Encyclopaedia of Poetry & Poetics,* 4th ed. Princeton, NJ: Princeton University Press.

Greenhalgh T, Hurwitz B (eds.) 1998. *Narrative Based Medicine.* London: BMJ Books.

Hegele A. 2017. Indigenous Poetics and Narrative Medicine. Synapsis, October 23, 2017. Retrieved from https://medicalhealthhumanities.com/2017/10/23/indigenous-poetics-and-narrative-medicine/

Hunter KM. 1991. *Doctors' Stories: The Narrative Structure of Medical Knowledge.* Princeton, NJ: Princeton University Press.

Hunter KM. 2005. *How Doctors Think: Clinical Judgment and the Practice of Medicine.* New York, NY: Oxford University Press.

Hunter KM, Charon R, Coulehan J. The Study of Literature in Medical Education. *Academic Medicine.* 1995; 70: 787–94.

Hyvärinen M. 2012. "Against Narrativity" Reconsidered. In: G Rossholm, C Johansson (eds.) *Disputable Core Concepts of Narrative Theory.* Bern: Peter Lang, 327–46.

Jones EM, Tansey EM. (eds.) 2015. The Development of Narrative Practices in Medicine c.1960–c.2000. *Wellcome Witnesses to Contemporary Medicine.* Vol. 52. London: Queen Mary University of London.

Kleinman A. 1988. *The Illness Narratives: Suffering, Healing and the Human Condition.* New York: Basic Books.

Kleinsinger F. Working with the Noncompliant Patient. *Permanente Journal.* 2010; 14: 54–60.

Lacquer T. 1989. *Making Sex: Body and Gender from the Greeks to Freud.* Cambridge, MA: Harvard University Press.

Launer J. 2018. *Narrative-Based Practice in Health and Social Care: Conversations Inviting Change,* 2nd ed. Abingdon: Routledge.

Lyotard J-F. 1979. *The Postmodern Condition: A Report on Knowledge.* Manchester: Manchester University Press.

McNamara P. Dreams and Narrative. Psychology Today. March 6, 2015. Retrieved from https://www.psychologytoday.com/gb/blog/dream-catcher/201503/dreams-and-narrative

Milosz C. 1968 "Ars Poetica". Retrieved from https://www.poetryfoundation.org/poems/49455/ars-poetica-56d22b8f31558

Milosz C. 1982. *The Witness of Poetry.* Cambridge, MA: Harvard University Press.

Mishler EG. 1986. *Research Interviewing: Context and Narrative.* Cambridge, MA: Harvard University Press.

Montello M (ed.) Hastings Center Report, Narrative Ethics: The Role of Stories in Bioethics. *Narrative Ethics.* 2014; S2–S6. Retrieved from https://onlinelibrary.wiley.com/doi/abs/10.1002/hast.260

Moody N, Hallam J (eds.) 1998. *Medical Fictions.* Liverpool: John Moores University.

Neilson, S. Caring Masked as Narrative Medicine. *Canadian Medical Association Journal.* 2009; 181: E93–94.

O'Mahony S. Against Narrative Medicine. *Perspectives in Biology and Medicine.* 2013; 56: 611–19.

Rilke RM. 2013. *Letters to a Young Poet.* Scotts Valley, CA: CreateSpace Independent Publishing Platform.

Sartwell C. 2000. *End of Story: Toward an Annihilation of Language and History*. Albany: State University of New York Press.

Shklovsky V. 1991. *Theory of Prose*. London: Dalkey Archive Press.

Spivak GC. 2008. *Can the Subaltern Speak?: Reflections on the History of an Idea*. New York: Columbia University Press. Retrieved from http://abahlali.org/files/Can_the_subaltern_speak.pdf

Strawson G. Against Narrativity. *Ratio*. 2004a; 17: 428–52.

Strawson G. Tales of the unexpected. *The Guardian*. January 10, 2004b. Retrieved from HTTPS://WWW.THEGUARDIAN.COM/BOOKS/2004/JAN/IO/SOCIETY.PHILOSOPHY★GALEN

Vaihinger H. 1924. *The Philosophy of "As If?"*. London: Routledge.

Warmington S. 2020. *Storytelling Encounters as Medical Education: Crafting Relational Identity*. Abingdon: Routledge.

White H. 1987. *The Content of the Form: Narrative Discourse and Narrative Representation*. Baltimore, MD: The Johns Hopkins University Press.

Williams WC. 1967. *The Autobiography of William Carlos Williams*. San Francisco, CA: New Directions Books.

Woods A. The Limits of Narrative: Provocations for the Medical Humanities. *Medical Humanities*. 2011a; 37: 73–78.

Woods A. Post-Narrative – An Appeal. *Narrative Inquiry*. 2011b; 21: 399–406.

Zaharias G. Narrative-Based Medicine 1. *Canadian Family Physician*. 2018; 64: 176–80.

3 What's the story behind narrative medicine? The shared epistemologies of narrative medicine and biomedicine

Is narrative medicine a handmaiden to biomedicine? Historically speaking, how could it not be?

Rita Charon (2006: 3) notes scientific medicine's tendency to objectify patients, aligned with the commodification of care, such that "Patients lament that their doctors don't listen to them or that they seem indifferent to their suffering". We mentioned in the previous chapter that this rhetorical stance unfortunately tars all doctors with the same brush, another example of the "general case". It is true that a body of evidence has accrued showing that, by their later years, medical school students show a measurable decline in empathy and a concomitant increase in cynicism as they are socialised into both objectification and commodification of patients (Peng, Clarkin, and Doja 2020). The standardisation of medical practice (grounded in the adoption of standard learning outcomes for medical education) has also long been seen as a source of such objectification (Bleakley 2014). These trends echo biomedicine's hold over what in everyday clinical practice extends well beyond the borders of both pure and applied science.

The powerful and often dazzling explanatory powers of quantitative biomedicine – reflected in Cochrane reviews privileging evidence gleaned from the "gold standard" of identity-hidden clinical trials – has, both in Charon's and our view, eclipsed a medicine of appreciation and qualities. Resistance against such biomedical dominance was inevitable, and came in the 1970s onwards in the shape of interest in qualitative research, patient-centredness and inter-professional team practices (Bleakley, Bligh and Browne 2011; Bleakley 2014). As explored in the last chapter, generic narrative medicine, a key pillar of the medical or health humanities, was also a part of this emancipatory movement. But the freedom came with certain conditions – a circumscribed freedom.

In the earlier days of the development of narrative medicine, Howard Brody (in Greenhalgh and Hurwitz 1998: xiv) used the metaphor of "the bridge" to link the narrative and biomedical approaches, suggesting that doctors "travel back and forth across the bridge", knitting together idiosyncratic patient narratives and best scientific evidence, such work described

DOI: 10.4324/9781003194408-4

through the additional metaphor of "shuttle diplomacy". (Brody also used the metaphor of "clinical equipoise" to describe achieving a balance between evidence-based and narrative approaches (Miller and Brody 1998)). But, as Brody (ibid.) recognised, the proposed back and forth across the bridge is halted in its tracks by a stubborn reality, where "modern biomedicine has ... tended to neglect the patient or the lived-experience side". In reality, proponents of a stricter biomedical approach stuck stubbornly to their side of "the bridge", effectively detonating the metaphor. For them, there was no bridge, no river to cross.

A better metaphor may be that biomedical purists retreated to their specialist burrows or bunkers (physiology, biochemistry, genetics, information science), alienating narrative through refusal, where science's love of quantities trumps the arts' and humanities' love of qualities. Thus there was no bridge for many, but instead the long shadow of what C.P. Snow (1959) had bemoaned in his landmark 1959 Reid Lecture as the ever-diverging "Two Cultures" (sciences and arts silos). [This sense of divergence between the disciplines was noted, and rejected, as early as 1928 – and again in 1952 – by the English philosopher and literary critic Owen Barfield (1973). Barfield argued that at the level of form or structure, poetry and science were equal partners – the difference was in expression, through poetry's more insistent use of metaphor. He described this as poetry's ability to transcend "knowledge" for "wisdom" – predating T.S. Eliot's similar distinction. Barfield thought it less important to concentrate on dividing poetry and science and more on explaining what made good poetry and good science]. To return to Snow's "two cultures", and contra Barfield, seemingly only a handful of concerned doctors would take the shuttle to fully integrate patient stories with biomedical facts.

Addressing the dilemma of science and art as mutually exclusive ways of thinking, C.P. Snow called this a symptom of a cultural illness:

> In our society (that is, advanced western society) we have lost even the pretence of a common culture. Persons educated with the greatest intensity we know can no longer communicate with each other on the plane of their major intellectual concern.

Literary scholars, in particular Anne Hudson Jones, Kathryn Montgomery Hunter, and scholar-doctors such as Rita Charon, noted that recognition of the value of narrative in medicine was not enough. One must cross over to literary departments to study narrative formally. Doctors should be formally educated in narratology in order to apply this learning to clinical practice. They must not only be hobbyists – already the bane of doctors' involvement in the developing field of the medical humanities at the time.

As noted in the previous chapter, Charon termed this "narrative competence", unwittingly doing damage to her cause, for competence is a reductive term literally meaning "good enough", where "capability" is a more elastic and adventurous descriptor of the outcomes of learning (Bleakley, Bligh and Browne 2011). In the wake of these developments in narrative medicine came a realisation that the approach does not pay due respect to the necessary core of biomedical science and its evidence-based medicine offspring (Ebell 2011; Meza and Passerman 2011). One might ask in response, "What are the central metaphors, epistemologies, and mythologies of 'biomedical science' and 'evidence-based medicine'?", but if you did that, then you weren't on the side demanding its due. The shuttle must be fully operational, the bridge must be crossed, and the burning question became "on whose terms?"

Where James Meza and Daniel Passerman (ibid.) entitle their 2011 book *Integrating Narrative Medicine and Evidence-Based Medicine*, so the metaphor of the bridge is now transcended by one of integration, a melding. Narrative must be drawn back from its impulse to wander. No more shuttling or footwork is needed back and forth between the two stations. Rather, the work can be done out of one common habitat. But this vision did not predict that maybe a basic biomedical approach melded with narrative studies would also serve to both dilute and blunt the previously concentrated and sharp borrowings from narratology – so that users no longer watched their metaphors and encouraged new forms, or let their poetic imaginations run free – reigning in the words in the service of functionalism and instrumentalism.

Ironically, it seems that Narrative Medicine (we capitalise the Charonian Columbia University approach to narrative medicine to distinguish it from other approaches) in such a milieu became a handmaiden to biomedicine, the very force it first resisted (Ebell 2011). As this marriage of biomedicine and narrative under the "evidence-based" banner proceeded, narrativists did not turn their eye to the potentially rich language of medical science, its metaphors and semiotics such as "sticky neurons" and "vascular degeneration". Rather, biomedicine turned narrative approaches to its own purposes, dulling narrative's blade. Narrative Medicine was persuaded that it needs evidential, research-based proof for its claims (the "evidence-based trap"); and second, the metaphor and image taps were turned off, drying out language to functional prosaic descriptors, so as to speak the language that instrumentalists understand.

As Peter Wyer and Rita Charon (2011: ix) say in their Foreword to Meza and Passerman's (2011) book, they support the latter authors' "joining of narrative ways of thinking in medicine with search, always, for the firmest and 'truest' thinking in the scientific foundations of clinical practice". We note "firmest" as a cousin to Charon's muscularities in her descriptors of Narrative Medicine, noted in the previous chapter. "Firmest" also resonates with the clinical "firm" (a long-standing term for a stable team) and a hint at the business model, where Narrative Medicine^{TM} is the "firm".

Meza and Passerman (ibid.: xv) further cite Charon:

> He [an evidence based medicine practitioner] came to us to say, 'Evidence based medicine lacks what you in narrative medicine know.' I was able to

say to him: 'Narrative based medicine lacks what you in evidence-based medicine know.' So we have formed a joint intensive study seminar. We call it narrative–evidence-based medicine, realizing that there is evidence to be had in narrative.

Confused, huh? Charon says that Narrative Medicine lacks what EBM experts know, but then realises that "narrative" already provides "evidence". Evidence of what? Or what kind of evidence? But this worry is a side issue to our main point that Narrative Medicine wants legitimacy and is prepared to align with EBM's manifesto, birthing NEMB. (This acronym makes us numb.) Returning to Charon's paradoxical muscular language for what is, after all, claimed to be a tender approach to patient care, we note a metonymic chain appearing: "firmest", "truest", "foundations", "intensive".

Again, Wyer and Charon (ibid.) argue for "a scientifically informed narrative medicine" that draws on "narrative evidence" just as it draws on "evidence based medicine". We are not sure that one can have it all ways. Our argument for scientific medicine's value from a poetic perspective is that good science is packed with interesting, generative metaphorical language that does important things. Instrumental and reductive science (distinguished from the ideal Science we've just described) is starved of such metaphor-rich language as the language dries out to be merely descriptive; or, it relies on hidden-in-plain-view metaphorical systems – often dead, but titanic, metaphor paradigms that structure the whole knowledge gathering enterprise (such as Kuhn's well-known shifting scientific paradigms).

In what is admittedly a very brief introduction, Wyer and Charon use only three functional metaphors: "a stereoscopic way of knowing", the well-worn "the fruits of our work", and "the firmest thinking" (the latter now forming a metonymic chain with other "hard" analogies quoted above, as we have noted, echoing with the well-used "hard evidence"). A stereoscopic way of knowing unwittingly mimics the "Two Eyed Way of Seeing" hermeneutic model of many North American indigenous peoples. Metaphors like these really can't coax science across the bridge, over the river, and into the territory of story. Science has one epistemology and art has another, but they are hardly alien; they are like sisters living comfortably in the same household under one roof of care.

Let us be clear that we are fed up with the science-art oppositional mindset. The English champion of "close reading", I.A. Richards (1926, 1955) (also the tutor of William Empson, whose work we encounter in Chapters 11–13) published *Science and Poetry* in 1926, where the two are reconciled as mutual ways to appreciate objects. Science describes and measures objects in themselves, where poetry accounts for human responses to those objects. We agree. Our issue is with metaphors and their quality. There can, on the one hand, be poor use of tired metaphors with little effort to generate new ones; and on the other, the fertile generation of metaphors that move the imagination and educate the senses. Thus, there can be metaphor paucity and metaphor generation in both science and art. Characteristically, we have used the qualifier "reductive" where we talk of metaphor and image paucity in science in particular.

We must nourish the living and productive metaphors and bury the dead ones in biomedicine if it is to flourish poetically (and then feed its development). In the Foreword to Meza and Passerman's book, Mark Ebell says, "Human beings are *hard wired* to hear and tell stories" (ibid.: x, our emphasis). The symptom of functionalism manifests in the choice of a dead metaphor straight out of this age's horrible hybrid: the biomedical songbook supplemented by the engineering manual. Metaphors like these amble awkwardly like revenants, emanating from a crypt of medical metaphors that reduce the body to a machine: 'nuts and bolts'. It does not tell a story – rather, it dishes up a cold fact so often that is no fact at all, other than to declare its status as received wisdom, as affirmations of the status quo.

We say, *No.* We say, *The brain is not hard but squidgy and sticky. The "wiring" is not wiring at all, but chemical inhibition and excitation resulting in patterned pulses of transmission.* We say *We recognise the value inherent in the machine metaphor but at the same time we recognise its status as instantiation of prevailing paradigm, of the body-as-machine.* We say, *Time for new metaphors.* We say to the poets especially, *Time for new metaphors.*

In Charon's (2016: 7) move to align narrative and evidence-based approaches, she notes that "The doctor who has accompanied her patient over a prolonged period of time will have the bank of biological knowledge about that individual necessary for timely and accurate diagnostic vision", but also they will have developed "the muscular therapeutic alliance necessary to engage the patient in effective care". Our questions, following from above, are first whether the assumed "bank of biological knowledge" is generative for imagination so that the diagnostic work itself is artful. And second, is the "therapeutic alliance" (itself a clunky, functional and frankly ugly term) aesthetically pleasing as well as ethically and politically sincere? A "muscular" alliance returns us to Charon's preferred metonymic chain of tough descriptors, where we had been promised an embrace of the tender such as Charon's (2016: 9) claim for "exquisitely attentive" (repeated for effect) reading and listening practices: "We hope readers will join us in recognizing close reading's exquisitely attentive reading practice to be the laboratory for the exquisitely attentive listening practice that is our goal in clinical work".

Also, through incarnation as a "muscular" option narrative is here protected from (perceived) science-based sceptics' criticism of it being a "soft touch". The rhetoric is clear – narrative is no longer a soft option. We do not sneer at such a practice of medicine – drawing on narrative to add aesthetic and ethical value to medicine is a good thing. Indeed, to us it offers a prototype of an ideal that we hope our text improves on by encouraging doctors to think poetically in biomedical encounters without feeling embarrassed or haunted by biomedicine's ghost, but rather fortified by biomedicine's strengths. We express reservations at the rhetorical strain to justify one thing, "narrative competence", in terms of another problematic, that of a "bank of biological knowledge" (this metaphor unfortunately adding to the commercialism we perceive in Narrative Medicine[TM]).

Furthermore, Charon's construction here is entirely outcomes-based and practical. If Narrative Medicine's point is solely to develop a "therapeutic alliance necessary to engage the patient in effective care", meaning, we think, to get them to agree to that which is "effective", meaning biomedical care most probably, then we wonder a bit about Narrative Medicine as a coercive instrumentalisation of the humanities. For our part, we are not so eager to fall into evidence-based medicine's trap, and we will explain our vision in subsequent chapters. We were both initially educated in pure sciences and so feel we have some experiential legitimacy to make our claims. We are also both proponents, as you might have gathered by now, of the aesthetics of science.

A key technique developed by Charon (2001, 2006) in her earlier work is the "parallel chart", where doctors keep informal notes about their responses to patients that are not formal descriptions of cases or treatments, but more qualitatively oriented, to include personal feelings and unique features about patients. But again, perhaps narrative has become biomedicine's handmaiden here too. Why a "chart" unless one is bowing down to standard medical practice? Would a novelist, a short story writer, a poet or even a journalist refer to her work as a "chart"? An astrologer does, but that's a different story. More, if Narrative Medicine is truly on a "parallel" path with biomedicine, then they will never meet (we're closely watching the metaphor trajectories in Narrative Medicine). How will dialogue and productive intermingling occur?

Meza and Passerman (2011: xv) continue to attempt to forge a single identity out of Narrative Medicine and Evidence-Based Medicine, although the claim is tentative: "there are hints that these movements will converge". But we thought they were on parallel paths and not on convergent routes? Let's get the metaphors right. Some would say that two differing epistemologies would never meet – as we have seen, this was C.P. Snow's verdict on the "two cultures" of arts and sciences, much to his dismay, and contra other commentators of the time such as Owen Barfield (1973). Charon (cited in ibid.: xvi) capitulates to science's need for evidence, where "narrative based medicine, *by definition*, is not meant to point to medicine that does not have evidence" (our emphasis). We find the qualifier "by definition" to be troubling. Narrative Medicine now appears, again, to be re-defined on biomedicine's terms as an evidence-based approach. We sense once more that Charon is pining for scientific legitimacy – that Narrative Medicine is only worthy of the name, only sanctioned in its official sense, if it is itself evidenced, proven effective.

But, for a qualitative method that purposefully invites complication, complexity and ambiguity, it is difficult to see how we can apply biomedicine's quantitative, measurement, and evidence-based research frames and directives to narrative approaches that are essentially qualitative, and claimed as self-evidently useful (the proof is in the pudding). Again this may be attempting a shotgun marriage of differing epistemologies. For us, the bigger danger is that narratives become capital invested in the aforementioned "bank of information"; that *narrative becomes data* rather than *data become narrative*, choking the parallel track of narrative at its source and restricting any crossings of the bridge and river to the "other" side. Charon et al. (2016: 105) promised us that "a story is something whose content cannot be reduced to analyzable data". But surely this is what Narrative Medicine does? At least, as we have seen, Johanna Shapiro (2009) eschews such obscurity in unashamedly treading the data path.

Narrative Medicine, once counter-bioculture revolutionary, could now be seen to have sold out for two reasons. First, a desire to appease the critical backlash of scientifically grounded, evidence-based medicine (see Belling 2010) has led, arguably, to a pact with biomedicine. Again, Wyer and Charon (2011: ix) describe the "stereoscopic way of knowing in clinical medicine" as the dual application of standard biomedicine and imaginative narrative approaches. As we have seen, this unconvincingly morphs into the ungainly descriptor "Narrative Evidence Based Medicine" (Charon and Wyer 2008). The authors claim that by not hyphenating this descriptor, "narrative evidence" and "evidence based medicine" remain distinct entities while working in parallel, but surely narrative approaches here are on the slippery slope to biomedical engulfment where they are seeking to label themselves as "evidence" at all? Isn't it an inherent risk in any human enterprise, when there is a junior and senior partner? This is a risk we are very conscious of as we wrote this book. We didn't want poetry to beat up biomedicine too much. It's not a David and Goliath thing (science is Big now but poetry has been a Giant too), it's more a "tough minded" science against "tender-minded" poetry, to draw on William James' distinction – the first outlook requires objective evidence beyond the readily disordered human sense, the second is the raw evidence of the senses.

Seth Vannatta and Jerry Vannatta (2013) attempt to resolve the dilemma of the differing epistemologies' refusal to cooperate by invoking Charles Peirce's "functional realism" as the yoke that can bind biomedicine with narrative medicine, the elusive bridge that we discussed earlier. Where the atomised event – such as the appearance of symptom – is dealt with by biomedicine's approach of measurement, narrative deals rather with the relationships between events that is best grasped qualitatively. There is no reason that these two cannot be yoked in the Peircean tradition. The population statistic (the general case) and the idiosyncratic presentation (the specific instance) can be entertained simultaneously. This is fine until we get an extraordinary event of marvellous intensity. Narrative's yoking with biomedicine is restraining. It is here that poetry can step in and that biomedicine's intrinsic fluorescence can be enjoyed; language blooms and deep metaphors multiply.

Maybe in a desire for credibility, Wyer and Charon (2011: ix) describe "scientifically informed narrative medicine" as one among a number of kinds of "evidence". Since when did story amount to "evidence" as a primary characteristic? Is this the way that James Baldwin, John Dos Passos, or Joyce Carole Oates think? This bounces us back to the "story as data" reduction (Bleakley 2005) that Charon explicitly refuses but implicitly reinforces. To be fair, it is the way that Montgomery Hunter thought when she suggested that stories offered by patients can be used as evidence for tracking down the cause of symptoms. But this appropriation of story may be seen as a primary way in which story's value – in creating surprise, tension, and uncertainty – is turned on its head as an instrumental device to reduce uncertainty, alleviate tension and avoid surprise by coming up with diagnostic answers.

We do not argue that story is not evidence. It can be. We worry about what is ultimately *claimed* as "evidence", and we worry about how the claim comes to be made. If a patient's story is only of diagnostic value, or a resource for coercion, then what, exactly, is being proven? There is no longer any narrative in the original sense other than lever-pulling and button-pushing on the narrativist's side. The absorption of patient story into medicine's narrative may potentially create an illness – one of mundanity – through the evisceration of quality, surprise, tension and danger. This potential instrumentalising of narrative approaches means again that they are no longer myth-busters, politically empowering, imaginatively dangerous, but simply techniques – as, again, is suggested in Charon's term "narrative competence".

Adoption of a poetic voice as key to diagnostic clinical work can be frustrated by a misunderstanding of what poetry does, or can do; but it is vital that we air poetry's concerns after many years of living in the shadow of narrative medicine; and in light of Narrative Medicine's desire to meld with evidence-based medicine for apparent legitimacy (thus potentially undermining much of its original revolutionary promise). To return to Meza and Passerman's (2011) book that promised an ill-starred integration of narrative and evidence-based medicines, the Introduction (by Mark Ebell) puts it that "[th]e language of evidence-based medicine is too often complex and opaque and almost always lacks poetry". So, if narrative medicine is aligned with evidence-based medicine, will the latter infect the former with its anti-poetic instrumentalism?

Our ears naturally prick up here at the mention of "poetry", but surely Ebell is misguided? Isn't it poetry that is (purposefully) more likely to be complex and opaque, where evidence-based medicine seeks clarity, concision and precision by placing stress on the importance of quantities and measure? Even where poetry, such as that of William Carlos Williams, is explicitly stripped back, draws from the lay conversational voice, and does not multiply metaphor, it is nevertheless imagistically complex. Its initial field is necessarily complex as architectural feature (line lengths and rhythm, voice effects, pauses, the look on the page). Poetry's measure is musical, beat based and rhythmical (concrete poetry is more so quantitative in spirit, as well as sculptural; conceptual poetry is often outright mathematical).

Is Ebell suggesting that poetry would *simplify* the supposed complex language of evidence-based medicine? In seeking transparency, surely the language of biomedical science that informs evidence-based approaches is more likely to be convergent, instrumental and reductive rather than divergent, open and creative? Poetry, of course, can be concise, but usually resists reduction to mere functionality. The language of poetry, replete with metaphor and image, soused in affect, is more likely to be complex and opaque in raising questions rather than giving answers. In short, isn't poetry too frustrating for minds inclined to seek "evidence"?

Schleifer and Vannatta (2013) usefully progress Charon's work. In particular, they incorporate more sophisticated accounts of clinical reasoning as an abductive ("reasonable best guess" or pattern recognition) process, as noted above (this is more fully explored in Chapters 6 and 7; see also Stanley and Nyrup 2020). This incorporates an ethically sensitive narrative approach, always attempting to recover meanings grounded in the patient's story rather than the doctor's interpretation. But the authors can be criticised as merely warming up classic generic narrative medicine fare through overgeneralisation, where medical "encounters almost always take the form of storytelling, and we propose the inclusion of an important new item in the patient record that is normally referred to as the 'History and Physical Exam', namely, the 'chief concern'". Is this, however, a recapitulation of Charon's "parallel chart"?

In conclusion to this section, generic narrative medicine (including narrative ethics) and its potent offshoot Charonian Narrative Medicine have been, and continue to be, powerful influences in what might be seen as a contemporary re-humanising of medicine. Recent contributions include our own work, such as the use of digital storytelling in medical education research (Bleakley, Wilson and Allard 2019; Allard, Wilson and Bleakley 2020) and close analysis of the work of metaphor in medicine (Bleakley 2017; Neilson 2019). However, it is of deep concern that poetry has been tucked in the back pocket of narrative medicine, relegated to a bit player. In the following section, we address what we see as a gap in the lineage of Narrative Medicine's use of "close reading" technique, central to its method. Their origin myth is I.A. Richards's masterful accounts from 1928 to 1929. Our origin myth is a decade earlier with the Russian Formalists from the beginning of the Revolution in 1917. We approach this, as ever, critically. The British literary critic and Marxist Terry Eagleton is our first stop.

The scientific aspirations inherent to Narrative Medicine's interpretive tool

Terry Eagleton (1983: xi) places the beginnings of modern literary theory in 1917 with Victor Shklovsky's "pioneering essay 'Art as Device'". Shklovsky is "the self-proclaimed 'founder of the Russian School of Formal method'" (Steiner 1984: 44) and has two major useful ideas: (1) a specific metaphorical orientation towards the accumulation and application of knowledge; and (2) the concept of "defamiliarisation".

Shklovsky defined the "Formal method" as "a return to craftsmanship" (ibid.: 45). His predominant metaphorical system for accumulating knowledge, as intimated in his definition, is a mechanistic one. As Steiner (ibid.) says, "Technology, that branch of knowledge pertaining to the art of human production, was the predominant metaphor applied by this model to the description and elucidation of artistic phenomena". We should note the parallels with medicine since Andreas Vesalius: medicine's key metaphoric system for structuring knowledge and guiding practice, as noted earlier, has been the "body as machine" (Bleakley 2017: 55 passim).

Steiner (1984: 45) relates some gossip from one of Shklovsky's colleagues, who called him a "fitter, a mechanic"; the case is made even more strongly with a comment made by Shklovsky to Roman Jakobson: "We know how life is made and how Don Quixote and the car are made too". Shklovsky's method is one that reduces wholes into constituent parts, which is also how biomedicine reduces the human into tissue, cellular, molecular, and chemical components and processes in order to understand the general case. Shklovsky (in ibid.: 46) is refreshingly explicit about this:

> The understanding man scrutinizes the car serenely and comprehends 'what is for what': why it has so many cylinders and why it has big wheels, where its transmission is situated, and why its rear is cut in an acute angle and its radiator unpolished. This is the way one should read.

In another instrumentalist parallel, Shklovsky's manifesto article, published in 1917 in the midst of the Revolution, was called "Art as Technique". This echoed the 1917 Revolution's aims to *engineer* an ideal society, part of which was transferring focus from a widespread agricultural base to a rapidly developing industrial base where the machine was made god in a humanist culture.

Importantly, the Revolution did not frame science, engineering and industry as objectifying, but as providing augmentation to, and expansion of, the senses. We will meet this view again in Chapter 7 as "Object-Oriented Ontology" (Harman 2018). It is critical to our understanding of how objects and artefacts (objects used to enhance the human senses in particular) are aesthetically encompassed by the fields of medicine and poetry. We use "field" here again in the same sense as Charles Olson and William Carlos Williams (as "projective verse"), as a "placing" of language (the clinic and the patient, the page and the reader) in such a way that defamiliarisation (see below) is encouraged. Objects are seen anew not just for utility but also for aesthetic value (thus, the patient is valued by the doctor, as the "Red Wheelbarrow" is cherished in the poet Williams's eye). We note that narrative medicine has extensively mined the personal and emotional, but rarely explicated an ontology of objects (a specialty for poets).

To return to the Russian Formalists, let us extend metaphoric understanding to biomedical terrain in again scrutinising the engineering metaphors. Shklovsky (1991) is less interested in a somewhat Romantic sum of what is called "the human" when performing thought, but more in the specific neural connections firing at a specific moment in time:

> In the theory of literature I am concerned with the study of the internal laws of literature. To draw a parallel with industry, I am interested neither in the situation in the world cotton market, nor in the policy of trusts, but only in the kinds of yarn and the methods of weaving.

Shklovsky's component part or constituent atom of literature was referred to as a "device", a creature of craft. The "device" itself is quite debatable as a useful, unique, and clear idea; in Eagleton's (2008: 3) summary: "sound, imagery, rhythm, syntax, metre, rhyme, narrative techniques, in fact the whole stock of formal literary elements".

The point is that Shklovsky tried to reduce entire wholes to their component parts and took a kind of satisfaction at his presumed ability to do so. This posture is not one uncommonly worn by – if we were to personify it – biomedicine. Michel Foucault (1970) argues that while we might expect such atomising – as a feature of regularities and classifications – of the "noble sciences" (mathematics, cosmology, and physics) during the Enlightenment, it also extended to disciplines such as economics and linguistics. This taxonomising impulse proved useful to the disparate contributors to Russian Formalists qua group as they conducted their investigations into poetry, just as it proved immensely useful to biomedicine as basic sciences grew knowledge through their use of the atomising experimental method. Again, for his part, Shklovsky intuited something truly important to understanding literature: "defamiliarisation" as a core practice.

Defamiliarisation – ironically given the use of engineering metaphors – is the idea that languages and practices used in art are deliberately artificial in order to prevent the reader from processing a text or performance as information in an automatised, or perceptually habitual, way. Put alternately, literature is language that calls attention to itself. More, returning to engineering, language must be tuned and we must be attuned to it. Eagleton (1983: 3) expands,

> what distinguished [literary language] from other forms of discourse, was that it 'deformed' ordinary language in various ways ... by forcing us into a dramatic awareness of language, [literature] refreshes these habitual responses and renders objects more 'perceptible.' By having to grapple with language in a more strenuous, self-conscious way than usual, the world which that language contains is vividly renewed.

To clarify this idea, the Formalists took further pains to distinguish between poetic and prosaic language. The difference was not in the presence or absence of symbols and imagery, for example, but rather that poetic language "was made artificially in such a way that perception lingers over it, thus reaching its greatest possible intensity and duration" whereas "[p]rose is normal speech: economical, easy, regular" (Steiner 1984: 147). Another Formalist, Jakubinski (in ibid.: 149), made a distinction quite useful for the current biomedical context:

> [l]inguistic phenomena ... should be classified, among other ways, from the standpoint of the goal for which the speaker exploits the verbal material in a given case. If he uses it for the purely practical goal of communication, we are dealing with the system of *practical language*, in which linguistic representations (sounds, morphemes, etc.) have no value in themselves but serve merely as a means of communication.

This describes in particular the realm of biomedically-framed communication in the clinic. In contrast, Jakubinski (in ibid.: 149) asserts, "Other linguistic systems are conceivable (and exist) in which the practical goal retreats into the background and linguistic combinations acquire a value in themselves .... I conditionally call this system verse language". Further,

> In practical language the semantic aspect of the word (its meaning) is more prominent than its sound aspect ... details of pronunciation reach our consciousness only if they serve to differentiate the meaning of words .... Thus various considerations compel us to recognize that in *practical language sounds do not attract our attention*. It is the other way around in verse language. There, one can claim that sounds enter the bright field of consciousness and attract our attention.
>
> ibid. (149–50)

Verse is "sound" prior to semantics, music prior to meaning, in a "bright field of consciousness" – resonating with Charles Olson's "Projective Verse" manifesto and Williams's underwriting. Auscultation and percussion are sound prior to diagnostic call in the physical examination (Bleakley 2020).

The "practical vs poetic language" oppositional trope has major currency in medicine amidst a current culture of burnout. If anyone reading this has attended a Narrative Medicine seminar and been taught "narrative competence", then your alarm bells should be going off, for what you're really being taught is Russian Formalism as a way to both improve your practice and, supposedly, to also revivify your working soul. This point is made explicit in a chapter devoted to "close reading" in Charon's (Charon et al. 2016: 165) *The Principles and Practice of Narrative Medicine* where she boldly declares: "We have shown at Columbia that rigorous close reading can be taught and learned in clinical settings, where its dividends have been found to enhance patient care". The science is included with purchase. She adds,

> But teaching healthcare professionals how to be close readers does far more than improve their interviewing skills. Here is where we find the

transformative potential of our practice of narrative medicine … [c]lose reading may be a threshold to a life fully lived.

ibid. (165–66)

We agree, but we're not sure that we would turn "close reading" into a quasi-religious (and mercantile) manifesto. We also note that biomedicine has its own close reading techniques that are perfectly legitimate. You wouldn't want a histopathologist who couldn't close read a tissue sample under the microscope; or a radiologist who couldn't read Multiple Images (Multiple Image Radiography or MIR).

We have noted that Charon's mini-history of close reading misses its origin point with the Russian Formalists (see Chapter 12) in 1917 because she begins with I.A. Richards, a British scholar active in the 1920s and William Empson's tutor at the University of Cambridge, as we shall see from later chapters (11–13) on ambiguity. We find this odd, for what Charon et al. (2016: 166) has been vending since her movement started (recall: "[r]igorous training in close reading – at least narrative medicine's version of close reading – improves readers' capacity for attention but also revolutionizes the reader's position in life from being an onlooker checking the log of past events to becoming a daring participant in the emergence of reality") sounds a lot like Shklovsky's promise. Again, grandiose claims, inflated language: not just engaging in life but "daring" and emerging from the fog of misunderstanding to face "the emergence of reality". Just like Shklovsky famously wanted to once more make the 'stone stony', so Charon wants to make the patient patienty again. Narrative Medicine[TM] can be conceptualised as two old ideas mixed together and branded as new compound: Freud's "talking cure" and Shklovsky's "defamiliarisation". This may be no bad thing, but some stated reflexive awareness of this and its limits seems sorely lacking.

We should note Richards's (1926: 14) alignment of poetry and science (see Klyce 1926). But rest assured, Richards had a similar approach to language insofar as he tried to systematise an approach. His *"Poetry and Science"* essay asks early on, "How is our estimate of poetry going to be affected by the sciences? And how will poetry itself be influenced?" The first paragraph of a review of the text in *The Sewanee Review* begins, "Happily blending scientific method and profound poetic insight, this brief book shows that both civilization and individual life, to be even tolerable, must satisfactorily reconcile science and poetry (or art in general)".

For our money, Richards was more so a synthesiser of art and science – that is, Poetry and Science is not terribly scientific, being (1) a mix of Richards's own philosophy of man, (2) a general commentary on the use of poetry for individuals and society, and (3) finally a mini – and originary – treatise on the marriage between cognitive psychology and poetry (something, of course, that we are attempting here). Science, in other words, is less a grand overarching god and rather a specific discipline, the one Richards trained in. There is much more to say about Richards's orientation towards science which it is

We may begin by adapting the conventional diagram of the communication engineer to our wider purposes.[1] In translation we have two such diagrams to consider as a minimum. There will be (say) a Chinese communication for which we find ourselves in the role of Destination; and we assume thereupon the role of Sources for a communication in English. But since other communications in

S   E   T   R   D   Dv

SOURCE → [ ]→[ ]→[ ]→ [ ]→[ ]→[ ] → DESTINATION

NOISE

S—Selector   R—Receiver
E—Encoder   D—Decoder
T—Transmitter   Dv—Developer

Chinese and other communications in English, having *something in common* with the present communication, come in to guide the encodings and decodings, the process becomes very complex. We have here indeed what may very probably be the most complex type of event yet produced in the evolution of the cosmos.

Between two utterances[2] the operative *something in common* whereby the one influences the other may be any

[1] Adapted with considerable changes from Claude E. Shannon and Warren Weaver, *The Mathematical Theory of Communication* (Urbana: University of Illinois Press, 1949), p. 5.

[2] I need a highly general term here, not limited to any mode of utterance, such as *overt* speech or writing. An act of comprehending may itself be regarded as an utterance, being a rebirth, after passage through the lifeless signal, of something more or less the same as the original which was transmitted.

22

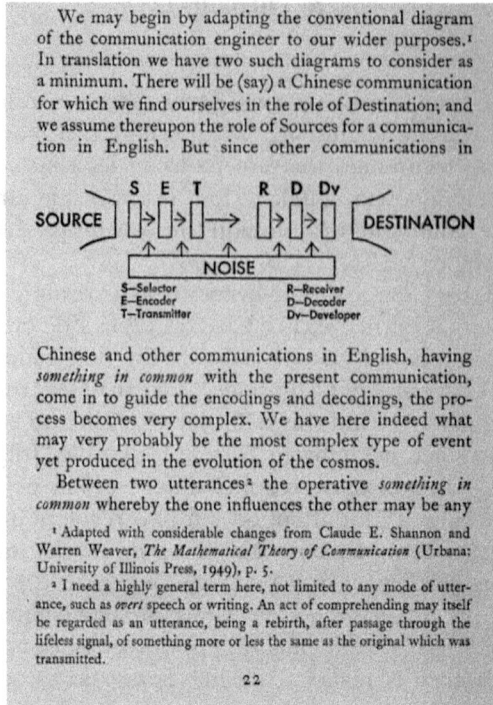

Figure 3.1 I. A. Richards' engineering model of communication.

beyond the scope of this text to provide – for example, there exist critiques of a perceived reductionist tendency to collapse New Criticism into "scientism" (Graff 1974) and "Behaviourism" (Barfield 1973: 34), which we find unconvincing. But we flag the disagreement for transparency of argument – while two more points are useful. The first is that Richards, like so many other critics of the day, did often try to concretise capital-S science and capital-E engineering concepts when it came to literature. For example, in *Speculative Instruments*, the following text and diagram appear, drawing on Shannon and Weaver, the fathers of linear communications theory, who first showed how "noise" can disrupt the flow of communication (Figure 3.1).

Our choice to work with the Russian Formalist approach to criticism is that we believe Charon already covered the supposed origin of close reading as it occurred in the West (Richards). But more importantly, we feel Russian Formalism's kind of close reading is more molecular, to use Nikolas Rose's (2007) terminology, in *The Politics of Life Itself*. Rose writes that "biomedicine visualizes life at … the molecular level" which "is itself enmeshed in a 'molecular' style of thought about life itself" (3; 11). In other words, biomedicine reduces biological wholes into constituent parts as its knowledge accumulation project. The goal is to render the body as data, so that data can be used to help the generic body; producing knowledge in this way results in encouraging people who live in such regimes to think of their lives not as unique wholes, but rather as a sum of situated parts. We feel that the Russian Formalist method of close reading is at the core of close reading as practiced now, and that it is also closer to the core of biomedicine than Richards's own method, which approached a truly scientific aspect when it pioneered reader response. The final reason for our preference to use Russian Formalism in this book is a major criticism of the health humanities' Eurocentrism. By focussing on the Formalists, we get out of the West. (We also depart from individualism to embrace social learning).

But our prods above are minor in relation to the central burning question: if Russian Formalism is the tradition within which Narrative Medicine largely works, or the historical well from which it draws inspiration, then why doesn't it consider poetry more often and in depth? Why is non-narrative poetry subsumed in narrative medicine thinking? As Pavel Medvedev, whom Steiner (1984: 139) calls a contemporaneous "Marxist critic of the [Russian Formalist] movement", suggested, the "hypothesis of the distinctness of poetic language is the basis on which the entire Russian Formalist method is built". It is worth scrutinising the attempts to science-ify Russian Formalism in this context.

Russian formalism aspires to science, I.A. Richards in its wake, Narrative Medicine in Richards's wake

The appeal of Russian Formalism for Narrative Medicine seems natural, for the Formalists were very much invested in transforming the study of literature into a science, while, as we have seen, Narrative Medicine has gradually adopted a practical orientation to prove itself in the image of evidence-based medicine. For example, Jakobson (in ibid.: 23) referred to what we would now call "literary studies" as a science whose objective was extracting (and abstracting) an essence: "The object of literary science is not literature but literariness, i.e., what makes a given work a literary work". Eichenbaum (in ibid.: 22), a member of the St. Petersburg-based Society for the Study of Poetic Language and a colleague of Shklovsky's, wrote,

> the Formal method, by gradually evolving and extending its field of inquiry, has completely exceeded what was traditionally called methodology and is turning into a special science that treats literature as a specific series of facts ... What characterizes us is neither 'Formalism' as an aesthetic theory, nor 'methodology' as a closed scientific system, but only the striving to establish, on the basis of specific properties of the literary material, an independent literary science.

In their enterprise to taxonomise language, the Russian Formalists again reduced language to its constituent parts, conceiving of it in mechanistic terms through engineering metaphors, so that the enterprise itself could be called a science, as a legitimising strategy: "What is significant about the Formal method?" Shklovsky wrote in his characteristic staccato style:

> What is significant is that we approached art as production. Spoke of it alone. Viewed it not as a reflection. Found the specific features of the genus. Began to establish the basic tendencies of form. Grasped that on a large scale there is a real homogeneity in the laws informing works. Hence, the science [of literature] is possible (in ibid.: 65).

Here, surely, is a logic for Narrative Medicine's desire for scientific legitimacy that it has overlooked: a striking similarity between biomedicine and Russian Formalism. Biomedicine's project is, as Lock and Nguyen (2010: 11) write in *An Anthropology of Biomedicine*, to bring about "a systematic and ultimately scientific approach to knowledge about the body and its management … grounded by knowledge produced by decontextualizing the body and subjecting it to an anatomical gaze". The authors update this epistemological formulation with a slightly more metaphorical version to the original text, writing that biomedicine is "a sociotechnical system" that is based "on biological sciences", the latter providing "a set of standards, protocols, and algorithms that enable the production of knowledge and practices to treat ailing individuals … Biomedicine, in theory then, is based on an assumption on the universality of human bodies that everywhere are biologically equivalent" (Lock and Nguyen 2018: 1). Vesalius redux, biomedicine boxed, body as information. Our technologies have allowed us to generate and process such information that is then abstracted into universalising principles; our "story technologies" (narrative purely as method) proceed accordingly.

For Shklovsky, the Formal method not only reduces language to its constituent parts and taxonomises but also discovers "basic tendencies of form" and demonstrates that there "is a real homogeneity in the laws informing works". It is the latter qualities that Shklovsky quite rightly identifies as the hallmarks of Western science. Where Russian Formalism and Narrative Medicine part company is in the former's rebellious embrace of art for art's sake, refusing to consider that art is a reflection of, for example, a sociology or psychology of the conditions that produced it. As Shklovsky maintained in what has been called "arguably one of the most well known paragraphs in aesthetic history": "In order to restore our lived experience of the world and feel things again, in order to make a stone a stone again, we have something called art" (in Yakubinski 2018: 16).

Russian Formalism was then the creation of an instrument of interpretation, and Narrative Medicine in its wake can be read as the instrumentalisation of art. Importantly, the project underwrites all current literary scholarship, no matter the tradition. The Formalist way of reading has proven a powerful hermeneutic. Moreover, we offer the scientific theme and aspiration of the Formalists as a unique connection, but in truth, the Formalists were part of the same cultural milieu inspired by the philosophy of positivism, which holds that, as Maya Goldenberg (2006: 2622) has stated, "only scientifically verifiable propositions" have meaning. Steiner (1984: 253), the definitive historian of the Russian Formalists, suggests that positivism circulating as far back as the 1870s was an influence. The Russian Formalists's "art for art's sake" rejected literature as reflection of "pseudo-religion, or psychology or sociology" (Eagleton 1983: 3). The Formalists and Biomedicalists adopt the mock political stance that art and medical science are both decontextualised, depoliticised, valueless enterprises (or rather they generate their own value), yet this is reflective of a larger cultural turn that cannot be isolated as egregiously abnormal or unique.

Shaking off the limitations of Russian Formalism and rescuing the notion of defamiliarisation, the latter allows us to slow down and appreciate that which can make a patient a human again. Patients were always human, of course; and so were we. We just needed a way to reconnect with the reality. Just as "the stone" is recovered *as particular stone* (and not as geology, generic building material, or obstacle), so humanity is recovered from reduction to symptom and underlying disease in addressing the homogenising provided by biomedicine (the individual caught in the generalising mould of the scientific model); and in addressing the instrumentality of Narrative Medicine (literature and literary studies used as a means to the end of "improving patient care", but what of "improving" literature to "improve" culture?). Art for art's sake is not a static stance of observation but one of continuous deliberation on what makes "art" – done for the sake of the art as object and not on behalf of the biography of the artist. Why? Because this feeds into an aesthetic sensibility and this is the oil that is needed to give the dry, homogenised, wood of biomedicine some nourishment, tone, and character.

In the following chapter we complete our running critique of Narrative Medicine, and the chapter after that returns to the Russian Formalists to also critique that approach rather than lionise it. This is again work of reclamation of Poetry Territory that we think has been colonised by narrative medicine of various persuasions. Our challenge to what we see as narrativism's overreach is necessarily political as well as aesthetic and ethical. We want justice for poetry where we see unjust repression of its voice. On poetry's behalf, we, again, have adopted tried and tested positions of resistance such as sly civility (Homi Bhabha) and empowerment of the subaltern voice (Gayatri Spivak). Hence, our often ironic stance and provocations.

In working slowly towards bringing poetry out of narrative's shadow, we have made, and will continue to make, Heideggerian "clearings" through critique, that the poet Peter Redgrove called "holes-in-the-day" (a pun on "holiday") as opportunities to break routines and stale habits; these are rents in the standard fabric. Narrativism has woven poetry into its being as prisoner and we want to spring poetry from jail. Part of our tactic is to use medicine as a means for bringing poetry's Being into focus. Our binocularism again is Poetry=Medicine. In time, we get to another question, one of application: how shall we "close read" a clinical encounter not only out of the orb of narrative medicine but also springing the normative psychological frames familiar to us from "communication skills" training in medical education? How shall we understand the "medical mind" as one invested in the "poetic imagination", in turn, understood by Aristotle to be the vessel within which poetry sits? Our wish is to see the clinical and poetic imaginations as equal partners in medicine and medical pedagogy.

References

Allard J, Wilson M, Bleakley A. 2020. Doctors Need Safe Confessional and Cathartic Spaces: What We Learned from the Research Project 'People Talking: Digital Dialogue for Mutual Recovery'. In: A Bleakley (ed.) *Routledge Handbook of the Medical Humanities*. Abingdon: Routledge, 410–18.

Barfield O. 1973/1952. *Poetic Diction: A Study in Meaning*, 2nd ed. Hanover, NH: Wesleyan University Press.

Belling C. Commentary: Sharper Instruments: On Defending the Humanities in Undergraduate Medical Education. *Academic Medicine*. 2010; 85: 938–40.

Bleakley A. 2005. Stories as Data, Data as Stories: Making Sense of Narrative Inquiry in Clinical Education. *Medical Education*. 2005; 39: 534–40.

Bleakley A. 2014. *Patient-Centred Medicine in Transition: The Heart of the Matter*. Dordrecht: Springer.

Bleakley A. 2017. *Thinking with Metaphors in Medicine: The State of the Art*. Abingdon: Routledge.

Bleakley A. 2020. *Educating Doctors' Senses through the Medical Humanities: "How Do I Look?"* Abingdon: Routledge.

Bleakley A, Bligh J, Browne J. 2011. *Medical Education for the Future: Identity, Power and Location*. Dordrecht: Springer.

Bleakley A, Wilson M, Allard J. 2020. Storytelling. In: P Crawford, B Brown, A Charise (eds.) *The Routledge Companion to Health Humanities*. Abingdon: Routledge, 397–401.

Brody H. 1998. Foreword. In: T Greenhalgh, B Hurwitz (eds.) *Narrative Based Medicine: Dialogue and Discourse in Clinical Practice*. London: BMJ Books, xiii–xv.

Charon R. Narrative Medicine: A Model for Empathy, Reflection, Profession, and Trust. *JAMA*. 2001; 286: 1897–1902.

Charon R. 2006. *Narrative Medicine: Honoring the Stories of Illness*. Oxford: Oxford University Press.

Charon R, DasGupta S, Hermann N, et al. 2016. *The Principles and Practices of Narrative Medicine*. Oxford: Oxford University Press.

Charon R, Wyer P. Narrative Evidence Based Medicine. *The Lancet*. 2008; 371: 296–97.

Eagleton, T. 2008/1983. *Literary Theory: An Introduction*. Minneapolis, MN: University of Minneapolis Press.

Ebell MH. (2011). Foreword. In: JP Meza, DS Passerman (eds.) *Integrating Narrative Medicine and Evidence-Based Medicine: The Everyday Social Practice of Healing*. London: Radcliffe Publishing, x–xi.

Foucault M. 1970. *The Order of Things*. New York: Pantheon Books.

Goldenberg MJ. On Evidence and Evidence-Based Medicine: Lessons from the Philosophy of Science. *Social Science & Medicine*. June 2006; 62(11): 2621–32.

Graff G. What Was New Criticism? Literary Interpretation and Scientific Objectivity. *Salamagundi*. 1974; 27: 72–93.

Harman G. 2018. *Object-Oriented Ontology: A New Theory of Everything*. London: Penguin Random House.

Klyce, S. A Review of I.A. Richards' Science and Poetry. *The Sewanee Review*. 1926; 34: 362–63.

Lock MM, Nguyen V-K. 2010. *An Anthropology of Biomedicine*. Hoboken, NH: Wiley-Blackwell.

Lock MM, Nguyen V-K. 2018. *An Anthropology of Biomedicine*, 2nd ed. Hoboken, NH: Wiley-Blackwell.

Meza JP, Passerman DS. 2011. *Integrating Narrative Medicine and Evidence-Based Medicine: The Everyday Social Practice of Healing*. London: Radcliffe Publishing.

Miller F, Brody H. Clinical Equipoise and the Incoherence of Research Ethics. *Journal of Medicine and Philosophy*. 1998; 32: 151–65.

Neilson S. 2019. The Practice of Metaphor. In: A Bleakley (ed.) *The Routledge Companion to the Medical Humanities*. Abingdon: Routledge, 144–54.

Peng J, Clarkin C, Doja A. Uncovering Cynicism in Medical Training: A Qualitative Analysis of Medical Online Discussion Forums. *BMJ Open*. 2018; 8: e022883.

Richards IA. 1926. *Science and Poetry*. London: Kegan Paul, Trench, Trubner & Co. (Republished as Poetries and Sciences, 1935).

Richards IA. 1955. *Speculative Instruments*. New York: Harcourt, Brace and World.

Rose N. 2007. *The Politics of Life Itself*. Princeton, NJ: Princeton University Press.

Schleifer R, Vannatta JB. 2013. *The Chief Concern of Medicine: The Integration of the Medical Humanities and Narrative Knowledge into Medical Practices*. Ann Arbor: The University of Michigan Press.

Shapiro J. 2009. *The Inner World of Medical Students: Listening to Their Voices in Poetry*. Oxford: Radcliffe Publishing.

Shklovsky V. 1991. *Theory of Prose*. London: Dalkey Archive Press.

Snow CP. 1959. *The Two Cultures and the Scientific Revolution*. Cambridge: Cambridge University Press.

Stanley DE, Nyrup R. Strategies in Abduction: Generating and Selecting Diagnostic Hypotheses. *Journal of Medicine and Philosophy*. 2020; 45: 159–78.

Steiner P. 1984. *Russian Formalism: A Metapoetics*. Ithaca, NY: Cornell University Press.

Vannatta S, Vannatta J. Functional Realism: A Defense of Narrative Medicine. *Journal of Medicine and Philosophy*. 2013; 38: 32–49.

Wyer P, Charon R. 2011. Foreword. In: JP Meza, DS Passerman (eds.) *Integrating Narrative Medicine and Evidence-Based Medicine: The Everyday Social Practice of Healing*. London: Radcliffe Publishing, ix.

Yakubinski LP. 2018. *On Language and Poetry: Three Essays*. New York: Upper West Side Philosophers, Inc.

4 Is narrative medicine just another story biomedicine tells before we go to sleep?

Problems of definition: narrative as Procrustes's bed

Rita Charon (2006: 9) says, where "narratives are stories that have a teller, a listener, a time course, a plot, and a point", then "narrative knowledge is what we naturally use to make sense of them". Because of the neglect of poetry in Narrative Medicine, we claim that Charon's generic "we" (universality) and the descriptor "naturally" (biological) are untested assumptions and employed rhetorically. A more interesting challenge to Narrative Medicine, perhaps, is to ask, What kinds of stories actually count as narratives? For example, Samuel Beckett's "story" "Ping" (http://remue.net/IMG/pdf/Ping.pdf) defies classification. It is a prose poem without explicit narrative elements, aspiring to the formal mathematical symmetry of some conceptual poetry while not blanching out affect (it raises a productive chill in us):

> All known all white bare white body fixed one yard legs joined like sewn. Light heat white floor one square yard never seen. White walls one yard by two white ceiling one square yard never seen. Bare white body fixed only the eyes only just. Traces blurs light grey almost white on white. Hands hanging palms front white feet heels together right angle. (Etc.)

The "character" is (literally as well as figuratively) suspended, made into a ghost and absorbed into the background ("never seen", "only just", "traces", "blurs", "almost white", "white on white"). The story is a whiteout but not a whitewash. Beckett was a modernist and so we could say that he subverts the whole notion of plot as an ironic gesture; and his characters are similarly disembodied embodiments (actually Beckett is smarter than this game-playing). We suggest in any case that spatiality-sensitive and image-based poetry is a better medium of appreciation and critical awareness with which to approach Beckett than classic narratology.

Is a postmodern deconstruction of 'story' (purposefully not developing character or plot for example) still a story? Is story the same as tale, and is tale different from anecdote? Vladimir Propp's (1968) classic analysis of folk tales in the Russian Formalist tradition reveals 31 dimensions. Move outward from the classic folk tale to other story genres and, as Cecile Alduy (undated)

DOI: 10.4324/9781003194408-5

suggests, "the word 'narrative' requires some elucidation", so that for narrative based medicine,

> what we really mean is a certain kind of narrative: not the picaresque, not the Joycean (in other words, neither the early nor the postmodern), but the good old Aristotelian (reincarnated nowadays in the Hollywood template, or even, the makeover reality show success stories, which by the way, fall perfectly into Propp's morphology of the folk tale, complete with opponents, obstacles).

Retreating then to Propp's morphology as a framework for narrative understanding and appreciation would be a little like relying entirely on classical anatomy to practice medicine – a rusting, reductive framework that by-passes anti-narrativists who write stories, such as Samuel Beckett (above), Clarice Lispector, Lydia Davis, Thomas Pynchon, David Foster Wallace, Angela Carter, Gil Orlovitz, and William Gaddis. These writers revel in paratext, subtext, intertext, dissolved text, but not in classical "story". We should add that we also perceive a high moral tone in the way that Charon and colleagues treat patients' accounts in forever and strenuously extracting the good. This clashes violently with texts such as Jean-Baptiste Del Amo's (2019) *Animalia* – the history of a modern French peasant family developing a pig farm – where the "health" of the farming family is judged not by how far it can metaphorically raise itself away from the soil, but by how deeply invested in that soil it can literally become, identifying with the animal life that sustains them through sets of manners that many urbanites may find grotesque.

Charon's case studies of metropolitan patients contrasts sharply with, say, John Berger's (1967) photojournalism account of a family doctor in rural England, and even William Carlos Williams's (2008) similar photojournalism account of his house calls in Paterson, New Jersey to less privileged households. Williams says of this: "When they ask me, as of late they frequently do, how I have for so many years continued an equal interest in medicine and the poem, I reply that they amount for me to nearly the same thing".

To return to what we might mean by 'narrative', Alduy (undated) recognises that we need to "release the grip" of the narrative impulse, otherwise: "some of the most fundamental of human experiences … are stripped down from their intensity, beauty, horror, and maybe their truth, when we try to make sense of them by forcing them into a narrative box". Packing all literature into the narrative suitcase (as Narrative Medicine *in practice* appears to attempt) we squash important differences between genres and styles of writing that convey different meanings and address differing life events and experiences. There are then, says Alduy (ibid.):

> texts which defy, almost forbid, a purely narrative reading: poetic collections like those of Scève, Jaccottet, or Deguy, which create as much silence and white between the poems as to force other kinds of reading response and other metaphors to describe them (constellations,

synchronicities, open ended repetitions that spiral in and out without coming back to center, even the "rhizome" dear to Guattari); picaresque novels or unfinished tales; fragments and elliptic aphorisms such as Pascal Quignard's; "grotesques" or "monstrous" essays as Montaigne describes them, where order is not a precondition for meaning...

We applaud Alduy's perceptive comment about creating "silence" and "white" in a text, as Beckett above illustrates so powerfully, and as Charles Olson's "field" process advertises. My goodness, how many times do "silence" and "white" appear in a clinical consultation as key moments (sometimes for despair, sometimes for insight, sometimes for grasping at loose threads)? These adventurous texts use narrative ironically, even parodically. Like poetry, Alduy suggests that such texts function as "devices crafted to open up new ways of thinking in multiple directions across or away from linear temporality". Narrative "force" – provided by plot structures that many see as story's main feature – may be missing in patients' presentations. This is in any case a kind of masculinising of narrative as per the 'heroic venture' category in Propp's taxonomy.

Recall that one of Charonian Narrative Medicine's key functions is the superimposing of plot structures on patients' otherwise disconnected accounts. We find this a methodological paradox at the centre of narrative medicine: that consciousness is nonlinear, and yet narrative medicine seeks to emplot that which is, in actuality, plotless; or in Beckett's world, an animated suspension, or a palimpsest. We might amplify Beckett's deconstruction of narrative by drawing on Jacques Derrida's notion of "striking through" where narrative is permanently suspended, a "narrative-to-come" or a receding horizon.

In summary of our concerns, and accepting that in Charon and colleagues' 2016 text, some authors do tackle a couple of more complex narratives (e.g. Spiegel and Spencer take on Alison Bechdel's graphic memoir), we are left with one thought: who is taking on the poetry in the Narrative Medicine camp? Irvine and Charon (2016: 113) mention, through a quote from Cleanth Brooks, a literary theorist, that poetry "cannot be paraphrased" but then compare such a poetry-sensitive insight with their concept of story: "In a like manner, a story is something whose content cannot be reduced to analyzable data". Well, if the patient tells the story and the doctor creates the plotmarks and the narrative forms, and then hands this back to the patient as an accurate diagnosis, but offered with a caring attitude, that in turn demands a biomedically based intervention from the thousands available – say a course of antibiotics – how exactly is this not paraphrasing and reducing the story to analysable data?

Pythonesque interlude: poking dead parrots for signs of resting (or, the worrying absence of lyric poetry in Charon's and colleagues' Narrative Medicine texts)

Poetry doesn't feature in Charon's influential 2006 text, but does have cameo appearances in the 2016 co-authored text. In Charon's (Charon et al. 2016:

186–89) own chapter on close reading, she analyses a poem by Lucille Clifton that was a chosen text for a seminar. We welcome this, but wonder why the poem was read for meaning, in a linear, puzzle-solving form, rather than close read in the Formalist/Richards manner as a holistic grasp of the complex. Though both approaches can treat poetry as an engineering problem, resorting to instrumental explorations and "explanations", it is the latter method that attempts to grasp the poem as a form of linguistic art interdependent with, but not necessarily determined by, sense. We understand close reading to attempt a phenomenological 'bracketing out' of the poem as object to be considered in its aesthetic self-display, free from hermeneutics or interpretation at this point. We applaud interpretation too, such as psychoanalytic readings of authorial intention, but we want that to be clearly signalled; and we insist that poetry be allotted its fullest life free from an insistence on meaning. Meaning is like the rain. Sometimes it rains.

More, the poem seems misplaced under the heading of 'Time' (narrative's domain) rather than 'Space' (poetry's particular concern), especially given that the matter of the poem is sited at the most intense *moment* of a death, and is not offered as story. Clifton's account of the last breath of Fred Clifton is a reverie on a phenomenological insight: "there was all around not the / shapes of things / but oh, at last, the things /themselves". We are reminded of *Revelation* 1:19 ("Write therefore the things which thou hast seen, and which are, and which must be done hereafter"). But this seems to be borrowed from Edmund Husserl's famous rallying cry for phenomenology: "back to the 'things themselves'". Strange too that this obvious connection is missed in Charon's group's analysis; and that the phenomenological instant is made equivalent to the last gasp of life (as opposed to the first breath) as an insight, a revelation. Here is an epiphany missed.

Craig Irvine and Danielle Spencer (ibid.: 105) handle phenomenology capably in their chapter on "Dualism". Poetry is considered as embodied text in an analysis of David Ferry's 'Soul' (https://www.pbs.org/newshour/arts/weekly-poem-soul). Like Charon's take on Lucille Clifton's poem, they offer a competent exegesis of Ferry's poem, but not a formal close reading. What we are missing, again, is their recognition that the poem does something different from narrative. For her part, Charon (ibid.: 188) inevitably circles back to the "plot" of Clifton's poem as if doomed to return to meaning, always an anchor for narrativists, while Irvine and Spencer (ibid.: 105–6) run to ground in biocriticism (in this case, a speculative one that entails the poet's imagined biography as an old man dying), thus imposing storyline on a poem that otherwise relies on marvellous spatial features – the anatomy of the lobster, both guts and carapace.

The poem seems to us ("… my feelers / Preternatural, trembling with their amazing / Troubling sensitivity to threat") to site the speaker in the body of the lobster as a spatial exercise and not necessarily a temporal one. Not "I am growing old", but more "this is what it is like in the body to become old"; here is a way to feel old; here, language enacts age. The metaphors are about the here-and-now "mess" of the innards ("… all digestion, and pornographic /

Inquiry …"), and articulation ("… embarrassed by my ways / Of getting around …"); articulation not of voice, for the poem is proof that this is working fine, but of bodily limits instead. And the realisation that one has perhaps not been open enough ("… I'm aware of … / … my protective shell".) Poor lobsterman, you are boiled in narrative even though you're on the menu as poetry!

In Irvine and Spencer's (ibid.: 106) analysis, one thing leads to another in an unfolding story of this man's "lost love". Properly, they note that the poem speaks of an ecological embodiment where "Our insides and our outsides are connected", but now the narratological habit kicks in: "We cannot tell our stories without telling the tale of our bodies and those who have touched us". This tic deflects from the beauty of the poem that is embodied in the place-based, aesthetic, self-exclaiming voice of the lobsterman in resistance of narrative plot and embrace of plot as field, as the soil of the lobster's innards: "Where is it that she I loved has gone to, as / This cold sea water's washing over my back?".

This plaintive cry is specifically apostrophised (water's) so that the missing woman (wife?) is represented by the apostrophised and absent "i" ("water is"). The lobsterman is pinned in the field of his bereavement. Indeed, it may be the absence of plot (his backstory) that creates poignancy in the poem. But why introduce emplotment at all into the analysis of the poem? We see it again as a habit of narrativism that is an expression of its unaddressed intention to colonise poetry. Poetry must be made to make sense to the narrativists, otherwise it has no use to them.

Charon (ibid.: 197–200) uses a poem by Galway Kinnell ("Wait": https://poets.org/poem/wait) with a group of clinicians and asks them to write about the poem in what amounts to a different kind of narrativistic "co-construction" of meaning. She again focusses on the poem as narrative and not specifically, for example, on its lyrical elements (of which there are many in the poem, such as "Pain will become interesting", a gnomic statement that invites unravelling). Charon (ibid.: 200) summarises the exercise, where "We learned to delve into a text, learning how to *find* the narrating act itself". The poem is read either as a meaningful narrative or a relational field to produce meaning – there is no way out. Yet Galway's poem deliberately stops us in our tracks, halting our desire to move through time, from the opening imperative to "Wait, for now". But Charon's imperative is narratological and so we are spun a storyline about "forecasts" and "fortune-telling" elements of the poem. These are there if you look for them, and we encourage 101 different ways of reading poems. (Some are more productive than others, though; and would the narrativists have more than just one way to read a poem?) For us, who are enamoured less of chronology and more of a nonlinear eternity, Kinnell's words stop us in our tracks and pin us to the place we are in: "Don't go too early. / You're tired. … // Only wait a while and listen". The poem demands that we savour the moment however difficult, as this "… will be the only time, / most of all to hear, / the flute of your whole existence, / rehearsed by the sorrows, play itself into total exhaustion".

Now we are stopped in our tracks, pinned to the moment, deepened in it. The questions of voice that Charon insists on as the frame for reading – more fiction's domain, for we tread closer to narrative when we consider poems as monologues – are overshadowed by the suspension of time. As in Kinnell's poem above, the "I" becomes an apostrophe, a missing element experienced as pause. The place of Being (Heidegger's Dwelling) is here perhaps more pressing than time that is paradoxically suspended. Might Narrative Medicine suspend its fixation on the temporal to allow poetry space to breathe?

Nellie Hermann's (ibid.: 251–53) Chapter 10, "Can Creativity Be Taught?", offers two poems written by students in workshops (hurrah! to the intention we say) describing a dead bird that one of the students had brought in. We couldn't help but recall the Monty Python 'Dead Parrot' sketch. Mr Praline has just bought a parrot from the petshop, half an hour ago, claiming the parrot is dead: "'E's dead, that's what's wrong with it!

Petshop owner: No, no, 'e's uh,…he's resting.

Mr. Praline: Look, matey, I know a dead parrot when I see one, and I'm looking at one right now".

In the classically supportive poetry workshop fashion, Nellie Hermann claims that dead bird poems shine on like crazy diamonds: "The poems were wonderful". We leave readers to respond in their own way, though we suspect you'll find signs of Pythonesque "resting" rather than hoped-for transcendence. In a lesser sense, our worry about such workshops is, where the poems are just left on the table like the dead bird they describe, they take on a kind of sacred, untouchable quality, they are put beyond critical reach. In a greater sense, we worry that poetry is being misrepresented as ventilatory aimlessness. Yet in the ultimate sense, what we crave is not superlative created content but more so competent, informed close reading of the content that understands poetry as poetry.

Back to Procrustes's bed

Abraham Verghese (in Dolan 2015), among the best of contemporary doctor-writers, describes how stories link events in our lives and invest them with meaning. They surprise, engage and satisfy, through creating tensions and resolutions as plotlines. They deepen understanding of character. They introduce metaphor and rhetorical devices to make language more gripping and engaging. There is epiphany, or sudden revelation of meaning, potentially changing the reader's viewpoint. So far, so Narrative Medicine, but, to his credit, Verghese has reflective awareness. Even as a narrative enthusiast he recognises that patients' "histories" as stories may have no resolution, epiphany, or significant use of dramatic forms. They may be flat as they are told. Further, the quality of the doctor-patient relationship is primarily achieved through the character and capability of the doctor's performance in the physical examination, using hands-on auscultation, percussion, and palpation, focussed on here-and-now acute use of the senses or what Verghese (1999) calls "the animal snout". Here, *topos* trumps *tempus*. Musicality and sound are prior to prose but not poetry, which is sound.

Verghese (2015) suggests that frustrating the patient's story may be a problem of medicine's own making: first as habitual rapid intervention, where the doctor typically interrupts 12 seconds into the consultation; and second as the engineered exchange of the physical examination to remote imaging (with the understanding that such testing is preferable because of its accuracy, one of biomedicine's supposed gifts. But what test is truly accurate if not informed by a whole clinical picture?). In particular, and unconsciously beckoning poetry, Verghese bemoans the lack of inventiveness in coining new medical metaphors – as we note throughout – thus falling back habitually on tired examples. This leads to "an atrophy of our imagination" (ibid.: 232–33). Here, we suggest that narrative medicine suffers from the symptom of "thick slicing", or lack of discrimination. This is the opposite of "thick description" that narrative medicine borrows from anthropology (Clifford Geertz in particular), where the patient's "thin" story is given body through narratalogical interventions and re-readings (Charon et al. 2016 22). In contrast, Verghese (2015: 234) warns against purloining the patient's story in the name of medicine, where "the voice of medicine" must not be mistaken for the "voice of the patient". The inherent problem is: who is in control of the narrative? It is still the doctors who have learned narrative medicine, despite their claims for co-construction of narratives?

Where narrative medicine models Procrustes's bed, utterances are stretched to fit a preconceived notion, missing in particular the extra-narrative intentions of lyrical verse. Let us give an illustrative example. Arguably the best of narrative medicine texts, *The Chief Concern of Medicine* (Schleifer and Vannatta 2013: 181–83) too forces poetry into the narrative mould. For example, the authors take William Carlos Williams's iconic and perhaps best known (it might be a tie with "This Is Just To Say") minimalist poem "The Red Wheelbarrow" and try to fit this singularly imagistic work into a storyline. Here, say the authors, "a significant feature of 'The Red Wheelbarrow' is that it implies some kind of narrative, a story with a beginning, middle, and end". As poets, we disagree. "Implies" is key here – lots of stuff can imply a narrative where the story is projected on to an event as an afterthought. What is captured here is a suspended moment in time: not only the event described in the poem, one comprising images (rain, chicken, wheelbarrow), but also the framing metareflection ("so much depends") on *these* objects, at *this* time.

The poem suggests something immense in a minimalist space (precisely what Minimalism promises), and it is the nature of the images and their connection that is this poem's meaning, if it could be called that. There is no narrative here except whatever plot is imposed on it. The speaker is undefined. Not coincidentally, nobody wants anything. There is no conflict. There is only an eternity, and this instantiation of Narrative Medicine has no apparatus to appreciate it. But the event itself may be best described poetically, as Williams does in the original text. We don't deride this narrativistic impulse, for it is speculative, and we salute the speculative. What we abhor is what is ubiquitous in the field: a resort to default (narrative) in the absence of the capacity or ability to analyse the poetry (as poetry).

Also, let's not interfere with the artistic credibility of the poet who wants to *show* and not necessarily *imply*. We described the phenomenological moment that so intrigued Husserl, of the object showing itself. Poems also thrive on implication, of course, but primarily they show or reveal, and in close-up as *ekphrasis* or close noticing. We note this as an ecological perception, a two-way process: the object displays as we display the object in words. Schleifer and Vannatta (2013), however, drawing on the detective genre, turn Williams's raw statements into a guessing game, a puzzle to be solved. As discussed previously, this is a common rhetorical tactic – as patients describe their symptoms, they do not necessarily do this with "detection" in mind, but the medical narrativist (like Kathryn Montgomery Hunter) may force what the patient has to say into the "detective fiction" mould.

Williams's poem runs,

> so much depends
> upon
>
> a red wheel
> barrow
>
> glazed with rain
> water
>
> beside the white
> chickens.

Schleifer and Vannatta stitch the consciously structured poem into one continuous line: "so much depends upon a red wheelbarrow glazed with rainwater beside the white chickens". Now this makes no sense as story and presumably Williams didn't write it with narrative in mind, but it does reveal a preference on behalf of the authors. There is mystery afoot perhaps ("so much depends") but the "characters" (wheelbarrow, rainwater, chickens) are undeveloped – even if the wheelbarrow is a striking red, more so because of the rainwater glaze – and there is no evidence of plot. Indeed, the strikingly plain speaking of the objects in their own right is the very poetic diction that makes this a brilliant minimalist poem as we claim above. The objects are simply there, radiant in their uncomplicated presence, one beside another. In other words, they are *placed*. Getting placed in space is, suggests the philosopher Ed Casey (2013), the primary phenomenological gesture. To say that the objects are the narrative (along with the metareflection "so much depends") is like calling the ocean floor a desert.

Yet Williams does poetically complicate the issue by three main devices of implication and explication. First, the opening stanza of implication sets a mystery. Just what depends on the wheelbarrow and chicken: the farmer's livelihood, or the self-worth of the wheelbarrow and the chickens in their own right? Further, Williams does not say, "much depends" but injects suspense, as "so much depends". The second device is one of explication – enjambment (from the French *enjambement* 'to stride over', 'to go beyond'). This is a much-used technique where a line is not punctuated, but falls away into the following line with a sudden surprise. We have more to say about enjambment throughout. Thus, "so much depends upon" is mild in comparison with the sudden step "so much depends / upon", making us eager to find out what the "so much'" refers to.

Third, and explicit, the poem is entirely removed from temporal reference. "So much depends" can be read as a reference to the future, but the poem is anchored in the instantaneity of the event, the bringing together of rainwater, glazing and wheelbarrow standing beside chickens grounded in space. Hence, the poem is purposefully structured through poetic diction as lyric poem and not as continuous narrative arc. We will now consider the poem as – (gasp) – a poem!, an ambiguous thing that need not be tamed, and in so doing, we prefigure Chapters 11–13 in which ambiguity is considered as the special property poetry offers to medicine as a relational tool.

Such poems do have medical implications, not just because Williams was a doctor-poet but also because this is an exercise in close noticing and witnessing, capabilities essential to the clinical encounter. We are completely on board with Charon's teachings in this regard. You might see Williams's poem as presenting a pretty slim noticing, stripped back to fundamentals. But isn't this precisely what medical students are taught to do, to boil down excess to dry essences as the hard tack of the diagnosis? We thereby highlight the special quality of Williams's work, in which a minimalist style seems to mimic the flattening quality of the biomedical epistemology, and yet analysing it as poetry seems to reclaim its richness, a richness that, in truth, was ineradicable. This is a paradox at the heart of the methodology of lyrical medicine. Now you can see why we subtitled this book "Towards a Lyrical Medicine". This has layered meanings.

One of these meanings is to "alter" the narrative, providing another voice. Plainly we want to alter what we see as narrative medicine's attitude to poetry such that it would sideline, distort, or quell its peculiar voices. This would alter the narrative of narrative medicine, and give an "alter" or another, where we have set generic narrative medicine and Charonian Narrative Medicine in particular as "other" in the mirror of lyric poetry. But also, as we have said, we do not want to worship at the altar of narrative medicine, if you will allow us the obvious pun. We admire secular narrative medicine, but we are suspicious of its evangelical wing.

Earlier, we drew on Wallace Stevens's use of birds as a metaphor for the imagination: "I am content when wakened birds, / Before they fly, test the reality / Of misty fields, by their sweet questionings" (from "Sunday Morning": https://www.poetryfoundation.org/poetrymagazine/poems/13261/sunday-morning). We like birds without evangelical wings that ask questions rather than make statements or preach "truths": we want to enter Stevens's discourse of democracy of imagination as "the green freedom of a cockatoo / Upon a rug". The cockatoo burns in our minds in a way Pythonesque parrots cannot: the cockatoo is alive. Really distinguishing the difference here might assist one in discrimination in the clinical encounter; not an outcomes-based improvement in observation but instead an apprehension of immanence, of realising that the defamiliarised moment is always on us in the presence of a work of art. This care – we do think it care paid to poems and poetry – can transfer to patients as medicine practiced with a poetic imagination.

To be fair, Schleifer and Vannatta (2013: 181–82) note that Williams's poem above, "The Red Wheelbarrow", "observes details in the environment and asserts value". But they simultaneously denature the poem by forcing it to take on the identity of narrative, admitting themselves from the start that this is perhaps a mistaken reading: "even when a poem does not present an explicit narrative, as in Dr William Carlos Williams's famous poem "The Red Wheelbarrow", it can help us learn to recognize and recover narrative knowledge". This seems like pretty slim pickings for narrative enthusiasts and, again, misses the poem *as poem*; in so doing, it abuses the work.

The rationale is that patients do not present whole narratives but bits of story that have to be pieced together. Thus, Williams's poem is taken as an example of fragmentary evidence of a wider story and is narrativised as exercise. Well, yes. The observations Williams makes are necessarily embedded in a wider scene, but again the whole point of making the poem may be to offer the frozen scene as exquisitely beautiful and right; as complete in itself. What is the point in doing the wrong exercises? Do we go to the gym to lift weights but somehow end up swimming instead? Williams offers a kind of moral about suspending interference. Time is explicitly suspended for a reason, so that things can show themselves. As we will insist, poets often like to dig where they stand.

Schleifer and Vannatta (ibid.) continue, "The story presents itself as a series of disparate facts, emotions, anecdotes" where "these elements of narrative and significance need to be gathered together to make a meaningful whole". Well, no: these are not "elements of narrative". What facts other than the possible physical fact of represented objects? We contend that there is not a single emotion named in the poem, and if there is an anecdote, we're at a loss. Pythonesque signs of resting are projected on to a poem that stands outside the limits of "story". But they are certainly "elements of … significance". The authors then assert, "practice and training in the interpretation of poetry is particularly useful in developing the competence of health care workers in recovering the information and meaning of a patient's story". Though we appreciate the advocacy for poetry in this instance, we point out that the authors are in a sticky position. Not only do they force poetry into the narrative box, but they also compound the problem by resorting to instrumentalism.

They mention "training" (from the Latin *trahere* 'to drag behind') not education; "competence" (meaning "good enough") and not capability or unfolding of potential; and "information" (poetry reduced to engineering metaphor) not knowledge or wisdom. These are our common bugbears in medical education. More, the advice is to give healthcare workers education in "interpretation" of poetry: informational meanings, not qualities. We prefer as noted to place appreciation before explanation, and the aesthetic before the instrumental.

Ultimately, after an understanding has been cultivated such that poems are appreciated as poems, then we cautiously endorse the application of this knowledge to clinical encounters. This is lyrical medicine. But skipping straight to the applied mode has wreaked such havoc in the medical/ health humanities. What if healthcare workers were introduced to poetry as a strangeness they never knew they needed, for their own selves; that they should cultivate their own relationship with poetry in order to cultivate their own relationship with themselves? What if a space were created between poetry and its application, again a plot that can be cultivated as field? What might happen then?

Schleifer and Vannatta freely admit that poetry helps us to deepen experience of phenomena, recognising that Williams's opening line "so much depends" orients us to value, rather than to information as objective fact. They derive a metaphor of their own, that Williams is telling us that the everyday is "glazed with value". Finally, a poetic insight, an epiphany! Such appreciation of poetry can alert us to the manner of presentation of patients and not just, in Schleifer's and Vannatta's words, "presented *information*" (italics in original), undermining their previous advice to recover the "information" of a patient's "story".

Patients' narratives as reconstructions and translations

The anatomy of the clinical encounter is not composed just of talk, yet imperial narrativism privileges the lexical, largely ignores sonics, the nonverbal (proxemics, gestures, tics, eye contact, touch, movement, paralinguistics) and semiotic, that Clifford Geertz (1973) calls "thick description". A range of gestures, intonations, silences, and accompanying signs and symbols largely fail to register in narrative medicine accounts. Rita Charon et al. (2016: 23) do note the importance of thick description on one occasion, but there is very little formal analysis and close reading of the nonverbal and semiotic in the 2016 text (read on to the following chapter for an extended example).

Maura Spiegel and Danielle Spencer (in Charon et al. 2016: 23), in the context of Narrative Medicine's "narrative competence", do note that understanding and reading patients' nonverbal gestures is important to intersubjectivity, where: "In the clinical encounter ... gestures, facial expressions, and body language can signal in such significant ways". Further, the authors note how nonverbal communications can both support and contradict the verbal, and can be ambiguous and are singularly contextualised.

But their account of the nonverbal is not adequate – we want to know about the rhythm and musicality of encounters; about lifting off the beat; about syncopation and silences. It took a graphic narrative for Charon and colleagues to insert the nonverbal into their narratology frame, which seems a little cheap. They could have learned so much from gapping words in the field *à la* Olson, or blocking words into concrete forms like Beckett, or exquisite phrasing from Louise Glück or Anne Carson. This after all is the way that we speak, especially in the pressing context of an emotionally stirred patient trying to describe symptom: sometimes sticking and stumbling over words, sometimes stunned into silence, and at other times eloquent and on point. Musicality is critical here: rhythm *and* blues, atonality and body melody, the sonic spaces into which words wander.

The 18th-century Viennese physician Leopold Auenbrugger, who first identified the potential for percussion of the chest, was a keen musician who once invited Mozart to play at his home (Bleakley 2020). Auenbrugger saw the potential for diagnoses not just in physical examination but also in lung and breath sounds such as crackles or alveolar rales. Our point is that patients' "talk" is extensive, embodied, and preverbal. Such preverbal and nonverbal elements "thicken" the story, and we need expertise to read such elements. The manner in which this is being theorised is akin to semiotics – signs and symbols in context, to include the world of objects and their significance in the clinical encounter (poets love to expand objects, while maintaining the stoniness of stone). We say "akin" because, in our view, nonverbal communication is not recognised as independent referents with a spatial and sonic character but rather intrinsically as part of the "narrative" in Narrative Medicine. All is sucked into meaning. Yet poetic/spatial awareness of the nonverbal is standard fare for the psychotherapist and clinical psychologist (and presumably for psychiatrists too), so Narrative Medicine's narrative competences may not be the best stop from which to alight from the bus for learning such "thick description" capabilities where they are thick sliced.

Doctors are semioticians before they are narrativists, users of signs and symbols grounded in biochemistry, and prompting for clearer information about symptom expression through formulaic means such as oppositional categories or semantic qualifiers (such as "is it a sharp or a dull pain?" "Does it hurt all the time or only at certain times?"). The patient will have a "frontstory" that is their discussion with the doctor, and a "backstory" that is just as important and is not revealed. The backstory is probably laden with affect that is central to the patient's care needs. The backstory is then no story at all, but a spatially sensitive constellation of half-explored and semi-articulated affect. Psychoanalysts will say that this unconscious backstory is actually shaping the encounter – but is it a back*story*, or a back*space*? We suspect it's both, a locker brewing metaphors and a storeroom of prescribed metonyms.

From our experience, often it is not the conversation between doctor and patient or psychotherapist and client that matters, but the space that has opened up in the place where differing foci fail to meet or only partially meet. Discontinuity and surprise regularly inhabit the accounts of patients consulting with doctors and clients with psychotherapists. Sometimes this adds up to a mistranslation. When patients describe symptoms – and events surrounding symptom appearance and development – are they, as the celebrated late 19th-century doctor and medical educator William Osler hints, telling "stories" ("Listen to your patient; he is telling you the diagnosis")? We say "hints" because Osler does not actually say "listen to your patient's *story*" but rather just "listen to your patient, he is telling you the diagnosis".

Charon (2006: 99) does recognise that spoken narrative may be absent in the clinical encounter, such as when working with a patient suffering from dementia; just as puzzling may be working through a translator, or with children, or with intellectually disabled persons. In cases such as dementia, suggests Charon, there is a "corporeal truth": "The nature of the body is such that patients cannot ordinarily just *tell* in words what needs to be heard about it". She is talking here of paratexts. Typically, a healthcare worker engages with a person suffering from advanced dementia through visual material such as photographs. In such an encounter, suggests Charon, a healthcare worker or a doctor engages in "listening for stories". But why would this be the case? Charon assumes that the adoption of narrative provides the context for the occasion of healing in the circle of patient story returned through doctor narrative for collaborative labour. But again, the "restorying" of the encounter seems to be the projection of the narrative will onto the patient who does not necessarily recognise, say in the case of dementia, photographs from the past in terms of story, but rather in terms of the power of the instant and of place. Here, recognition is not the same as recall.

We think that doctors should recognise the common inability of people to actually say what's happening, a failure of language or of vocabulary for them. In other words, a story they can't quite tell, not completely anyway, and with missing things they aren't privileged to detect. The clinical encounter is usually not single, even the one-off, but rather one-over-time, in which a mutual lexicon is developed and patient and doctor educate each other relationally to discover what's happening. (We recognise relative exceptions, such as in Emergency Medicine). And to remember what is happening, memories compound to influence the newest encounter. This is a kind of narrative medicine, if applicable that we think is vastly more complex than the emplotment kind that Charon vends.

Steal the story?

The leap from the doctor "taking a history" to the patient "recounting a story" is long established and now habitual, as a tic. Here is Robert Centor (2007) from the University of Alabama (feel free to make a drinking game with the appearance of the word "story"):

> ... the great physicians differ from the good physicians because they understand the entire story. Only when we understand the complete story do we make consistent diagnoses. Each patient represents a story. That story includes their diseases, their new problem, their social situation, and their beliefs. How do we understand the story? We must develop excellent communication skills and gather the history in appropriate depth. We must perform a targeted physical examination based on the historical clues. We must order the correct diagnostic tests, and interpret them in the context of the history and physical exam. Once we collect the appropriate data, we then should construct that patient's story. The story includes making the correct diagnosis or diagnoses. The story must describe the patient's context. ... Understand the full story.

History and mystery are key components here, but whose mystery is this? In Centor's account, the long-established *empirical methods of the consultation* fill the mould of the *patient's story*. As Centor's words disclose, "we then should construct the patient's story". This ambiguity is telling – Centor presumably means that the doctor *re-constructs* what the patient says in the consultation (as a gathering of the history) in light of the physical examination and test results: the patient's story, near death, is somehow resuscitated by the doctor. It is, of course, a representation once it is returned to the patient as medical narrative and all narrative medicine texts recognise this, but they fail to unpick the dilemma. The story is now untethered from ownership and has become both metaphor and "free-floating" signifier.

But also, in a Marxist frame, the patient's labour has been exploited and her capital has been appropriated by medicine. At this point, medicine has an ethical duty to restore ownership of the means of production of that capital (patient's story) to the patient, but this ethical responsibility may show slippage, where in medicine and medical education for example "cases" are regularly presented without permission from patients. To add to the appropriation, the patient's story reappears as medical education academic capital within the industries of research and inquiry: conferences, papers, and books on narrative medicine.

Returning to the status of "story", again, in narrative medicine circles, "story" seems to embrace any utterance. A physician, John (2013: 57), makes a plea for a shift from doctor-centred to patient-centred practice, first drawing on another of Osler's maxims that runs, "it is much more important to know what sort of patient has a disease than what sort of disease a patient has". John goes on to say, "The patient should always be allowed to describe his symptoms and sensations using his own words" – this, says John, is the patient's "story". But inevitably:

> The doctor then duly moves on to closed questions, which are used to confirm specifics and understand the cause of symptoms in a more technical context. Indeed, as the consultation progresses closed questions can be used successfully to focus specific areas that maybe do not emerge from the patient's *story* during the initial open-question session.

Two issues emerge from this: first, again, is the patient necessarily telling a story in recounting a number of disconnected issues, facts and feelings every time she speaks? And second, what will the tactics of representation be and how will the patient's labour be rewarded and honoured?

In terms of the first issue, Charon (2006: 99) wants it both ways, where, "[u]sually, the story of sickness comes out chaotically, achronologically", and then proceeds to recommend imposing "plot" in order to restore chronology. Well, as Abraham Verghese noted earlier, there can be achronological stories. But where does imposition of plot end? In the service of diagnosis, such an imposition may seem justified, but this appears to compromise authentic patient-centredness, again as reflected in co-construction of meanings between doctors and patients. Practically speaking, making sense of things is important. But what are the limitations to emplotment? And when does emplotment just not apply? We suspect the imposition is vast, for Narrative Medicine has a poor understanding of what poetry is and can do. We are nervous about claims for patient-centredness that are actually doctor-centred emplotments. Stories are returned to patients with interest say the narrativists, but such "returning" surely remains doctor-centred even if the intentions are good? Indeed, there are echoes here of well-intentioned colonialism.

Hans Duvefelt (2016) is also wary of "storying" medical encounters as literalising:

> Sir William Osler wasn't exactly wrong when he said, "Listen to your patient, he is telling you the diagnosis." But he didn't mean it literally. His patients did not offer up esoteric and complete medical diagnoses on a silver platter. They left him clues in plain language that he listened to carefully in order to make the correct diagnosis. He penned his words in an era when medical information was scarce among non-medical people. There was no Dr. Google, Dr. Oz or Dr. House to educate the public about diseases or medical terminology a century ago.

An apocryphal story from the same author (in the age of Dr Google) also shows that when stories are told, they may actually be unhelpful in reaching a diagnosis:

> Mrs. LaVerdiere made an appointment for nausea some time ago. As soon as I walked into the exam room, she started telling me about how she must have eaten a spoiled crab sandwich on her trip to a coastal fishing village the weekend before. Her conversation was full of theories as to why she was feeling unwell and her husband wasn't. I finally got her to describe in great detail exactly what she felt, and the gnawing pain that radiated to her back did not fit with a simple case of food poisoning. Her CT scan showed the smallest pancreatic cancer ever diagnosed at Cityside Hospital, and she underwent a Whipple procedure as easily as any routine minor surgery.
>
> (ibid.)

As an aside on the veracity of the account, Whipple procedures are known to leave patients very ill, something Duvefelt omits. However, the procedure may be the only chance a patient has of a cure. Further, patients sometimes do not tell *their* stories faithfully, but rather recount incidents in a lay "medicalese" that they think will suit their doctor's mindset:

> Mrs. Waller describes ordinary bodily sensations in the most dramatic terms and throws terminology around that rocks me out of my country-doctor way of plain-talking. She has, over the years, described ordinary itches as "you know how it feels when you've been bitten by a thousand fire ants," headaches as "I felt like I was about to pop a berry aneurysm" and indigestion as "pyloric stricture." I have the distinct impression she is always trying to make my job easier by describing things in more or less medical terms in case I forgot to speak English.

In an analysis that describes the three main ways in which patient "stories" can be confounded, Duvefelt (ibid.) explores the above example of talking in medicalese – often picked up from the Internet – as if this will please the doctor. Such acquired patient-speak thus offers theories and diagnoses rather than plainly describing symptoms. This can frustrate doctors. As for the other ways, some people are simply unable to recognise what they are feeling (as sensations), or to adequately describe emotions. Instead, they report what other people observe of their behaviour. In this way, they are strange collateral historians of themselves. The final way comes when bodily sensations are described rather than the emotions that accompany them, such as anxiety. In this case, we have a so-called physical focus with emotions either un-narrated or, as is more often the case, shunted onto a physical target. We do not find in Narrative Medicine's version of close reading adequate ways to deal with these sublimated and sideways narratives.

To this, we might add that in psychiatry it is obvious to all that the way a patient tells a story is filtered through their presenting psychological conditions – thus a persona labelled as "hysteric" tells a story flamboyantly; an anxious person stutters and fumbles her way through an account; a depressed person relates a story as if under a thundercloud; a paranoid person tells a story larded with suspicion or unjustified accusation; a person labelled as "psychotic" offers a mass of bizarre and disconnected detail to the normative hearer. These examples are given non-judgementally. Here, *the manner in which a "story" is told is probably more important or revealing than the story itself.* We are not convinced that Narrative Medicine adequately addresses this question of tone or style.

A psychoanalytic muddle

We have raised objections to Narrative Medicine that question its potential for "slantwise" reading (rather than reading of slantwise symptom expression). We are not sure how inventive Narrative Medicine is in re-inventing its close reading methods. As an example of our claim, we will look at Narrative Medicine's use of psychoanalysis as an aid to close reading.

We are puzzled by the relatively thin slicing of psychodynamic approaches, especially as Charon et al. (2016: 1) has expertise in this area, claiming that "psychoanalysis" is among the practices that "supply the clinical foundations of our work". The drumbeat throughout *The Principles and Practices of Narrative Medicine* is consistent: baldly, listen closely to the patient's story, recast in more complex and insightful terms through narrative competences, and return the tale to the patient in a collaborative re-storying that honours both biomedical readings and the humanity of the context. Now the first fly in the ointment concerns methodology. According to purist (either New Criticism or Russian Formalist) brands of close reading, we are in trouble invoking psychoanalysis, because the first rule is that "there is nothing outside the text". The second concern is veracity, or the status of the story. If, as psychoanalysis tells us, the patient's story is in the "backstory", the repressed content now eking out in the clinical encounter and being read analytically by the practitioner, where does Narrative Medicine site the "story" (and more, in terms of countertransference and counter-resistance the practitioner's quality of narrative reading)?

Freud was interested primarily in subtext and its slantwise reading (and secondarily in intertext through the transference dynamics) (recall that Freud never won a Nobel Prize, but did receive the Goethe Prize for literature). In Charon and colleagues' (2016) Chapter 12, a case study is reviewed psychoanalytically. Charon's long-time patient is diagnosed as diabetic and reactively switches into a state of high anxiety and self-blame. She makes an appointment to see Charon (carrying a bad viral infection), who later writes her a letter, a narrative that "recasts" the consultation in reflective, caring human language. Charon uses this letter to advertise the value of the narrative approach.

The patient comes for a follow-up visit and says that every time she reads Charon's letter, she cries. She sees the letter as getting to the heart of the matter, fully embracing her emotional concern. Yet, as we read the letter, acknowledging its heartfelt intent, what we see at its core is that Charon says "the diagnosis may be wrong, let's get you tested again". In the third person, and after a cavalcade of cloying praise for the patient's perceived goodness, Charon says, "Perhaps, the doctor ventures, the elevated sugar was caused by this bad viral infection. That happens regularly. Perhaps we might first let you fully recover from the viral illness and then see if the sugar levels off". Is this not the biomedical voice of reassurance, speaking in the language of diagnostics? Why the overblown fuss about narrative? Was narrative merely a wet blanket thrown on affect, with the real business left to biomedicine to do? Or was writing a "narrative" to this patient a patronising move such that the final arbiter, biomedical diagnostics and reasoning, could weigh in with finality?

We don't want to be cynical, because this was clearly a touching moment for both doctor and patient, but the medical issue when foregrounded may be readily addressed as chief complaint. But it is not, according to Charon, the medical issue that is the patient's chief concern. Rather, it is emotional distress about being ill at all. And yet we are told that this woman, for example, had "a history of severe asthma and allergies in childhood", and "a total knee replacement through which she sailed". But her mother had treated her as a sick child, or, she played the "sick role" in the family. The current diagnosis of diabetes had re-stimulated the distress locked up in this childhood experience, seeming "to reawaken the voice of her mother". Charon's strategy in dealing with the distress is threefold: in clichéd ("dread disease") and overwrought ("This diagnosis of diabetes, such as it was, catapulted her into an unadulterated face-off with aging and death") prose, she (1) ignores the data right in front of her face (sick role), (2) hypervalidates the emotional distress through a larded affirmation, and (3) is all on the way to offering medicine the final word. The means to get to actualise a lengthier version of "Perhaps the doctor was wrong, I'll test you again" was – cue music now – *story*.

But the gaping hole in Charon's account from a psychoanalytic perspective is an adequate account of the transference dynamics between a doctor and a patient who identify with similar values as apparently comfortable New York (sub)urbanites, returning to a point we made earlier. The countertransference from Charon seems to be one of wanting to provide the mother figure. The narrative balm draws not at all on the lessons of family dynamic one might gain from a writer such as Lucia Berlin (2015) who wrestles openly with emotions such as bitterness rather than sublimating them for more positive affect, or disguising them with saccharine overlay. Berlin shows the acute (therapeutic and medical-diagnostic) insight of a literary writer in the double meaning of the title to her collection of stories "Manual for Cleaning

Women". As a feminist and a long-term alcoholic in and out of recovery, "cleaning women" becomes a jibe at both the patriarchy and the addiction recovery programmes; but also Berlin did work as a cleaning lady, among many jobs, including an administrative assistant in a medical practice.

In the same chapter, Eric Marcus then proceeds to analyse Charon's narrative account, but in doing so compounds its presumptions. Marcus gives Charon's letter the status of a transitional object that may be used by the patient to work through lingering, unresolved issues with her mother (the patient is in her sixties, we don't know if the mother is dead or alive). The "transitional space" created by the Narrative Medicine artefact – Charon's letter – becomes a magical object. Marcus imagines (the reader is never told what happened to the patient) that the Narrative Object,

> Within the transitional space, the patient's dark and terrorizing fantasies about the existential dilemmas of the illness can be held at bay from contaminating the space of identity. … Now the illness can become merely an illness, to be dealt with in practical ways, and not as a representative of a terrorizing, depressive experience of a scolding mother.

Well, first, poor mother – she doesn't get a voice or a look in (no wonder – Charon has replaced her symbolically, as all-forgiving mother figure). More importantly, on a biomedical note of clarity, we still have no idea if the diabetes diagnosis was a misdiagnosis. It isn't clarified in Charon's follow-up account later in the chapter. And to add to the misery, how can the psychological issues be so neatly divided from the somatic, so that psychoanalysis might clear up one, while we can deal with the diabetes diagnosis "in practical ways"?

Of course, in psychotherapy, especially psychoanalytic approaches, a co-construction of a meaningful story is the chief purpose of the clinical encounter, where the healing is in changing the nature of the patient's story. James Hillman (2019) goes further by suggesting that the purpose of psychotherapy is to restore meaning to stories themselves, to the larger myths that shape character and life events within which the local stories are told (such as the multiple mother archetypes looming in Charon's case study). But the re-structuring of myth is precisely what poetry promises, and is, in fact, assisted in delivering on that promise because it is composed of the substance of myth. In a radical challenge to psychotherapy's goals, Hillman suggests that therapies fail where they are taken literally, in other words when they become dogmas or are applied without due recognition of the role of metaphor and image.

A therapeutic approach from any school of thinking is a "fiction", a conjecture. Perhaps, in this line of argument, narrative medicine too is in danger of falling foul of literalism. "The story", once concretised, is mistaken as explanation for symptom, rather than exploration of that symptom or symptom set. Looking at that another way, the literal symptom has a literal cause (biomedicine's domain); but the way that the cause is registered, discussed and then understood or given meaning by the patient is linguistic and conversational (both narrative's and poetry's concerns), and metaphorical and imagistic (the main interests of poetry). Furthermore, a purpose of concretisation is to solidify meaning, to gather together an ur-sense of a tale. Poetry is about multiple readings, about an endless, unfixed series.

Is Narrative Medicine ever wrong?

We are further concerned about idealism: that narrative medicine generally, and Narrative Medicine in particular, consistently paints pictures of successful interventions (this is why we urge readers to explore the autobiographical "fictions" of, for example, Lucia Berlin, where medical narratives are often disturbing, ambiguous, or unresolved, and set in underprivileged or excluded communities). The run up may be shaky, but the leap is made and the intervention is steady and good. Rarely do we get accounts of failures, misdiagnoses, clinical errors, poorly managed narrative interventions, miscalculations, patients falling between the cracks of services. When these do come, they are never systematic. Or even dull and pedestrian accounts – where are they? Occasions when nothing happened, there was no resolution, the patient refused to cooperate, there was a personality clash between the doctor and the patient, the diagnosis was too fuzzy and so forth.

We don't have to seek accounts of medical work in resource-poor countries of the South globally. It is here on the doorstep in the otherwise privileged global North. See again, in North American settings, William Carlos Williams's and Robert Coles's (2008) photojournalistic *House Calls*, or Abraham Verghese's (1995) *My Own Country: A Doctor's Story* about the first AIDS patients in a rural backwater in eastern Tennessee. And in a rural English setting, again, John Berger's (1967) photojournalistic study (with Jean Mohr) of the family doctor John Sassall, *A Fortunate Man*.

How about this staple of real life: after being badly injured in a fistfight, the patient was brought in an ambulance to the Emergency Department, drunk and falling over. His first utterance on entering the Department was to puke. He then let out a string of obscenities and refused to allow anyone to touch him. A wound on his face reopened and gushed blood, a telling semiotic. And so on …. Of course, "plot" can be superimposed on this, but at what expense for other forms of understanding and engagement? Or, when is plot wishful thinking, an overreach not on what is poetry, but what is dull and basic? *Better to defamiliarise such encounters than emplot them.*

While narrative medicine's reach increases, it seems that there is a directly proportionate inability for self-critique. It is a standard rule of academic work that one recognises limitations and objections to theoretical conclusions and subsequent practices. Without such critique, approaches smack of self-congratulation. An irony inherent to *The Principles and Practices of Narrative Medicine* is that its critique of biomedicine as conducted masterfully by Craig Irvine and Danielle Spencer never meets its partner in self-critique.

Hey, Godot's here again! But in name only

We must say again that poetry does nothing useful in medicine or anywhere else, but a good start in appreciating its uselessness in medicine is to separate it from the utility claims of narrative medicine. Samuel Beckett (1966) is a good guide. In "Ping", a "short story" mentioned previously, Beckett deconstructs the classic "narrative" account and in the process offers us a poem-like thing. We give you the beginning again because it's so instructive:

> All known all white bare white body fixed one yard legs joined like sewn. Light heat white floor one sure yard never seen. White walls one yard by two white ceiling one square yard never seen. Bare white body fixed only the eyes only just. Traces blurs light grey almost white on white. Hands hanging palms front white feet heels together right angle. Light heat white planes shining white bare white body fixed ping elsewhere.

"Ping" (https://astrofella.wordpress.com/2020/12/30/ping-samuel-beckett/) is just 908 words long, repeating phrases such as "light heat white" and words such as "traces". Striking out on a wholly associational, idiosyncratic direction here, we feel that "Ping" is as close as literature comes to orthopaedic surgery's "white out" arthroscopies. This is the art world's "white cube" (the gallery space) that strips space back to a bare minimum as a background to allow objects (such as sculpture, paintings, or installations) or activities (such as performance art) to be *placed* or foregrounded. Time here is suspended. Beckett's room too is the white room of the clinic as imperium. Beckett brings the body to place in the descriptor, but then does something remarkable – he dissolves the body against the white of the background. It is an imperialism of white caught in its own box, but it is the opposite of colonising. The white spectre dissolves itself in its own substance. Deleuze and Guattari (2004a, 2004b) call this a "de-territorialising" and dissolution of patrolled borders.

Beckett often claimed that his work meant nothing, and was designed to signify nothing but failure. In *The Unnamable* (1953), he says, "… you must go on. I can't go on. I'll go on", and in the story "Worstword Ho" (1983), one that unpicks "story" from within, so that we are left with Beckett saying, equally famously, "Ever tried. Ever failed. No matter. Try again. Fail again. Fail better".

What we have plotted in these opening chapters is a view of "narrativism" as an imperialistic ideology that has arisen from the bread and butter work of narratology. We would not wish to brand most narratologists or literary scholars as craving such lofty ambitions to be crowned. They are far more humble. Have we unfairly caricatured generic narrative medicine and its commercial apogee in Narrative Medicine[TM]? Readers can decide. From our roost in poetry pulpit, we recall Samuel Beckett's comparison of his own work with that of James Joyce from an interview in *The New York Times* (Shenker 1956; see also Gates 1996): "He's tending towards omniscience and omnipotence as an artist. I'm working with impotence, ignorance". We leave "knowing" to narrative medicine as we proudly side with impotence and ignorance, defamiliarising clinical encounters so that they are made strange, comprised in ambiguity and recognised as such. With Beckett at our shoulders, in the following chapter and then Section 2, we move away from critique and towards a cumulative argument for a different medicine, one of qualities as well as quantities. We example and illustrate at every point, bringing Beckett's receding figure into focus and then letting it recede again, in good gestalt fashion.

References

Alduy C. (Undated). Against Narratives III. Or a Certain Kind of Narrative. Blog. Arcade: Literature, the Humanities & the World. Retrieved from https://arcade.stanford.edu/blogs/against-narratives-iii-or-certain-kind-narrative

Beckett S. 1953. *The Unnamable.* London: Faber & Faber. Retrieved from http://s3.amazonaws.com/arena-attachments/1675308/7bbd95bc63562c1b18ecf816568d9bd6.pdf?1517359229

Beckett S. 1966. Ping. Retrieved from https://astrofella.wordpress.com/2020/12/30/ping-samuel-beckett/

Berger J. 1967/2016. *A Fortunate Man: The Story of a Country Doctor.* Edinburgh: Canongate.

Berlin L. 2015. *A Manual for Cleaning Women.* London: Picador.

Bleakley A 2020. *Educating Doctors' Senses through the Medical Humanities: "How Do I Look?"* Abingdon: Routledge.

Casey E. 2013. *The Fate of Place: A Philosophical History.* Oakland: University of California Press.

Centor RM. To Be a Great Physician, You Must Understand the Whole Story. *Medscape General Medicine.* 2007; 9: 59.

Charon R. 2006. *Narrative Medicine: Honoring the Stories of Illness.* Oxford: Oxford University Press.

Charon R, DasGupta S, Hermann N, et al. 2016. *The Principles and Practices of Narrative Medicine.* Oxford: Oxford University Press.

Coles R, Roma T. 2008. *House Calls with William Carlos Williams.* Brooklyn, NY: Powerhouse Books.

Del Amo J-B. 2019. *Animalia.* London: Fitzcarraldo.

Deleuze G, Guattari F. 2004a. *A Thousand Plateaus.* London: Continuum.

Deleuze G, Guattari F. 2004b. *Anti-Oedipus.* London: Continuum.

Duvefelt H. Listen to Your Patient's Story: It's Their Diagnosis. Hans Duvefelt MD/Physician. December 14, 2016. Retrieved from HTTPS://WWW.KEVINMD.COM/BLOG/2016/12/LISTEN-PATIENTS-STORY-DIAGNOSIS.HTML

Gates D. He Couldn't Go On, He Went On. May 26, 1996. Retrieved from https://www.nytimes.com/1996/05/26/books/he-couldn-t-go-on-he-went-on.html

Geertz C. 1973. *The Interpretation of Cultures.* New York: Basic Books.

Hillman J. 2019. *Healing Fiction: On Freud, Jung, Adler.* Washington, DC: Spring Publications.

Irvine C, Charon R. 2017. Deliver Us From Certainty: Training for Narrative Ethics. In R Charon, et al. (eds) *The Principles and Practices of Narrative Medicine.* Oxford: Oxford University Press, 110–36.

John M. From Osler to the Cone Technique. *HSRC Proc Intensive Care Cardiovascular Anesthetics.* 2013; 5: 57–58.

Propp V. 1968: *Morphology of the Folktale.* Austin: University of Texas Press.

Schleifer R, Vannatta JB. 2013. *The Chief Concern of Medicine: The Integration of the Medical Humanities and Narrative Knowledge into Medical Practices.* Ann Arbor: The University of Michigan Press.

Shenker I. Moody Man of Letters; A Portrait of Samuel Beckett, Author of the Puzzling 'Waiting for Godot'. *New York Times,* May 6, 1956. Retrieved from https://www.nytimes.com/1956/05/06/archives/moody-man-of-letters-a-portrait-of-samuel-beckett-author-of-the.html

Spiegel M, Spencer D. 2016. Accounts of Self: Exploring Relationality through Literature. In: R Charon, S Das Gupta, Hermann N, et al. (eds.) *The Principles and Practices of Narrative Medicine.* Oxford: Oxford University Press, 15–34.

Verghese A. 1995. *My Own Country: A Doctor's Story.* New York: Simon & Schuster.

Verghese A. 1999. *The Tennis Partner.* London: Chatto & Windus.

Verghese A. 2015. The Physician as Storyteller. In B. Dolan (ed.) *Humanitas: Readings in the Development of the Medical Humanities.* San Francisco: University of California Medical Humanities Press, 224–35.

5 What can Russian Formalism do for us lately? And other unapplications

Defamiliarisation redux

Poetry can give us frames for making sense of medical encounters, as we shall explore in subsequent chapters. But literary techniques such as close reading of texts also offer fruitful frames. In this chapter we draw on the literary technique of defamiliarisation, already introduced and hopefully now familiar, to illustrate how clinical exchanges can be appreciated and understood as an aesthetic exchange, beyond the usual instrumental readings provided by "clinical communication skills" lenses. Defamiliarisation may be better known in medical education circles as "making strange" and "thinking otherwise". Readers may find it ironic that we engage with a "technique" yet criticise instrumental readings of poetry for example, but we are here engaging with Russian Formalism critically.

How might we treat a medical interview, a consultation, through the practice of defamiliarisation? (Actually a praxis – a theory in action.) In Lichstein's (1990: n.pag) *Clinical Methods: The History, Physical, and Laboratory Examinations*, an instructive chapter called "The Medical Interview" begins,

> The medical interview is the practicing physician's most versatile diagnostic and therapeutic tool … Interviewing is often considered part of the 'art' in contrast to the 'science' of medicine. There are many reasons to dispute this distinction. Perhaps the most compelling is that labeling it an 'art' removes interviewing from the realm of critical appraisal and suggests that there is something magical or mysterious about interviewing that cannot be described or taught. This chapter will demonstrate the validity of interviewing as a clinical science based on critical observation and analysis ….

Strong and angular words demystify synthetic and fuzzy "mystery" for "validity", "science", "critical" work, and "analysis" – you feel the elbow in your ribs. Thus unruly and dynamic processes of interaction between human beings have, in a common move inspired at least in part by logical positivism, become a clinical science. Anyone familiar with medical school pedagogy is also familiar with the quasi-systematisation of interview techniques, and

DOI: 10.4324/9781003194408-6

this in turn is embedded in formulaic, instrumental "clinical communication skills" frameworks. The above quotation only mildly hyperbolises a core desire of clinical practice: to be, once and for all, *truly* biomedical and scientific. True to Russian Formalism, the systematising of interviewing occurs at the level of method as well as content.

We will later analyse an interview transcript of a consultation not for information (a biomedical imitative), or for the cultivation of empathy (outcomes are biomedical or at least instrumental goals, in search of verifiable information rather than wisdom), but rather to radically transform the way one sees any clinical encounter. It is the pure tool itself that is the thing of value: the means of making language strange unto itself, the de-practicalising of language that paradoxically can give the clinical exchange a radical spiritual freedom. Seeing the world in this way, the world is no longer only biomedical and the values of functionalism are wholly transcended in critique. Importantly, it is also formal and beautiful. In moving beyond measurement (that may be an important element initially) it embraces qualities. We must defamiliarise ourselves from automatised practice, perhaps even defamiliarise basic biomedical imperatives while still reaping their benefits, if we are to be well or to live well within the constraints of our illnesses.

Slow jamming the medical interview, Russian Formalism style

The heterogeneity of Formalists necessitates that we choose a single Formalist's approach in order to demonstrate the value of the whole. Osip Brik's work seems ideal to analyse a text, where Mandelker (1983: 335) called his method the "ultimate model for the Formalist approach to versification study". Unfortunately, Brik's major essay *Sound Repetitions* has yet to be translated into English despite the passage of over a century, so we decided to use Victor Shklovsky's seminal essay "Art as Device" (https://warwick. ac.uk/fac/arts/english/currentstudents/undergraduate/modules/fulllist/first/en122/lecturelist2017-18/art_as_device_2015.pdf). The essay is recognised as a driving stimulus for Russian Formalism and provides a guide to close reading of texts, looking at how poetic language adopts an ornateness, a difficulty, an obliquity, rendering what used to be generally described as "imagery" a technique to de-automatise object relations, making us see the depicted thing or action as if for the first time.

Since our objective is to defamiliarise medical work such that it becomes strange and beautiful, or something other than automatic, Shklovsky's method is a good first step. Physicians have more work in a day than is possible to compress into linear, flat, chronological time – a circumstance that naturally encourages us to automatise clinical work. As Shklovsky (1991: 4–5) explains,

> If we examine the general laws of perception, we see that as it becomes habitual, it also becomes automatic. So eventually all of our skills and

experiences function unconsciously – automatically. If someone were to compare the sensation of holding a pen in his hand or speaking a foreign tongue for the very first time with the sensation of performing this same operation for the ten thousandth time, then he would no doubt agree with us. It is this process of automatization that explains the laws of our prose speech with its fragmentary phrases and half-articulated words.

Gaining medical expertise is also gaining habitual practices without reflection, and this includes both practical skills and clinical cognition. What if we slowed medical work down into a closely rendered simultaneity as "adaptive" expertise? Might it jostle us out of the habituated mode and into something that, admittedly, can't practice modern medicine with the efficiency demanded by the prevailing neoliberal regime, but which might give the little biomedical cog of the individual physician a gift, that of opening up a gap between automaticity and imagination?

Our question is not a novel one, and indeed has a historical answer in the medical literature. In "Making Strange: A Role for the Humanities in Medical Education", Arno Kumagai and Delese Wear (2014: 974) introduce Shklovsky's key idea. Informing the authors' use of literature, movies, art, and interactive theatre to engage students and faculty in reflective exploration and discussions, "making strange" becomes a key pedagogical tool, that of provoking a state of cognitive and affective disequilibrium. This describes the sense of discomfort one may feel when encountering a person, an experience, or a perspective that is unfamiliar, and turns this into a practice. The question for the doctor is, do you fall back into habitual practice or do you question that practice to inhabit the gap created by the questioning?

Kumagai and Wear (ibid.) want "to trouble one's vision and assumptions by making "natural" relationships appear unusual or even bizarre and by forcing one to look on them anew". At the end of the article, they claim, "This ability of art to provide health care professionals an 'open space' to explore, bear witness, and engage with other individuals who are in the midst of becoming is perhaps art's greatest gift of all" (ibid.: 977). Yet the instances of art Kumagai and Wear provide are of a surpassing defamiliarisation, a "strong" kind that cannot help but work their aggressive artifice on the reader such that her perceptions are jostled. (In addition, their survey-type close reading is light-touch and cannot do the job of defamiliarisation in situ; the technique is pointed at but not enacted.) Our objective is not to see art "out there" in other things, which is equally important, but instead to recognise the inherent art occurring in all things, at all times, *including* routine medical practice; or, to make the stone stony (by expounding its stoniness). Our focus is defamiliarising everyday work. By doing something specific – ironically, we invite you to call this a technique, an instrumentalisation of self-care – we may see medicine as if for the first time, over and over again. This is love. And, we freely and comically admit, it is also Narrative Medicine by another name, minus its "competence" tag, moving rather to capabilities and expressions.

We will expand the technique into the poetic once we have taken this first step.

Before demonstrating the technique, we provide a rationale for our particular substrate. Genuine raw patient transcripts are not easy to find. YouTube has a vast selection of display and demonstration interviews (display being interviews conducted with an audience present, watching, with real patients; demonstration interviews are with simulated patients) but no authentic interview transcripts for analysis. The reason for the absence of such material is obvious yet the absolute absence of them in favour of inauthentic simulations or contrived spectacles is strange, resulting in the medical work available to be viewed being somehow a fictional product. This follows medical education's increasing reliance on simulation and the simulacrum, a worrying trend (Bleakley, Bligh and Browne 2011), echoed now in the emergence of the virtual consultation. Yet this is not an impediment for the task we set ourselves; the same technique can be applied to the actual.

Psychiatric interviews exist in the literature, such as the one in Lawrence Kirmayer's (2000) lovely chapter "Broken Narratives: Clinical Encounters and the Poetics of Illness Experience", but these tend to already be quite well picked over at the level of the close reading method. Kirmayer (ibid.: 156), for example, prefers to challenge traditional narrative approaches and offers a version of "rhetoric" as his lens to understand clinical encounters:

> If we think of rhetoric as the verbal art of persuading others, we see it at work in clinical conversation and interaction as patient and healer try to influence each other to reach a mutually satisfying conclusion or way to continue. Studies of rhetoric suggest that much argument and effort to influence others rests on the poetic/evocative use of language.

Kirmayer is unusually attuned to poetry in his analysis. In this chapter, he close reads a clinical encounter as we might – one rendered as text, incidentally, without gestural or intonation cues provided. Tellingly (and, note, two decades ago), Kirmayer (ibid.: 156–57) critiques narrative medicine as reductive:

> the act of telling one's story, no less than the act of "reading" implicit in diagnosis and therapeutic interpretation, occurs in a social context radically different from that of the writer carefully composing a text for publication. Everyday stories are more fragile, inconsistent, and incomplete than a self consciously constructed text. The clinician, as reader, is heavily constrained by the institutional context and the necessity to act based on his reading of the situation.

At bottom, Kirmayer's technique is close reading, albeit situated in a larger interactional matrix denoted by him as "social" and "world". The "pure tool" has been applied to achieve a practical anthropological understanding of the medical encounter. He collapses huge amounts of it into single sentences of summary in order to prompt a rich piece of dialogue for analysis so as to show a fundamental disconnect between patient, doctor, and their mutual contextual factors. We use the same tool as Kirmayer, albeit for different ends. Kirmayer wishes to show the larger social world in which any medical encounter always occurs, as well as emphasising some common pitfalls of the metaphors under which these encounters are predicated.

What we do is to dialectically rejoice in the uselessness of the work on the one hand, while recognising its imaginative and spiritual necessity on the other. That a useful clinical by-product might occur is itself the iatrogenic good. We do not want to interpret anything for a practical purpose, but wish to read the encounter as poetry alone, as the Russian Formalists would. The text alone contains everything that you need. Your task, reader, is to decide on that text. We think that any patient encounter afford such a self-contained text for doctors. For our example, we thought it best to select something available publicly so that you could watch it unfold, too; so that you could have an attempt to be visually defamiliarised as we were. In essence, we can do this together.

We eventually settled on a YouTube example after viewing several dozen candidate videos: "Building Efficiency and Effectiveness through Patient-Centred Interviewing" by Auguste H. Fortin and colleagues (Fortin 2012, 2014), who uploaded the video to promote the book *Smith's Patient-Centered Interviewing: An Evidence-Based Method, 3rd ed.* We found the "evidence-based" descriptor irresistible. Any "evidence-based" candidate worth its salt needs a non-evidence-based counter-technique in order to counter burnout in the profession. For us, all the interview needed to be plausible and competent (there are a lot of bad interview / good interview dyads that irritate since the contrast is an easy trick, formally speaking. As the rhetoric does its work, a reader or viewer is less inclined to be critical of the tandem "good" interview). A few frills put Fortin's faux interview ahead of the rest: the setting was realistic (so many simulations are bare bones and "clunky"); and, rare in this subgenre of YouTube, the medical interviewer enters a closed-door room with a patient in a ward bed. Rather than start with questions, we get to see the doctor make an entry as a character. The interview is aware of itself as a drama. This is a kind of formal awareness that the Russian Formalists themselves might cheer.

The first intervention: meticulously writing out the interview

Either search YouTube for this video or type <https://www.youtube.com/watch?v=_wuTXZ7yvDs> into your browser. Skip to 9:09 of the video and try to write out the medical encounter yourself, in your way.

Now that you have done so, take a look at what we have done:

> A door opens. A medical individual by appearance, male, moustached with goatee, in white coat, enters a hospital room and closes the door behind him. In bed with the head at a 40 degree angle is a middle-aged

woman, nasal prongs properly affixed, one pillow behind her head. She appears somewhat worn. The bottom quarter of a telemetry monitor appears showing no identifying information. The man takes a couple of steps forward and pauses.

Camera focussed on man in white coat, woman in foreground, man in background.

MAN IN WHITE COAT: Hi. Mrs Ward?

Lag to camera switch to focus on woman directly ahead, man seated to her right. Camera switch occurs on this fashion back and forth whenever the speaker changes.

MIDDLE-AGED FEMALE: [In a hoarse voice]: Yes.

MAN IN WHITE COAT: Hi. I'm Dr Fortin. [Extends hand to shake.]

MW: [Shakes hand while saying, still in a hoarse voice that continues for the rest of the interview] Hi.

DF: [Sits down in an adjacent chair on the right side of the bed saying] Hi. Nice to meet you.

MW: Nice to meet you.

DF: Huh. I'm one of the resident doctors here on the medicine team. The emergency room called me and said, uh, that you were going to be admitted to the hospital.

MW: [affirmative noise] Mmm-hmmm.

DF: And they mentioned that you had a pneumonia.

MW: [Nods, almost makes a sound, doesn't.]

DF: Yeah. Well, if it's okay with you what I'd like to do is learn more about what brought you into the hospital. I've got a lot of questions to ask you, to kind of get to know you, so that we take the best care of you here, and, uh, then I'll examine you. Does that sound okay with you?

MW: [nods, makes a welcoming gesture with hands]: Sure.

DF: Great. Again, I understand from the emergency room that you came in with a pneumonia. Was there something else also caused you to come in today, just so we know how we're spending our time together here?

MW: It was mostly just the, uh, coughing up blood ...

Transcribing this brief encounter was laborious. Though only 59 seconds elapsed on the video, the amount of time taken to write out this version was over 20 minutes. The method was to closely synchronise movement with dialogue and to provide stage direction as description for how the dialogue came across in performance. In essence, the encounter was rendered formally as a play, a dramaturgical framing following Erving Goffman's (1959) work on "impression management" in communication exchanges. One then marvels at how beautiful the slight hand gestures are, the occasional pause as denoted by a comma, then small conversational noises that solder our speech together. The video had to be replayed time and time again in order to get the dialogue completely right, to get the synchrony of movement and interplay of speech correct. In other words, the material was worked with in the guise of artisanal reconstructor, renderer, or translator into text. The scene was defamiliarised. (As we transcribed it, we couldn't help but wonder in our restless defamiliarising fashion: What would happen if, rather than its translator, the interaction was rendered in the genre of fiction; or as poetry; or as psycho-sociological transaction? Each time, another defamiliarisation no doubt – keeping this particular technique from becoming habituated.)

Let us look, borrowing from Shklovsky's playbook of automotive analogies, a little more under the hood of the reconstruction in formal terms. Note the character names and how they are designated at the beginning. The name "DF" is not retrospectively designated to represent Dr Fortin at the beginning of the drama. Instead there is "Man in White Coat" because he is exactly that until he is introduced or foregrounded by naming. Once introduced, he becomes Dr Fortin. Similarly, "Mrs Ward" is initially "Middle-Aged Female" until her identity is known after her affirmative response to the doctor. Paying attention to the mechanics of the drama in this way, even the conversational niceties and otherwise automatised or "well-oiled" protocols of greeting, brings us closer to the complexity that passes by our consciousness, and sometimes bypasses our consciousness as tacit recognition. The process of naming is of course a humanising gesture; and its opposite is true: withholding a name can appear as dehumanising and insulting.

In the same vein, let us pay attention to the scene. It is important to notice the strange wooden door frame, which is useless to notice and yet informs the verisimilitude. It is there; it is meaningful, not just scenery, but as we set out in a subsequent chapter, an object in the environment that affords something important – entry and exit, privacy, dwelling, and so forth. We notice the two cameras and the lovely lag that followed each change in speaker, and metaphorised this lag as like the slow pause we should bring to our lives on occasion, but this camera did it epically – and, in another irony, in an automatised way.

The method of close attention produces more than transcription, although that is all it might seem to anyone who merely read the account herself. What it does is produce a means of relating to interviewer and patient that is participatory and not passive; the words work, doing well in the imaginary encounter; so invested, the speech becomes the viewer's somehow. Scooped up in the scene are all our efforts to do good, to make a difference, to identify and ameliorate suffering – which, we think, will be the same kinds of encounters transcribed by other physicians if they took up this technique and used it on their own (receptive, consensual) patients. Recording a virtual conversation in a virtually secure environment once informed consent is obtained, with deletion of the conversation immediately thereafter, is reasonable. Explain that you are conducting the activity to improve your care. That's true enough. This mirrors an established research method of "video ethnography" in ward and surgical theatre settings pioneered by one of us (AB) in medical education (Bleakley 2001).

It is our fervent hope that you will see yourself in an automatised mode, which is ideal, since that is the mode that requires exposure. Dr Fortin had a script to do well on camera, but you won't. In the automatised mode, you use the general structure and relational techniques provided during medical school. You'll make what you do into a script, and in so doing, you'll see as if for the first time yourself. Not for the purposes of evaluation and improvement, but rather for being benignly confronted with the fact that you care about the work you do. You will have to write out this realisation over exquisitely drawn out minutes. You'll come to see the work you do as a front-stage drama, with a host of backstage issues (how do you act out of character and away from script, for example?). Qua Shklovsky, your perceptions (we are addressing this to medics at this point) will be refreshed and the meaning of what you do – for it *is* there, it *was* why you entered medical school and it *is* why you stay in the profession – is paradoxically reinforced and refreshed through the affirmation of its perpetual presence as a habit. We claim this as poetic ground. As we will claim the actual words themselves as part of poetry's firmament in the following section.

The second intervention: poetry alone (text only transcript)

The basic principle underwriting this intervention – that sound is an important part of communication, in excess of denotation – is ancient, something poets have known for forever. Pre-Homeric performers sang the epics accompanied by the lyre where tone was central to performance; Mandelker (1983) thought this principle was perhaps most memorably articulated in the modern era in English by Edgar Allan Poe in several literary essays, including in "The Philosophy of Composition". In this essay, Poe claims that the entirety of his long poem "The Raven" extended systematically from his need for a refrain. Here is a snippet of his reasoning:

> Having made up my mind to a refrain, the division of the poem into stanzas was of course a corollary, the refrain forming the close to each stanza. That such a close, to have force, must be sonorous and susceptible of protracted emphasis, admitted no doubt, and these considerations inevitably led me to the long *o* as the most sonorous vowel in connection with *r* as the most producible consonant.
>
> (n. pag)

What ensues in Poe's essay is an extended self-compositional memoir progressing out from the sonic and image-origins that extend from the word "nevermore". The reasoning is profoundly idiosyncratic yet it also represents the way a poet thinks about language and sound, which is of course at a variance to that of those who engage in practical speech. Poe's sound-based reasoning is also substantiated in much modern work on human vocalisations and their emotional ramifications (see Myers-Schulz et al. 2013) that extends back to the early 20th century.

Brik massively expanded upon Poe's enterprise in his essay "Sound Repetitions" in which it is said by Natasha Kurchanova (2010: 57) that he analysed hundreds of individual examples from Pushkin's and Lermontov's verses to illustrate the argument that in poetry, repetitions of sounds and "sound combinations" that did not carry any semantic charge stood on a par with imagery and "served not only as euphonic additions, but were the results of an independent poetic striving", "anchoring the work structurally". We reinforce here the importance of charting paralanguage in communication: silences, hesitation noises, unconscious repetitions, intonations, pitch and speed of talking, guttural voicing, and so forth.

In other words, sounds and their repetitions contribute to meaning in both extra-sensical and supra-sensical ways, beyond denotative meaning and towards connotative meaning. An English edition of Brik's original work is, obviously, impossible to reproduce based on the sonic pattern analysis of Russian poetry; nevertheless, the close attention to sound in a semi-systematic fashion is what can be brought forward in keeping with Brik's vision as articulated earlier. Complete lines of dialogue follow, alternating with sonic and metrical interpretations.

(11:50 start) MW: I guess I'm feeling tired because the cough wakes me up in the middle of the night. So, uh, just … exhausted. Being kind of a crabby mom lately.

> *Perhaps the most obvious sonic concentration here is the concentration of k sounds, a plosive consonant, in the first sentence: "because", "cough," and "wakes" enact a kind of coughing fit at the level of language. There is spluttering too focussed on the s consonants: "guess', "because", "wakes", "just", "exhausted", after which "Being kind of a crabby mom lately" is a welcome syncopation (iambic pentameter count). Moreover, the largely trochaic metre at the beginning of the first line "I guess I'm feeling tired" matches the emotional tone of the patient and the content of her speech, as the falling rhythm of trochaic metres have long been associated with a tone of despair. The line changes midway into an iambic pattern with an extra syllable. Now a rising rhythm, this fact can – if one can't analyse stresses – be intuited at the quickening of the pace ("wakes me up in the middle of the night").*
>
> *The second line's vocal fry ("uh") in addition to the pause denoted by the ellipse also enact the exhaustion just described.*
>
> *The terminal sentence fragment of dialogue lapses back into a trochaic rhythm, making the point that there is a despairing impact of the illness on MW's family.*
>
> *The cough takes on the role of an independent being with its own will, waking up the mom in the middle of the night. In this role it is a disrupter of sleep rhythms and of rhythm in general. The woman has lost her beat because of the cough's insistence, and is dead beat, exhausted by it.*

AF: Crabby mom. Say more about that?

> *Here we have a basic repetition to start, which is not worth analysing except if one is commenting on interviewing technique. Despite its brevity, it is the second*

sentence that is telling. For one sees the long heavy play of vowels here in the midst of attempting emotional identification with the patient. Some research points to the particular sadness of the "o" sound over that of the "i" sound (Rummer et al., 2014), meaning that the interviewer's emotional tone seems to match that of the patient's (and not be inappropriately lighthearted, say, with an "I'm so interested in this. Fill me in"). The tone of voice of course would be the main indicator.

MW: I've got my two young kids that are home with just me. And uh, I feel bad. You know, you don't want to be crabby or anything, I've just been so exhausted and not feeling well that … I just … I guess I snap very easily at them. I don't mean to, but I do.

The obvious metaphor here is that of the "crab" as it brings forward MW as mother, elaborated on with the subsequent "snap". At the level of language, though, the ultimate sentence and its initial iambic rhythm that is disrupted with the "but" that verbally evokes the self-lacerations of the crab's own claws: "don't"/ "do", a pincer effect.

AF: Okay. Mmm. Yeah. So you're really not able to be the mom you want to be because you've been feeling so sick. How has that been for you, emotionally? **(end 12:44)**

These lines heavily rhyme. "Able to **be**" / "mom you want to **be**" / "**been**" / "**been**" / "emotionally." That the rhyme occurs using the adverbial form of "emotion" is of significance, but more so using the copula form of "to be", for the close repetition of sound and verb in past, present, and future tenses makes for a strong aspirational chime.
There is upbeat in the glossing of how the woman feels ("the mom you want to be") followed by the downbeat of "feeling so sick". These are ascriptions but they probably match the woman's overall rhythm of rise and then collapse, rise and then despair.

Admittedly somewhat idiosyncratic, this analysis attends less to the speech as insight to be mined and more so to affect to process at the level of its sonic expression. To accomplish the analysis, one has to, again, write out the dialogue and then defamiliarise it further by considering it less on a making sense level and more on a sound sense level. This is always a useful first step, and then to adding a metrical analysis keeps what otherwise might become a rote transcriptional exercise properly defamiliarised.

We are converts to the poet Emily Dickinson's notion of thinking "slant" or slantwise ("Tell all the truth but tell it slant": https://www.poetryfoundation.org/poems/56824/tell-all-the-truth-but-tell-it-slant-1263) where,

The Truth must dazzle gradually
Or every man be blind –

As Dickinson puts it, this is an ethical gesture – it frustrates the desire to hammer home your point and works in a much more subtle, caring way. For example, "breaking bad news" is "taught" to medical and healthcare students as a technique/protocol/skill/competence – or brutally instrumentalised. This "general case" instrument can become hopelessly inadequate when students meet the specific case that has its unique uncertainties. Our drawing on the Russian Formalists here is a way of applying their method to see clinical encounters slantwise, but it is also, we hope, a valuable contribution to both research methodology and non-instrumental (or aesthetic and ethical) clinical practice and bedside manner.

We have escaped Narrative Medicine's reach

In bringing this chapter and this opening section of the book to a close, we recognise the unlikely outcome that this analysis will win converts to the cause of metrically analysing patient speech. However, the practice is worthwhile as advertised; that Narrative Medicine's valorised "close attention" is at least as valid through this means as through another; also, that paying attention to sound is to pay attention to one's own relationship with sound and with speech (see Myers-Schulz et al. 2013). There are other, obvious, connections – sound is central to diagnostics as are its metaphors (rasping cough; rattling, bubbling, and clicking rales) (Bleakley 2020). At a minimum we have introduced a lexicon into the clinical encounter that embraces musicality, something that "narrative competence" may have excluded. (We leave it to you the reader to judge whether or not we have made a sound argument.) It is, in other words, to be in alignment with a poetic way to think; and it is this alignment that is at such odds with biomedicine, an opposition that might be useful in the Late Capitalist Days of Physician Burnout.

Having sounded out limits to narrative, we plunged you headlong into sonics in poetry. This is partly to remind you of poetry's pre-Homeric, pre-written language, origins in vocal intonations and then in song, for these origins can meet medicine's bottom-line diagnostic techniques. Consider a symbiosis in the physical examination, where auscultation and percussion become a body sonics informing the blunt expressive subtexts of discomfort, illness, distress, despair, and pain. The dispiriting exhalation of an exhausted person can tell as much as their exhausting "story" and in a fraction of the time.

We have thinned out the narrative overgrowth to reveal the soils of poetry – the allotment plot that replaces the emplotment plot. In subsequent chapters, we cast off our narrative chains. We start more clearly to link medicine with poetry, or the poetic imagination with the medical mind. In the following chapter, we thoroughly investigate the question: *What is the "medical mind"?* How do doctors think; but more, how do they imagine? And how do poetry and the poetic imagination engage with the thinking and imagining that starts with a patient consultation, in its turn kick-starting diagnostics?

We will not be pitching poetry against biomedicine (a lost cause, where they do different work). Nor will we claim that poetry is a cure-all (another lost cause and a symptom of narcissistic inflation). Poetry's uselessness is perhaps its greatest asset and we will put that to good use. We like Sun Tzu's *Art of War* strategy that the art of combat is to defuse combat, to not go to war at all – medicine's martial metaphors undone.

References

Bleakley A. 2001. Using the Ward Round for Teaching and Learning: How do Junior Doctors Learn from Consultants through Ward-based Teaching? Conference Proceedings, 2nd International Conference on Researching Work and Learning. July 26–28, 2001. Calgary, Alberta, Canada. University of Calgary, Faculty of Continuing Education.

Bleakley A. 2020. *Educating Doctors' Senses through the Medical Humanities: "How Do I Look?"* Abingdon: Routledge.

Bleakley A, Bligh J, Browne J. 2011. *Medical Education for the Future: Identity, Power and Location.* Dordrecht: Springer.

Fortin AH. Building Efficiency and Effectiveness through Patient-Centred Interviewing. YouTube. May 7, 2014. Retrieved from https://www.youtube.com/watch?v=_wuTXZ7yvDs

Fortin AH, Dwamena F, Frankel R, Smith RC. 2012. *Smith's Patient-Centered Interviewing: An Evidence-Based Method,* 3rd ed. New York: McGraw Hill.

Goffman E. 1959. *The Presentation of Self in Everyday Life.* New York: Anchor Books.

Goldenberg M. On Evidence and Evidence-Based Medicine: Lessons from the Philosophy of Science. *Social Science and Medicine.* 2006; 62: 2621–32.

Jakubinski L. 2018. *On Language and Poetry: Three Essays.* New York: Upper West Side Philosophers.

Kirmayer L. 2000. Broken Narratives: Clinical Encounters and the Poetics of Illness Experience. In: C Mattingly, L Garro (eds.) *Narrative and the Cultural Construction of Illness and Healing.* Berkeley: University of California Press, 153–80.

Kumagai A, Wear D. "Making Strange": A Role for the Humanities in Medical Education. *Academic Medicine.* 2014; 89: 973–77.

Kurchanova N. Osip Brik and the Politics of the Avant-Garde. *October.* 2010; 134: 52–73.

Lichstein PR. 1990. The Medical Interview. In: KH Walker, DW Hall, JW Hurst (eds.) *Clinical Methods: The History, Physical, and Laboratory Examinations,* 3rd ed. Oxford: Butterworth-Heinemann, 29–36.

Mandelker A. Russian Formalism and the Objective Analysis of Sound in Poetry. *The Slavic and East European Journal.* 1983; 27: 327–38.

Myers-Schulz B, Pujara M, Wolf RC, Koenigs M. Inherent Emotional Quality of Human Speech Sounds. *Cognition and Emotion.* 2013; 27: 1105–13.

Poe EA. Undated. The Philosophy of Composition. Poetry Foundation. Retrieved from https://www.poetryfoundation.org/articles/69390/the-philosophy-of-composition

Rummer R, Schweppe J, Schlegelmilch R, Grice M. Mood is Linked to Vowel Type: The Role of Articulatory Movements. *Emotion.* 2014; 14: 246–50.

Shklovsky V. 1991. *Theory of Prose.* London: Dalkey Archive Press.

Part II

Theorising lyrical medicine

6 Re-visioning diagnostic reasoning, or stepping out from the skull

Clinical reasoning: a dialogue

"We had that sewn up years ago", say the cognitive psychologists.

> The novice has to make deliberate, rational judgements based on best available evidence from physical examination and testing, backed up by their biomedical science knowledge. In a process of differential diagnosis (helped by algorithms such as Bayes' theorem), they gradually pare down options to the best judgement and seek confirmation from seniors.

"What if the diagnosis is complex?"

> Then they seek help as early as possible. This is called Type 2 diagnosis. Experts use this rational process too when a diagnosis is tangled or difficult. The experienced, or expert, doctor however mainly uses what's known as Type 1 reasoning. This is pattern recognition. Even before examination: The clinician might say, *I've seen this before*; or *I'm pretty sure what it is*; or *In fact I'm certain*. Tests will confirm. This is seeing a whole picture, a gestalt.

"Well, ok. But when an expert makes a Type 1 pattern recognition decision, what's the thinking process?"
    "Well. That's largely a black box".

> What? You mean the fruits of years of hard slog at medical school are told to go away and have a drink at the bar, or worse, are locked away in a cellar? And another thing: how can all this (the black box stuff especially) be going on inside the skull of the doctor? What about context, meaning, the patient, colleagues and tests?

"Oh, yeah, of course this goes on in a context, but the real thinking is done by the doctor".

DOI: 10.4324/9781003194408-8

OK, but there's lots unsaid there. Again, what's in the black box? Is it mostly memory? And what about the effect of the environment on thinking? I've heard artificial intelligence people talk about "predictive processing", where you think ahead (like intuition) and act on this, but this is in constant feedback loop with memory, so that the thinking ahead is being adjusted moment by moment.

"Yeah, I'm sure. But I've got enough to do just treating patients".

In this chapter, we open the black box that is clinical judgement in the head, and we account for the role of context or environment in that judgement process. We take a big leap and suggest that this diagnostic clinical reasoning process in the round has strong similarities with poetic composition. Further, this is not just an accidental overlap.

The undercut edges give an apple-core appearance

A couple of decades ago, one of us (AB) set up a research project in which he matched up experienced doctors in visual specialties (radiology, dermatology, histopathology) with established visual artists to exchange ideas about how doctors and artists "notice", "look", and "see". The doctors focussed on visual cues for making diagnoses through radiology images, photographs of skin presentations, and histopathology specimens, where the artists focussed on how they made aesthetic judgements in drawing, painting, photography, and sculpture from illustrative examples. Conversations and practice exchanges were filmed and analysed, where the artists visited clinics and laboratories and the doctors visited studios and gallery spaces (Bleakley et al. 2003a, 2003b). The project was then presented in a high profile gallery (Tate St Ives UK) to a public audience for dissemination and reaction.

One key finding was that artists looked at how doctor's clinical images concentrated on aesthetic detail such as colour differentiation and form (shape, placement). This finding applied in reverse, but the doctors talked about forms or patterns in more instrumental ways, by-passing the aesthetic. Recognising a form turned out to be a step towards diagnosis. Outcomes surfaced: doctors looked habitually (even while highly experienced) and errors could occur from this familiarised, "tired eye". The artists refreshed the doctors' looking by pointing out subtleties of colour and form that the doctors were missing.

Generally speaking, we think that poetry is useless; in fact, it escapes capture if an attempt at pure instrumentalism is made on its person. Based on its life in our own practices, we suspect that it could have an applied function in refreshing doctors' ears in appreciating not only patients' words but also their own descriptions as they think diagnostically, often drawing on patterns (fields) from imaging or tests. The distinction is tricky but real: live a certain way and particular habits are refined, but try to engage in a "poetry activity" directly and one is often left looking for signs of resting in a dead parrot. In the previous chapter, we provided an example of how a poet's ear may help to educate for appreciation of sound expression in the clinical encounter. We provide lots of examples throughout the book of how the poetic imagination and the medical mind might cohabit.

To return to the research project described above, a welcome by-product of this research was to look carefully at the language that physicians use to describe diagnostic reasoning in action, to close read their 'think aloud' accounts. For example, the seasoned radiologist put up an X-ray showing a restriction in the colon (specifically, the last section of the bowel or sigmoid) that could be recognised by its uncanny appearance or pattern as an apple-core shape. Indeed, it attracted the metaphor-likeness attribute (a simile) of "apple core lesion". The radiologist summed up the diagnosis in a trio of terse statements:

> There is an area of narrowing in the sigmoid.
> The undercut edges give an apple core appearance.
> This is colonic carcinoma.

Now the first sentence appears to be prosaic description using technical language, a biomedical reduction. But there is poetry here too: "an area of narrowing" is more pleasing than "a narrow area" because it is in process rather than static (not at all pleasing to the person progressively suffering from the constriction, of course). The second sentence is poetic. The "undercut edges" consonance plays on the hard "d" consonant; "edges give" plays on the hard "g"; while "apple core appearance", playing on the vowel "a", is lighter and gives a lilting tone to the statement's closure as an alliteration. The third statement is one of fact, a definitive diagnosis, period/ full stop/ closure (actually a little worrying as other diagnoses may be possible).

Given that this is somebody's colon and here is a serious cancer, we appreciate the ethical difficulty of discussing this in terms of poetry and beauty. But throughout, as we link poetry and medicine, necessarily language will have suffering and disease as its topic, as well as recovery and hope. We hope readers won't be too put off by our resolute focus on beauty, for to forsake the recognition of it amidst great difficulty in the name of "ethics" is to close a mind as surely as insistence on biomedical utility does.

Therefore: as an advert for the beauty and complexity of language, the origin of the word 'colon' is the Greek *kölon* meaning "the pause before the clause". It signifies taking a breath. In anatomy and physiology, colonic movements are like clauses, breaths, as waste matter moves through.

We give this example to show how diagnostic reasoning and poetry can collide unexpectedly, or are always already there if noticed; and, if noticed, there is the possibility that the diagnostic process itself can be defamiliarised, made sharper. The remainder of this chapter will map this in detail. In a roundabout way – slantwise – as we provide the hard evidence sceptics crave where they ask the question, "What's the use of poetry in medicine?"

In Part I, we articulated an argument that questions narrative medicine's imperialism and shows how poetry does different things than narrative. In this chapter, we explicitly link the poetic imagination to clinical thinking at a granular level, primarily to diagnostic reasoning, but also including prognostics and overall treatment and care. Our unit of analysis is first psychological (the cognitive process of clinical reasoning and its poetic resonances) and then ethological (the behaviour of doctors in their natural habitats). We will show how poetry both feeds, and feeds on, medicine. As we show alignment between poetry and the cognitive psychology of clinical reasoning, we explore radical new perspectives in clinical reasoning that have developed over the past few decades, but have never been brought into conversation with poetry as far as we know. We show how diagnostic reasoning *is* poetry, a claim that may seem ridiculous at first sight.

We will anatomise the processes of clinical diagnostic reasoning as this is defined by a world-orientation – an immersion in the social world and its significant objects and artefacts. This perspective challenges the previous psychological hegemony in which clinical reasoning is explained as an individual's internal psychological process: inside the head of the doctor. First, reasoning is explored as distributed across persons, events and objects in immediate and immersive contexts, which is after all a "common sense" perspective. The ethologist Jakob von Uexküll (1934/2010) called this the machinations of *umwelt* or local habitat. Second, where clinical reasoning has been described in narrative terms, or narrative has been imposed on clinical reasoning events (another hegemonic event as our previous chapters illustrate), we point out that such events need not be framed as linear, progressive and temporal. Rather, they may display as nonlinear and complex, messy, sporadic, and place-based. They can perhaps be reconceived using the resources of poetry.

King Offa is the Dyke

At this point we hold up a 'Poetry Welcome!' sign. Wherever possible, we now use poetry to illustrate the argument we are making, but more, to act as a clinical intervention in its own right. Poetry will illuminate the body's work and medicine's work on the body (including affect, mind and imagination). Our argument will be embodied, poetically.

To illuminate clinical reasoning as a distributed process, and not confined to thinking-in-the-head, we draw on the arch-English post-WWII poet Geoffrey Hill, often called the poet's poet, admired for his complexity. There are many poets who might have served us for analysis; Hill is not alone among poets who conjure a tremendous social world for their own intersubjective creations. Dionne Brand, for example. We would add George Elliott Clarke's *Canticles* series too. Robert Lowell. But we stick with Hill because he is the signature name in complexity. And whom else is a better fit for credentialist, subspecialist-preferring biomedicine? In an interview in *The Paris*

Review (Phillips 2000) Hill is asked about his poetry often being viewed as "difficult":

> We are difficult. Human beings are difficult. We're difficult to our-selves, we're difficult to each other. And we are mysteries to ourselves, we are mysteries to each other. One encounters in any ordinary day far more real difficulty than one confronts in the most "intellectual" piece of work. Why is it believed that poetry, prose, painting, music should be less than we are? Why does music, why does poetry have to address us in simplified terms, when if such simplification were applied to a descrip-tion of our own inner selves we would find it demeaning? I think art has a right – not an obligation – to be difficult if it wishes.

Hill demonstrates the powerful organising force of poetry as well as paying it proper respect, for it will tell you better than we can what it might do for you, in its difficult ways. We draw specifically on Hill's (1971) *Mercian Hymns*, an account that bounces back and forth between the times of Offa – an 8th century King of Mercia, a kingdom of Anglo-Saxon middle England – and an imaginary contemporary childhood, perhaps Hill's own. In this text, Hill shows that reasoning is necessarily stained by the world in which that rea-soning is immersed and to which it is subject. Reasoning is not purely of the subject but also 'in' and 'of' the world.

Offa, the anti-hero of *Mercian Hymns*, was King of the English Midlands from AD 757 to 796 and also conquered much of southern England. He might have remained a footnote in English history had he not built 'Offa's Dyke', which is a large earthwork following the modern border between England and Wales, or Anglo-Saxon Mercia and Welsh Powys. The beauty of Hill's poem is that it enacts his overall project for lyric poetry's purpose: elegantly by-passing knee-jerk personal-confessional styles to engage with the world lyrically; in other words, to step out from the skull and embrace the context for living. Here, we part company with strict close reading to invite context back to text. Actually, the text is a product of its immediate context where language affords an ecology, and we extend this ecology to the house the poem inhabits: the poet's *umwelt* and readers' and listeners' surrounds. This returns us to William Carlos Williams' (1967) metaphor of the housing of poetry as a necessary architecture for the poem's stability, described in our Introduction: the house of the poem built in the projective field.

Cognitive reasoning models have exposed what was previously 'black boxed' as a tacit dimension to thinking. They uncover the memory of bi-omedical information plus the unconscious use of heuristics by which that information is applied to 'cases'. Recall our example of the radiologist's di-agnosis at the beginning of this chapter: "There is an area of narrowing in the sigmoid", a light biomedical reduction; "the undercut edges give an apple core appearance" (simile), a heuristic. However, this model in turn 'black boxed' the *umwelt* or social context for reasoning. The radiologist 'speaks aloud' to give us entry into his cognition, but what speaks first is the artefact – the X-ray, that is the radiologist's primary *umwelt*. In a distributed, ecological cognitive model, this black box is opened and described. Of course, as a kind of poetic justice, radiologists' clinical lives are spent largely inhabiting black boxes of images in black box rooms.

The step from the 'hard' mechanics of the mind to the 'soft' *umwelt* is also one from linearity to uncertainty and nonlinearity. It is to lose one's name and identity as anchor (in Cartesian terms, thinking as the only certainty) and to drift amongst the mintings of metaphors contributed by surrounding objects as we attempt to name them.

In Hill's poem – another black box opened through close reading – Offa's identity is served by bathing in nature as "King of the perennial; holy-groves, the riven sand- / stone …". The spacing between words is intentional. Hill is creating a field, allowing each word elbow room and leg space to show its worth, and breathing space for contemplation. He is gradually weaving a habitat – taking us back once more to Olson's Projective Verse and the poetic field where the poem is *placed*.

Through virtuoso technique, Hill prevents the poem from being reduced to the personal, as identity check. It provides a model for the power of resistance to reductionism; and here, we use Hill's model as a reminder that cognitive reasoning is extra-cognitive, both 'situated' and 'extended' to engage with context, worldly objects and above all, other persons. Thinking is always social and object-oriented. Being is made through language (the object of objects, or meta-object), whose purpose is to re-invent Being.

The poem opens by Hill pitching Offa's self-interest against the worldly Other of objects:

> … overlord of the M5: architect of the his- / toric rampart and ditch,
> the citadel at Tamworth

and so forth. Then Hill brings the person Offa, rather than his worldly associations, into focus:

> saltmaster: money- / changer: commissioner for oaths; martyrologist: /
> the friend of Charlemagne.

"'I liked that,' said Offa, 'sing it again'". Offa sees himself in the mirror narcissistically where the reader sees Offa in the mirror of worldly things. Having set this frame, Hill's poem continues to anatomise Offa, never psychologically (too predictable after Freud) but through Object-Oriented Ontology (Harman 2018) (explored later in this chapter as a fully blown philosophical position akin to Russian Formalism's "stoniness of the stone"), an understanding of being as "situated" in worldly things and activities, including other persons of significance. Developing from the initial "stoniness of the stone", it is not so much the object in its own right that matters, but rather how the object (and its stoniness) comes into being through relationship to other objects.

This is Freud deluxe, as developed in the object relations school of Melanie Klein and Donald Winnicott. Here, (M)Other-child relations are expanded to material others, "transitional" objects such as toys and artefacts (these days televisions and computer screens, action hero models, Barbie dolls and Pokemon cards). Objects become our other "relations" (family) as we use them to stand in for family and friends. They are naturally both subjectified and objectified simultaneously. Hill has Offa doing the same in his poem. Identity is *of* the world, where we are accommodative to the world rather than assimilating it, to draw on Jean Piaget's (Inhelder and Piaget 2006) distinction.

Wine, urine and ashes

As Offa's childhood is recounted (it could be any childhood, as Hill switches between 8th and 20th century Anglo-Saxon England and his own childhood and its object relations), so first we know Offa by what he gives off and not what he is:

A pet-name, a common name ...
... A laugh; a cough

and then: "A syndicate". He joins a collective, is syndicated. This is a group known by a collective name. It is a worldly family group, objects giving subjectivity as family members, our object 'relations'. These are things of nature. Hill refuses psychobiography for object-oriented biography and object relations psychodynamics. We know Offa not by personality, but only as "A name to conjure with". The conjuring is of the world in which he is immersed. Offa is identified with:

badger and raven
... Orchards
fruited above clefts ... honeycombs of
chill sandstone.

Identification is complete. The personal body is the body of earth. The boy's "toys" (objects as relations) are things of nature:

Candles of gnarled resin, apple-branches, the tacky
mistletoe.

Immersion in the natural world becomes identification with that world: "Milldams, marlpools / that lay unstirring. Eel-swarms. Coagulations of / frogs" that the boy attacks while he "battered a ditchful; then sidled away from the / stillness and silence". Unhinged, he lures his childhood friend "down to the old quarries, and flayed / him". Hill notes (with a wry smile?): "the mad are predators".

Offa is mad, in both senses, angry and displaced (his [M]Others are multiple, worldly). He is constantly searching for placement. He finds it temporarily in minting new silver coins with immaculate impressions of his head, fixing his likeness, nailing his identity. But he knows that this is also a metaphor, where over time handling of the coin would gradually efface his likeness. "He reigned forty years" but Hill gives no detail of his emotional development, only that "Seasons touched and retouched / the soil", where

> ... the boar
> furrowed black mould, his snout intimate with
> worms and leaves.

Again, we come to know Offa by the things around him. What he observes is how we observe him: "a snail sugared its new stone". He mocks his family by drinking their health only sporadically because his extended family is now the forest, where "Tutting, he wrenched at the snarled root of a dead crab- / apple. It rose against him" and he is "lightly concussed". Skin to skin, nature speaks back to Offa and moulds him: "retribution entertained"; his world is "Wine, urine and ashes"; "... he left behind coins ... and traces of red mud".

Hill draws the reader's attention to what Offa does with matter (ecology) rather than what's the matter with Offa (psychology).

Are we not talking about every doctor here and his or her relationship to patients (as world-orientation), and how that doctor conceives of his or her clinical reasoning and prescribing (augmented by objects such as tests and pharmaceuticals)? Every medical encounter is necessarily an object relations exercise. Do they situate this inside their heads or do they engage with the wine, urine and ashes of their patients' worlds and their "traces of red mud" that we will take as a metaphor for symptom, as well as worldly objects such as the doctors' drug formularies? If the latter is the case, and it patently is, why in Offa's name has medical clinical reasoning been hamstrung by personalistic psychological models for over (at least) four decades that situate clinical reasoning in the skull and not in the world? This hegemony seems to us as troublesome as that of narrative medicine's suffocation of poetry.

Let us temper our initial outrage. We introduced this chapter with the historically constituted tensions between differing epistemological frames of reasoning: one situated in the person, the other a distributed phenomenon where the world or context affords or sets the scene for decisions. But surely we can have both? Yes, of course, they work as a whole and to oppose them is silly (they should never have been separated in the first place, Monsieur Descartes!), but we are again attempting to come out from the longstanding epistemological shadow (or treat the Cartesian stain) of individualism to engage with the collective.

Hill successfully melds Offa the bully and deranged child with his transitional object – the world at large, with which he eventually fuses. His Dyke is like a marker between the two territories, but can be read as Offa's submission to the world of soil and stone. He becomes earth rather than being earth. He identifies not just as territorialist (ego extension) but finally as territory itself. There is one final step that Offa cannot take. He has moved from cognition owned (personalism) to cognition distributed (claiming the land, situating in the field). Now he needs to release the land to realise cognition as a visiting swarm, a shaping force. For Hill, as a devout Christian, this is the force of deity. Offa as child "wormed my way heavenward for ages", but always with the soil as mother: "amid barbaric ivy, scrollwork of fern". Note the language that Offa learns is that of the natural world: he speaks the stuff of the forest and soil. For humanists, the equivalent is the force for collective good, or democracy. This is the force that science in medicine squeezes out in its search for "objectivity". Biomedicine must reclaim this touch with humanity – it doesn't have to lose its search for objectivity in the process. Can medicine engage fruitfully with this force of democracy (human rights, equity, equality)?

Hill has a generic answer: restore science to natural history. Our equivalent in medicine would be less work in the laboratory and more in the observation of patients in their natural habitats, with the eye of the ethologist (lots of role models here: Chekhov, Williams, Nawaal El Saadawi, Perri Klass, Danielle Ofri). Offa says, "I was invested in mother-earth, the crypt of roots / and endings". Even in combat, the fruits of the earth shine through: "Metal effusing its own fragrance, / a variety of balm". Offa moves about his own clinic of earth tending to the health of it:

> Primeval heathland spattered with the bones of mice
> and birds; where adders basked and bees made pro-
> vision, mantling the inner walls of their burh:

So the doctor inhabits the poetry-rich clinic as *umwelt* as both habitat dweller and natural historian, with a keen eye for distortions of nature and how these might be attended: "to cradle a face hair-lipped by the searing wire". Here, "Tumult recedes as though into the long rain".

Hill's work has been referred to as an "aesthetics of history" (Wootten 1998). Could the work of the clinic be revisioned as an aesthetics of medicine?

From tic to tick (or vice versa)

We continue with our theme of doctors and poets as ethologists, working in an ecosystem, and extend our questioning of narrative's over-reach and imperialism. We have dwelt a lot on story and its discontents. Here is another story that turns out to be something else, a piece of natural history that we render as unnatural and ahistorical. In the opening pages to his masterpiece on ethology *A Foray into the Worlds of Animals and Humans* – first published in 1934, a decade before his death – the German zoologist/ethologist and bio-philosopher Jakob von Uexküll (2010) recounts the life history of the humble, blood-sucking tick. The female tick, having copulated, "climbs ... to the tip of a protruding branch of any shrub in order to either fall onto small mammals who run by underneath or to let herself be brushed off the branch by large ones". Blind and deaf, the tick identifies her prey through smell – strictly limited to that of butyric acid given off by the skin glands of all mammals. If the tick, brushed off the branch, meets the skin of the mammal, it buries its head beneath that skin and "pumps a stream of warm blood slowly into itself". This is the tick's first and last meal, after which she falls to the ground, lays her eggs, and dies.

Given the fact that a mammal might only come by every so often, the tick must be able to survive without food of any kind for a long time. And here is the remarkable thing about the tiny predator's blood feast: von Uexküll reports that under laboratory conditions, ticks have been kept alive for 18 years, suggesting that such a lifespan also occurs in the wild. This remarkable fact turns time into something beyond the ready grasp of humans, for it is, in effect, a dead, empty, or suspended time; certainly a warp. As time is cast as thin and elastic, so space for the tick is collapsed to what von Uexküll calls *umwelt*, met earlier – a perceptual lifeworld with the dimensions of the immediate environment, a place or placement. For the tick, we're talking a restricted bubble (a term that is now irritatingly familiar in times of Covid-19 restrictions).

The tick's life experience amounts to just seven sequential events: climbing a branch; waiting on that branch; smelling an animal beneath; falling on the animal or being brushed off the branch; preying on the host's blood; falling off the host; then laying her eggs and dying. Von Uexküll refers to these as "perception marks", thus switching attention from time (lifespan) to place (*umwelt*). Space is collapsed into a small, confined area bounded by the promise of one particular smell: a particular place where the tick leaves its mark. Time, the tick's lifespan, is marked by vacuous suspension, practically inanimate, in effect cancelling itself out. These seven events may constitute a narrative arc as life history for the diachronic biologist, but not for the episodic tick.

Following von Uexküll's second-hand narrative (the first hand narrative account is self-evidently obscure to us, for it involves the tick's accounting of its own life cycle in words), what we present here is a third-hand account, possibly even an anecdotal "story" about two other "stories". We remind the reader that a narrative is a spoken or written account of connected events. Typical features of a narrative are, again: embellishment of a natural event as a series of events unfolding in time, involving a plot that creates some kind of tension with a peak and resolution (denouement), and well-drawn characters. The Booker Prize winning writer George Saunders (2021) says that the key to a good story is "escalation" – a constant ramping up of tension to keep the reader engaged.

What gives narrative characteristic style and body is the appropriate use of genre: tragedy, comedy, epic, lyric, science fiction, magic realism, and so forth. The first re-telling of the tick's life by von Uexküll and the subsequent re-telling of von Uexküll's story by us provide some of these features of narrative. There is even a sense of personality or character ascribed to the tick (to anthropomorphise for a moment, she is undoubtedly "patient"). But in naturalistic reality, there is little of narrative substance save quiet continuous being that does not make for fulsome exposition. Indeed, the tick's "story" (as tick) is largely hollowed out where much of it, in a human analogy, is like waiting at the bus stop for the unlucky #13 bus that never arrives.

The ticking of the clock for the tick is an all-too-human metaphor. Ticks are, presumably, time-senseless, but place-sensitive, making an analogy flare in our minds. The tick non-story presents as a readymade poem if we follow Marilyn McEntyre's (2012: 1) distinction between narrative and non-narrative poetry, the latter "emphasizing in its singular way discontinuity, [and] surprise". In the potential lifespan of the tick we have no idea when the fateful moment will arrive – that of the warm-blooded animal brushing the branch. Hence, discontinuity and surprise define the event. The desire to turn events into experiences through storytelling may be seen in its own right/rite as a habit, a tic. Good habits (as skills for example; even, dare we say, competencies) should be encouraged, while bad habits should be challenged, and treated, as rust. We suggest that poetry is a good habit of practice and of mind.

How language thinks the doctor

Returning to Geoffrey Hill's *Mercian Hymns*, we suggest that the poem offers a compass for navigating clinical work as a natural historian in three ways: the poet first teaches close noticing; second, witnessing (watchful waiting) as a natural historian; and third, humility. To this we can add a fourth element: poets teach us how to think with science in artful, graceful, and creative ways. We pick up on this point later when we discuss Peircean abductive reasoning, where adaptive expertise in clinical reasoning is explained as a "holistic grasp" (gestalt) of the context (presenting symptoms). This reflects Gaston Bachelard's poetic view of science as "a continual interplay between intuitive, experiential (subjective), and rationally discursive (objective) forms of knowledge" (in Tiles 1984: 57). This is the natural historian's ecological grasp of a presenting context, a symptomatic occasion in the environment (one factor out of kilter necessarily affects a number of other factors in its vicinity). For this activity, in the clinic, the knee-jerk response need not be "clock the patient's story". Rather, it may be a poetic grasp of the occasion as a whole, the patient *in place*. We illustrated this through the close reading of a patient encounter in our previous chapter.

In the context of these insights, we will discuss a historical sea change in how medicine thinks about clinical reasoning, shifting from linear models to nonlinear approaches. Gustav Freytag famously described the conventional narrative arc of: 1. Exposition, 2. Rising action, 3. Climax, 4. Falling action, and 5. Dénouement. Narrative medicine has borrowed this arc and applied it literally rather than figuratively. Consider this example from Silverman and Freya (2019):

Exposition: Patient is shovelling snow
Rising Action: Develops severe chest pain
Climax: In the emergency room find ST elevations and troponin of 20
Falling action: Catheterisation
Denouement: Gets better and leaves the hospital

How much closer can narrative medicine get to biomedicine? And how much more instrumental can narrative get than this? We lose narrative entirely to biomedicine. But isn't this what Rita Charon et al. (2016: 2) promised all along, where, "The goal of narrative medicine from its start has been to improve healthcare"? We hope you don't think we're being uncharitable. It's just that this is so raw (as in uncooked): is narrative, which we insist on considering as art, there to "improve" anything, let alone healthcare? We see its role as far more complex and troubling.

Indeed, a primary purpose for literature as a whole is to question optimistic terms such as "improvement" simply through its resplendent being. Complexify, interrogate, refract beauty, yes. Just for a while, can we suspend the notion that poetry *does* anything specifically while keeping our minds open to the possibility that it has a general effect? Poetry is like the dark matter of the cosmos – it permeates without pressure (what Wallace Stevens calls a Presence rather than a Force – see Bleakley 2017); yet in the presence of dark matter, our universe expands.

Poetry challenges such linear reductions ("improvement") because it thinks in such a different way from the temporal narrative arc, bringing activity into place. Primarily, lyric poetry would identify with nonlinear, complex, open adaptive systems thinking. However, closed and linear techniques are imposed on the open poetic imagination to give form to what otherwise may slip from complexity into chaos. Lyric poetry, nevertheless, largely remains plotless, refusing Freytag's arc and embracing Hill's detailed sketch of Offa as an (object-related) identity delineated by a world of objects, a creature of the soil, allotted a place in the field. The poem can be improved, but not for general "improvement".

For object relations psychology, the "cure" is gaining adult autonomy by resolving the role of transitional objects such as favourite teddy bears and abandoning toys for a loving relationship with persons after trust has been developed. See how Offa turns this on its head in growing transferring object-identity from cruelly tormenting others to identification with the natural world, ascending through the twisting ivy, descending to handle the soil: such identification in turn leading to a turn in identity. But Object-Oriented Ontology says, "multiply up your object relations" and "place trust in your world of extended objects (artefacts)". For us, the poem is a central object in such an expanding world; but we would push this further and say that we, persons, are objects in the poems' worlds. They visit us and transfer curiosity, excitement and sensuality. Let us not analyse that out of the window and exhaust poetry. Some think it is a formidable source of nourishment.

Following the Russian Formalist imperative for the effect of poetry (see Chapters 3 and 5), we will defamiliarise or make strange standard psychological models of clinical reasoning in the head through consideration of how language forms, or "thinks", the doctor and how reasoning occurs as a future-focussed event as well as relying on memory. In reasoning, unconscious life, flow of affect, and imagination are in conversation with conscious shaping of language and embodied communication.

The Will and the Well

Medicine and poetry are alike in having a tacit store of rules (a "Well") that is shaped by a conscious process (a "Will"). For medicine the Well is a web of biomedical knowledge; a number of heuristics or short cuts such as aphorisms, metaphors, Art of Memory images; both singular and common case exemplars; and semantic qualifiers and illness scripts. For poetry this Well of rules is diction: rhythm, metre, rhyme, tropes, lines, stanzas; guidelines for metaphor generation; referencing other poems; and so forth. This Well can be reinforced – poets typically keep notebooks, jottings, and inspirational ideas. Coleridge famously kept voluminous notebooks, picking over books he had read for idiosyncratic or startling insights (especially natural history observation) and memorable phrases (Lowes 1927), or noting what he had observed on his famous long walks with Wordsworth and the latter's sister Dorothy (Nicolson 2019).

Jonathan Livingston Lowes (1927), the American scholar and literary critic who died in 1945, famously traces every image in Coleridge's *The Rime of the Ancient Mariner* and *Kubla Khan* to the poet's notebooks that, for Lowes, acted as a "Deep Well" of inspiration. The "Will" was termed "The Shaping Spirit". Through this model, Lowes set out to demystify the architecture of poetic imagination and to note that imagination was always based in sense images, or that metaphors are embodied. The modern poet Peter Redgrove (AB personal communication) used a technique he called "sealed writing", where he kept notebooks, often illustrated, with seeds of ideas for poems. These would then be "sealed" or put away and not opened for several years. On re-examination, the contents will be largely dross, but some will have "fermented" and some hardened to gems to offer brilliant insights, starting points for poems, often a whole stanza, and certainly a structural idea (field) for a poem.

The tacit rules of medicine (including, importantly the anatomical/ biomedical web of memorised information and connections) inform and shape reasoning by adaptive experts through pattern recognition or clinical gestalt, commonly referred to as "Type 1" reasoning, as described at the beginning of this chapter. Type 2 reasoning does not draw on such a tacit store of rules, information and images, but is conscious, logical, rules-based reasoning. Poets in turn again set their poem's shape in a field, or set down words and dig them over and over, on the basis of an initial tacit form.

Let's start in the head, revise this, and then move out to the world.

The Art of Memory or super-mnemonics

What's placed first in the head, or taught up front in the undergraduate medicine curriculum, is anatomy and biomedical science. This is memorised for recognition and recall. Retrieval of this information depends however on how it becomes linked to pathologies or presentations of symptom in specific (memorable patients) and general (types and classifications of diseases) cases. The most basic tactic of clinical thinking is retrieval of significant information. But this can be enhanced.

Memory is key to the medical mind, so much so that medical schools might be thought of as memorising fact(st)ories. Biomedicine necessitates the mastery of information, but this ability can be imaginative, following poetry's turning of the literal into the metaphorical. Pre-existing medical analogies are the obvious example, where something is said to be like something else (apple-core lesion, violin string adhesions, pear drop breath, etc.). The analogy isn't to amuse, but exists as a stirring mnemonic.

Speaking historically, these mnemonics have always been. Before writing was invented, memory was key. *The embodied improvisation around memory produced poetry.* Prior to Homer, lyricists took epic narratives and reformulated them in song with strong elements of improvisation. Songs were "stitched together" (the pre-Homeric Greek singers, *rhapsodes*, literally translates as "stitchers together of songs") through memorising large sections of story and adding new elements. The traditional (apple)core of the epics had repeating themes (heroes die young), images and metaphors ("wine dark sea") and epithets for characters ("wily Odysseus"), thus taking the burden off memorising a ton of ugly facts (Marshall and Bleakley 2017).

Our own capacity for memorisation without aids is dismal by contrast to the ancients. The Greeks put the blame for this squarely on the advent of writing just as we post-postmoderns place the blame squarely on the Internet. Plato, in the *Phaedrus*, tells the story of an Egyptian sage introducing writing to his king. It will, he says, make the Egyptians wiser and will improve their memories. The king disagrees. Writing will: "produce forgetfulness… because they will not practice their memory…. You have produced an elixir not of memory but of reminding".

Medicine draws on the same formats. Biomedical knowledge is the backbone epic story (the conquering of disease as its shaping force) that is re-told according to new information. As expertise increases, a store of illness scripts, semantic qualifiers, and heuristics are built. Such expertise is a contemporary version of an ancient poetic tradition of the Art of Memory whose history is expertly traced by Frances Yates (1966). In the age of Google, memory is becoming increasingly less important to learning. Returning to the pre-Homeric example above of lyric singers, imagine how important memory must have been to the circulation of knowledge prior to the printing press and ready availability of books.

Yates (ibid.) details the historical rise of mnemonic techniques, noting a peak during the Renaissance. Here, something is remembered by literally re-membering it, by associating the thing to be remembered with a fantastic, pathologised, or bizarre (and then readily memorable) image. We re-member the thing we want to recall by fleshing out its body through association with a rotting or fantastic body or object. Somebody with a bad memory for names recalls 'Leo' by associating the name with an image of a flaming lion. Without the association, life would be reduced to information, a state suffered by Funes in Borges's (1962) story "Funes the Memorius". The information is all there but the meaning is missing. This is how raw medical students feel before they have had some clinical experience and seen a number of illustrative "cases". Things start to stitch together. Recognition starts to trump recall.

Where the Art of Memory's basic method is to associate a striking, often pathologised, image with the object or fact that is memorised, striking images of pathology are used as resemblances in medicine for diagnostic purposes – such as an X-ray image of a "bamboo spine" (showing ankylosing spondylitis).

A gentler use of the Art of Memory – without explicit reference to this technique and written in ignorance of it – is shown in Ed Schwartz and Tomos Richards's (2019) *Cases of a Hollywood Doctor*. This is an exam preparation book for medical students and junior doctors centred on case-based learning. The authors offer 52 cases across specialties, presented "in a readable and enjoyable" way "to combat the dullness of your average textbook". Without explicitly acknowledging the link, each case is presented with vivid memory associations – typical of the Art of Memory technique – to aid recall and recognition. For example, a person falls off a wall and sustains a suspected cervical spinal injury. The diagnostic choices include whether or not this person requires investigative imaging. The suggested mnemonic is Humpty Dumpty (triggered by story and graphic).

The case information is as follows: The patient had been drinking heavily and fell backwards off a two metres high wall. He is not able to walk and complains of neck pain. On examination he has cervical spine tenderness, bruising around the eyes, and clear fluid draining from his right ear. CT imaging of the head and neck is advised where a base of skull fracture is indicated.

Yet the poetry inherent to the case lies in conjuring up the Humpty Dumpty image so as to trigger the mnemonic association; also, the "bruising around the eyes" has a striking metaphoric formulation as "raccoon eyes" that stimulates the unfolding of the larger story as an aid to make diagnosis. From diagnosis, clinical implications proceed.

Elsewhere in the book, an acute, severe asthma case is memorised as the big bad wolf blowing the house down, now breathless. The wolf appears again, biting Little Red Riding Hood as she walks home through the woods. She has serious wounds to her forearm and the mother brings her in to A&E thinking that she needs stitches – the case focusses on whether or not the wound should be sutured. The answer is no, as the wound could get infected if sutured directly. Instead, it should be cleaned; checked for any underlying damage to tendons, blood vessels or nerves; tetanus status should be verified; finally antibiotic treatment should be prescribed and the patient referred to the operating theatre for debridement of wounds. All of this is, of course, more readily memorised through the Art of Memory using an image of Little Red Riding Hood as the visual trigger. Previously memorised information tumbles out as the trigger is envisioned. Note that in both cases – Humpty Dumpty and Little Red Riding Hood – the folk story is secondary to the poetic image. The image becomes the mnemonic as a form of metonymy. You don't need the narrative for the isolated image to strike home. Mnemonics are like mastery of information in biomedicine, and yet some mnemonics, image-based, are not. There is complexity lurking in the seeming simpler mastery of information.

Affordance

Art of Memory techniques account partly for what is in the black box between a doctor seeing a patient and immediately knowing the diagnosis: again, Type 1 reasoning, "direct route" pattern recognition – you see it and you know. It just happens, and so the black box normally need not be explored. Nobody asks herself while driving a car: "how do I do this?" Such reflexive dwelling would interfere with the automaticity of driving and you would lose concentration. It needs somebody from outside to map out how you learned to drive, how it has become automatic, and what happens cognitively. Psychologists are experts at this, explaining for example how a senior doctor or surgeon has gained "Adaptive Expertise" through years of practice, where variations in presentation are tolerated and easily accommodated (that's the "adaptive" bit) (Kneebone 2020). However, even in adaptive expertise, pattern recognition can lead to error, where habit overrules subtle cues and cues that can be missed.

Psychologists, however, like other specialists, work within habitual frames that limit their horizons. Unless they are social psychologists, or ethnographers, their unit of analysis is the individual and her interior states. In studying perception, psychologists typically modelled individuals picking up information from the environment through the senses and then making sense of this information in the brain. This is an inside-out view: the work of making sense of the environment is done by individual cognition. James J. Gibson (1979) famously turned this view on its head by suggesting that the environment does work for us in presenting patterns of information that offer "affordance" – what the environment offers – or "affords" – the individual. The senses in turn do not work independently (a category error) but act as a system that is attuned to the immediate context by whatever that context affords. Gibson took the idea from Jakob von Uexküll's notion of *umwelt*.

In Geoffrey Hill's poetry earlier, the poet has Offa shaped not by personality impulses from within, but by the world's whim. At every turn, Offa, the bully, is tempered by nature's affordances until his authority is entirely absorbed. This is a compensatory gesture for Offa's narcissism. Hill was not interested in poetry itself as personal confession or autobiography, but as an ethical social engagement with culture and the things of the world. By identification with the objects that shape us, poetry becomes a democratic force. Poetry is a complex environmental affordance in its own right – we stand in its presence and we are changed. We do not write poetry, but poetry writes us. Hill, again as a devoted Christian, framed poetry as an act of grace. Having said this, we do think that poetry has a function in shaping character and identity as it reflects back to us some strange unknowns. We think we are shaping a poem but it has its own purpose in speaking back, again as "field". As lines begin to "work" so they work on our characters. Poetry creates fermenting cultures and these feed us.

Offa stands as case study of personality cult dislodged through worldly engagement. This is often achieved through memorial. A big figure engages in a grand gesture to project a personality, but the product comes to overshadow the person. In Offa's case, Offa's Dyke is an earthwork consisting of a wall and ditch 20 metres in width, 2.5 metres tall, and running for 132 kilometres. It is a massive earth and stone construction. Offa leaves a poetic imprint, a kind of monumental poetry legacy as earthwork. Its modern equivalent is the M5 motorway running from Exeter to Birmingham in the UK that parallels Offa's Dyke along its route on the Wales and England border.

Frances Salter (2016) notes that Hill "argued that poetry is not entertainment, or self-expression, but a public service of the most crucial kind" speaking "to and for the culture it resides in". Here, we might substitute "medicine" for "poetry". Hill was clear that confessional aspects of poetry did not speak of idiosyncratic concerns but of the confessional voice itself, the shared public voice of ethical concern – how should we live a life in a collective, public sense? How might medicine better serve this public, cultural calling? Poetry and medicine must serve democracy, investing in social justice as previously noted. This is necessarily complex. For poetry it involves freedom of expression and the release of words from imprisonment in cliché and pedestrian, normative prose of the "engineering manual" variety (suspend applications of Russian Formalism here for a minute, that's a special case and not the general case).

For medicine, it involves dismantling hierarchy within its own institution to model equity as a prelude to a humane medicine. This requires "deterritorialising" (Deleuze and Guattari 2004a, 2004b) of both poetry and medicine, or the dissolution of Offa's Dyke as border. It is also the part-dissolution of Offa's ego boundary (Freud's notion of defence mechanisms such as denial) in identification with nature, something that we have trouble with in clinical encounters, where a fine balance is struck between identification with the patient ("empathy" doesn't capture this, but that is the crude term we use) and emotional insulation to prevent burnout.

A first step is to release clinical reasoning from private ownership in the head of the lone clinician and return it to collective ownership across clinical culture (including the contributions of patients). This is what Rita Charon and colleagues (Charon 2006; Charon et al. 2016) map out as a project for Narrative Medicine, as we have seen from previous chapters, through a "re-storying". New thinking in interdisciplinary academic studies is helping us to re-conceive the "black box" of personal clinical reasoning as a web of affordances in the clinician's immediate context that design or shape the reasoning from without. We will summarise this new thinking, as it feeds poetry as much as medicine. Offa's territorialism, symbolised by the Dyke, and his conquering of much of Mid- and Southern England is replaced by a nomadism ("de-territorialising") that we think of as a good umbrella metaphor for lyric poetry and medical reasoning.

A better metaphor is love: permeating and permeable, resisting boundary and restriction. As love is not a thing in itself but a connection, a love of something, an inclination, so we will review our insistence on poetry's strength of close noticing of objects (a strength also of diagnostic clinical observation). Deleuze and Guattari's (2004a, 2004b) sense of "nomadism" is to reject fixed territory for connections between places. So we see value in reformulating the "stoniness of the stone' as how the stone differs from other objects, and "object relations". Or the stone is known in difference from .... I.A. Richards (in Nowottny 1965: 142) says,

> The mind is a connecting organ, it works only by connecting and it can connect any two things in an indefinitely large number of different ways. Which of these it chooses is settled by reference to some larger whole or aim. ... The reader, I would say, will try out various connections, and this experimentation ... is the movement which gives its meaning to all fluid language.

In the following chapter, we show how cognitive psychology, as this can be applied to explore clinical reasoning processes, has only recently caught up with Richards's ideas from the 1920s. In modelling thinking as an ecological process (mind in world) rather than an egological process (world in mind), clinical reasoning is concerned with connections between things (patient-context, patient-doctor, patient-treatments) rather than things in themselves (organ or systems biomedical focus). The poetic imagination models such object connectivity.

References

Bleakley A. Force and Presence in the World of Medicine. *Healthcare.* 2017; 53: 58.
Bleakley A, Farrow R, Gould D, Marshall R. Making Sense of Clinical Reasoning: Judgement and the Evidence of the Senses. *Medical Education.* 2003a; 37: 544–52.
Bleakley A, Farrow R, Gould D, Marshall R. Learning How to See: Doctors Making Judgements in the Visual Domain. *Journal of Workplace Learning.* 2003b; 15: 301–6.

Borges JL. Funes the Memorius. Retrieved from http://vigeland.caltech.edu/ist4/lectures/funes%20borges.pdf

Charon R. 2006. *Narrative Medicine: Honoring the Stories of Illness.* Oxford: Oxford University Press.

Charon R, DasGupta S, Hermann N, et al. 2016. *The Principles and Practices of Narrative Medicine.* Oxford: Oxford University Press.

Deleuze G, Guattari F. 2004a. *A Thousand Plateaus.* London: Continuum.

Deleuze G, Guattari F. 2004b. *Anti-Oedipus.* London: Continuum.

Gibson JJ. 1979. *The Ecological Approach to Visual Perception.* Boston, MA: Houghton-Mifflin.

Harman G. 2018. *Object-Oriented Ontology: A New Theory of Everything.* London: Penguin Random House.

Hill G. 1971. *Mercian Hymns.* London: Andre Deutsch.

Inhelder B, Piaget J. 2006. *The Psychology of the Child.* New York: Basic Books.

Kneebone R. 2020. *Expert: Understanding the Path to Mastery.* London: Penguin.

Lowes JL. 1927/ 1951. *The Road to Xanadu: A Study in Ways of the Imagination*, 2nd ed. London: Constable.

Marshall R., Bleakley A. 2017. *Rejuvenating Medical Education: How Homer Can Help.* Newcastle-Upon-Tyne: Cambridge Scholars.

McEntyre M. 2012. *Patient Poets: Illness from Inside out.* San Francisco: University of California Medical Humanities Press.

Nicolson A. 2019. *The Making of Poetry: Coleridge, the Wordsworths and Their Year of Marvels.* London: William Collins.

Nowottny W. 1965. *The Language Poets Use.* London: The Athlone Press.

Phillips C. The Art of Poetry No. 80: Geoffrey Hill. *The Paris Review.* 2000; 154. Retrieved from https://www.theparisreview.org/interviews/730/the-art-of-poetry-no-80-geoffrey-hill

Salter F. The Long View: Geoffrey Hill and Why Poetry Matters. *The Oxford Culture Review.* October 16, 2016. Retrieved from https://theoxfordculturereview.com/2016/10/16/the-long-view-geoffrey-hill-and-why-poetry-matters/

Saunders G. 2021. *A Swim in a Pond in the Rain: In Which Four Russians Give a Master Class on Writing, Reading, and Life.* London: Bloomsbury.

Schwartz E, Richards T. 2019. *Cases of a Hollywood Doctor.* Baton Rouge, LA: Taylor & Francis.

Silverman E, Frayha N. Storytelling in Medicine. 2019. Retrieved from https://www.hippoed.com/pc/rap/episode/dudewheresmydea/storytellingin.

Tiles M. 1984. *Bachelard: Science and Objectivity.* Cambridge: Cambridge University Press.

Von Uexküll JJ. 1934/2010. *A Foray into the Worlds of Animals and Humans: With a Theory of Meaning.* Minneapolis: University of Minnesota Press.

Williams WC. 1967. *The Autobiography of William Carlos Williams.* San Francisco, CA: New Directions Books.

Wootten WG. 1998. The Aesthetics of History in the Modern English Long Poem: David Jones's the Anathemata. Basil Bunting's Briggflatts, Geoffrey Hill's Mercian Hymns and Roy Fisher's a Furnace. Doctoral thesis, Durham University. Retrieved from http://etheses.dur.ac.uk/4782/

Yates F. 1966. *The Art of Memory.* London: Routledge & Kegan Paul.

7   Out from the skull and into the world

Reclaiming biomedicine from the narrativists: abduction

Recall from previous chapters that Narrative Medicine first set itself up as a counter to what it perceived as a reductive biomedicine (Charon 2001). Then it sprang to, making friends with the evidence-based medicine movement to call for an evidence-based-narrative-medicine, where Wyer and Charon (2011: ix) describe a "scientifically informed narrative medicine". Then it published a recent update that acknowledged the ease of the "biomedical reductionist" label without changing direction, where Charon (Charon et al. 2016: 8) extols "the beauty of human encounters, a place where mysteries abound". Here, science surely fears to tread.

Too many splices! Biomedicine should not have been cleaved so readily from narrative approaches in the first place; and we are cautious about the stance that the medical/ health humanities habitually adopt – that they provide a counter to biomedicine's imperialism.

Biomedical science should not be a hindrance to the kind of delicate, imaginative yet responsible and responsive medicine that poet-physicians call for. Biomedicine, grounded in the history of science, is a necessary substrate for clinical reasoning as we have seen. Biomedicine is part of the Well of knowledge, a complex web, that reverberates, rejoices, and tunes to "recall" and "recognition" as the back-space and backstage of tacit knowing that feeds the Will of clinical activity. We need the biomedical as a necessary level of complexity, a key unit of analysis, but we do not need to habitually reduce other units of analysis such as the social, cultural, and ecological, to the biomedical substrate. Poetry works beautifully with science as its lens, but poetry cannot be reduced to science (or principles of engineering). Medicine works beautifully with science, but cannot be reduced to scientific knowledge only.

Challenging reductive science (patients as symptoms, symptoms as chemistry) is a primary task of science teachers at medical schools who could re-imagine their sciences poetically. Such creative science teaching can learn from history. Returning to the "two cultures" debate, the historian of science Fernand Hallyn (1987: 24) attempts to heal divisions between science and humanities, describing a historical "poetics of a scientific enterprise" in the

DOI: DOI: 10.4324/9781003194408-9

harmonic visions of Copernicus and Kepler. Hallyn here is taking "poetics" in its widest sense, to refer to the exercise of "abductive reasoning" in science. Ascribed to the American philosopher Charles Sanders Peirce (1839–1914), the founder of Pragmatism, abduction is the primary way in which major scientific insights (as paradigm shifts) occur, and is also the characteristic way in which medical experts make decisions. While we love poetry in its own right, we also like the way that a poetic imagination can be applied to science through re-visioning language, increasing metaphor use and developing new metaphors, and so forth. Both thinking scientifically and representing science are open to a number of aesthetic, abductive mouldings.

Where induction refers to the development of theory through gathering data from experiments, and deduction to the testing of a theory, abduction is the process by which hypotheses fall into place, prior to their testing or the gathering of data, as insight, intuition, illumination, serendipitous meeting of elements, or holistic apprehension ("gestalt"), the latter the hallmark of pattern recognition in clinical reasoning. Hallyn's description has science re-covering the poetry of the natural world (the wonder of phenomena such as the natural order of the Periodic Table), but it needs the scientist to exercise a poetic imagination for this to occur.

Hallyn (ibid.: 8) describes the process of major scientific insight as "enigmatic". It may come from a dream, a daydream, a sudden inspiration, a coincidence, an intuition or penetrating insight – forms of epiphanies. But abductive reasoning can be seen as "everyday epiphany", as pattern recognition or clinical gestalt based on adaptive expertise. Abduction is based on preparing the ground (the Well) through storing memories, cases, memorable instances, anecdotes, cognitive short cuts such as "old saws", semantic qualifiers and illness scripts, metaphors (often as resemblances), and prompts based in mnemonics or Art of Memory techniques. These in turn are further grounded in a cognitive process of feedback that is at once both anticipatory (the Will) and based in memory (the Well).

Again, these compressed codes are the exact fabric from which the poet cuts her cloth (Well shaped by Will; images and affect shaped by conscious application of poetic diction). Both poets and doctors have to learn to be "stitchers-together-of-songs" like the pre-Homeric lyricists as singers that we have referred to earlier (Dalby 2006: 174–75). Abduction can then describe 99% perspiration (experimental evidence gathering) and 1% inspiration (insight, epiphany), but this quantified example does not match the intensity of the qualitative experience, where the 1% inspiration may be explosive.

The philosopher Karl Popper described primary insights in science as "poetic intuition" whose frame is literary and artistic. The work of science rests with the inductive or deductive processes post-abduction, post intuition. Hallyn (1987) describes abduction as "instinctual", thus comparing it to the work of the animal snout and limbic system (where emotions and "felt" visions are both registered) rather than the human cortex (where intellect fizzes and logic presides). With neurology as the rhetorical frame, the work of the frontal lobes is central to abduction, as the site of forward planning and self-monitoring (damage to the frontal lobes primarily leads to impulsivity – an inability to monitor behaviour). The frontal lobes may also do the guess-work of imagining a future event a split second before it happens based on previous patterns of activity, that Andy Clark (2016) refers to as "surfing a wave of uncertainty". Primarily, says Hallyn, work of abduction that frames scientific logic is metaphorical or feeds on and develops metaphors, again as work of the poetic imagination. By "poetic" Hallyn is casting the net wider than actual written and spoken poetry, and wider than Aristotle's "poetics".

Gino Soldati and colleagues (Soldati, Demi and Demi 2019: 15) describe poetic abduction at play in bedside diagnostic approaches to patients with respiratory disorders that echoes Hallyn's model of poetics above. They also describe such procedures as semiotics and "manipulative abduction". In pal-pation, auscultation and percussion extended to use of ultrasound as "ampli-fier", "soft, hidden, unexpected and strategic signs" are encountered often as moments of "serendipity". Here, the abductive process is one where "physi-cians are able 'to think through doing' to get the correct diagnosis". In other words, hypotheses are formed, tested, and reconfigured as collapsed in space "instants" rather than over time as narrative, these instants best described as "poetics". The authors insist on the affective dimension to such bedside diagnostic work and do not bracket this out as standard medical education dictates: "Abductive inferential path originates with an emotional reaction (discovery of the signs), step by step explanations are formed and it ends with another emotional reaction (diagnosis)".

There is a nod to the "sleuthing" model of diagnostic work where, "In this searching for signs doctors act like detectives". The "step by step explana-tions" can be configured less as following a trail and more as a choreographed dance around presenting symptoms and their context. Any description of such activity must resort to new metaphors for understanding as innovative explanations emerge at levels of brain, behaviour, and context.

Our metaphors of Well and Will applied to these complex contexts are, of course, crude and generalised. We admit to the fragility of the metaphors and would not want them to appear as opposed, but to work by the notion of enantiodromia, in which one end of a continuum can tip and resolve itself as reappearance at the other end of the continuum, a reversal. Well can trans-form into Will and vice versa as rapidly as backstage becoming frontstage (and vice versa) in human encounters. We refer you back to the simulated clinical interview analysed in depth in Chapter 5, where a see-saw effect is created in the dialogue between patient and doctor caused by differential weighting of verbal, nonverbal, imagistic, and semiotic events. These would pool or puddle, causing weight; and then lift suddenly, causing release and swing:

DF: Huh. I'm one of the resident doctors here on the medicine team. The emergency room called me and said, uh, that you were going to be ad-mitted to the hospital.

MW: [affirmative noise] Mmm-hmmm.

DF: And they mentioned that you had a pneumonia.

MW: [Nods, almost makes a sound, doesn't.]

DF: Yeah. Well, if it's okay with you what I'd like to do is learn more about what brought you into the hospital. I've got a lot of questions to ask you, to kind of get to know you, so that we take the best care of you here, and, uh, then I'll examine you. Does that sound okay with you?

MW: [nods, makes a welcoming gesture with hands]: Sure.

DF: Great. Again, I understand from the emergency room that you came in with a pneumonia. Was there something else also caused you to come in today, just so we know how we're spending our time together here?

MW: It was mostly just the, uh, coughing up blood…

(ibid.)

In this last utterance, the see-saw weighting towards the doctor that has been created by the gravity of his attentiveness is suddenly changed into its opposite. The patient, in recounting symptom, metaphorically enacts symptom, and in the re-membered coughing up of blood there is a release of burden, a weight off the mind, an intimacy as revelation. The patient is not revealing a secret in recalling a symptom, but is expressing an inner pathology now revealed in image (recall) of the event (actual coughing up of blood). Backstage is suddenly frontstage; previous privacy is now revelatory, as blood takes on three forms at once: literal (coughed up), imagistic (recalled), and metaphorical and symbolic (symptom).

In pattern recognition, the whole picture of symptom presentation is recognised quickly and may be grounded in a resemblance ("strawberry tongue" in paediatrics, or culinary metaphors such as "honey crusts" in impetigo and "Victoria plum lesions" in Sweet's disease) (Tucker and Lewis 2004). Here, the doctor does not engage in either developing or testing a theory but entertains a process (largely intuitive, unconscious or tacit) of clinical gestalt, delivered whole. The figure emerges from the ground. Poetry too follows such a system that is primarily not of normative rules, but of an exercise of style and composition, described by Hallyn (1987: 15) as "a unique configuration". Again, a figure emerges from the ground.

But these poetic ways of diagnosing, based in abduction, are not passive. They do not just arrive out of the blue. The intuitive part only flowers on the back of preparing the ground and planting the seeds through gaining expertise. This is another natural example of foreground/ background or frontstage/ backstage conversation. The poet Seamus Heaney describes the revelation following such poetic abduction, where: "The world is a different place after it's been described by a poet" (in Sharma 2020). Geoffrey Hill (2019) describes poetic abduction, the sacred appearance of the poem from its own depths, through a medical analogy, where writing poetry is a "bold pioneering type of spinal tap into nature" that is "in the hands of an / amateur liable to fatal mishap". Back to our (sub)standard medical student poetry as advertised for example in Johanna Shapiro's (2000) text, quite a contrast to Geoffrey Hill's sublime offerings.

Externalism, the "new realism", or enactivism

Where personalistic psychology has opened the black box of cognitive process, it has blacklisted ventures beyond the territory of the skull. Until recently, overall learning – rather than just clinical reasoning – in medicine was dominated by theories focussing on individual behaviour and cognition. This has now changed to a focus on social context (socio-cultural theories) and extension of cognition through use of artefacts (socio-material theories), constituting a paradigm shift (Bleakley 2006; Sparrow 2014). We see a similar paradigm shift – from an individual to a collective and artefact-enriched focus – in accounts of diagnostic clinical reasoning (for a different slice through this same paradigm shift, see Bleakley 2021b). We are now opening the black box of environmental affordance, appreciating more deeply the complex fabric of von Uexküll's *umwelt* and Heidegger's place of Dwelling, and seeing that connections are as important as things-in-themselves. *This is, in short, a phenomenology of place that poetry craves, paralleling narrativism's phenomenology of time.*

In adopting social learning theories in medical education, the price we must pay for this leap is both increased tolerance of ambiguity, and learning how to utilise contradiction as resource in expansive learning (Engeström 2018). With such increased tolerance and mobilisation of contradiction as resource, we have the basis to move from linear/closed systems to nonlinear/open systems. For the instrumentalists, evidence shows that intentionally distributed, collaborative healthcare (the adoption of democratic habits to challenge unproductive hierarchies) improves quality of patient care, patient safety and worker satisfaction (Hughes et al. 2016; West et al. 2017). We must adequately conceptualise medical reasoning as a distributed, materially augmented, semiotically enhanced phenomenon. We see this as poetic work, again as theoretically mapping place through phenomenology, but more, of expressing experiences of place through ontologies, or states of being and their connectedness.

Poetry for us can represent and articulate the states of being of the medical mind as it discovers the meanings and qualities afforded by its natural habitats of consultations, examining, treating and prescribing, and aftercare as clinic settings. These are Dwellings for poetry, open spaces for work of reclamation. We must be clear again, we are not saying that poetry leads to better healthcare. Rather, poetry is a fermenting culture that is *implicated* in expanding life.

This paradigm shift from the personal to the world (as local context) can be understood as an effect of the confluence of historically disparate yet contingent intellectual and practical processes. These include the overarching philosophical frame of phenomenology (Sparrow 2014) with its interest in the shaping of the self as an effect of looking into the mirror of the Other, or the stranger, including the Other of the natural and built surroundings. This has spawned two radical streams of thought: Externalism (Rowlands 2003) (also termed "new realism" and "speculative realism", and including within it an approach called "enactivism") and Object-Oriented Ontology (Harman 2018) that we introduced earlier. We discuss these approaches below, in the spirit of delineating the field that will contain our poetic/abductive reasoning lines.

Externalism

Externalism explores experience not as an individual looking out on the world, but as forces in the world creating the conditions for experiences and identities to emerge. This follows James J. Gibson's (1979) "ecological perception" model – that the environment *prepares and shapes* the senses as a system through affordance of properties, rather than perception acting on the environment. In contrast, egological stances have historically been privileged in medical education, driven especially by North American individualism. This is built in turn on a long historical tradition of Protestant and Capitalist self-sufficiency and male gendered heroism. In contrast, collectivist and distributed learning theories are grounded in liberatory Marxism and more recently in collaborative feminisms (Bleakley 2021a).

Enactivism

Within this stable of distributed, externalist models is "enactivism". In *The Embodied Mind*, Francisco Varela, Evan Thompson and Eleanor Rosch (2017: 173) challenge the tradition of placing "mind" in the head through the notion of "enaction". Here "perception consists in perceptually guided action" and "cognitive structures emerge from the recurrent sensorimotor patterns that enable action to be perceptually guided". In other words, activity and mind are co-dependent and mutually productive, where cognition is embodied and extended. Cognition is shaped through feedback from the effects of action as these impinge the environment. Here, "self" is not lost, but identity reconstitutes itself as identification with context.

In "The Man Whose Pharynx Was Bad" Wallace Stevens (http://bactra.org/Poetry/Stevens/The_Man_Whose_Pharynx_Was_Bad.html) imagines somebody who has lost their personal voice and must regain a voice of some kind:

I was the world in which I walked, and what I saw
Or heard or felt came not but from myself;
And there I found myself more truly and more strange.

Back to "making strange" or defamiliarisation. The "other" voice is the world soul, speaking strangely. Here, as personality is overpowered by Presence of worldly activities, Geoffrey Hill's Offa becomes the wall and ditch that he has built, and is also wholly identified with earthly things as "wine, urine and ashes". Or the relationship to the object is one of *identification* and not objectification. Doctors have to identify with their patients in an open-ended roaming across an ever-changing population, resisting objectification.

Bahar Orang (2020: 33) describes this self-effacing nomadism, a breaking out from subjectivity into identification with the Other and world, as porosity, an "open bracket" – openness to surroundings, to soaking in beauty:

> Beauty, I imagine, is desire twice, is all at once, is delight,
> the open bracket, something asking to be touched.

We need these elastic metaphors. In comparison, the "extended" and "situated" metaphors to theorise cognition from the models mentioned above are technically fine, but imaginatively we are back to Wallace Stevens's "Cat's milk is dry in the saucer". Orang's "desire twice" is a richer description of an embodied and embedded cognition instantiated through desire to be touched – literally, or just brushed against, or metaphorically as touched by an idea.

Again, Orang's "open bracket" has a double meaning – a physical bracket now loosened, and a linguistic bracket now suspended. Clinical reasoning for doctors in practice has been bracketed out (and even placed under erasure as permanently suspended) but we think that, via poetry, clinical reasoning can be re-viewed and re-stored as a visible practice, albeit nomadic. It is a chronic condition of medicine, historically shaped, where doctors identify as heroes and personal responsibility is paramount. This has often resulted in inflation. Contemporary medicine however has inverted this stance and turned worldly, where medicine is both feminising and democratising, as a caring and tender-minded practice and as team effort.

From our brief survey of the history of clinical reasoning, we see what poetry can bring. Bahar Orang's "desire 'twice" describes an awakening of Borges's Funes from a life of information (reductive biomedicine and linear systems) to a life of meaning and wisdom (medical practice guided by a poetic imagination embracing metaphor, necessarily more complex, adaptive, nonlinear and porous than a linear type). This moves us from Stevens's "cat's milk is dry in the saucer" to Orang's "open bracket" necessary for "soaking in beauty". At last, some nourishment, balm, and liquidity – dry speech transformed as eloquence. Orang's phrase has the double meaning of bathing in beauty and taking beauty in. J.J. Gibson's "ecological affordance" is the beauty of the world shaping our perceptions, knowledge and decision-making. Clinical reasoning is now efflorescent and in ferment. Reasoning finds its home in the world and not the mind. Beauty is no longer a human invention but a "readymade", a found worldly gesture. And this gesture is the revelation of a web of effects in which we are implicated and through which we sense, feel, reason and imagine.

Peter Stilwell and colleagues (Stilwell et al. 2020) employ the enactivism model to make sense of an individual's experience and management of pain. Pain is not reduced to neural process, but is a worldly enactment best described through metaphor (Neilson 2016). Pain is understood in the context of historical, cultural and social meanings such as employment of images and likenesses; and in the context of feedback from others that modulates pain episodes. The reader is referred to SN's (ibid.) work on pain that ties together meticulous historical research with scientific modelling and confessional poetry in an auto-pathography. As doctor, poet, and scholar, Neilson examines pain and its "management" through this triangulation as a dark poetic force of tangled metaphors meeting the languages of science and best clinical practice. There is a big difference between a doctor asking a patient to "please score the intensity of your pain on a 1–10 scale" and asking the patient to describe the pain experience in detail. The register, from de-personalising instrument to personal testimony, encompasses a major cultural power shift from doctor-centred to patient-directed talk. Patients inevitably bring fresh metaphors – and as we have explained already, new metaphors are desperately needed.

Readers are also referred to Deborah Padfield's (2016, 2021) "Perceptions of Pain" project (https://deborahpadfield.com/Perceptions-of-Pain). Padfield has produced a set of "pain cards" that visually illustrate and discriminate differing kinds and levels of pain. These can be used in consultations to better articulate a patient's pain experiences. Eula Biss (https://www.snreview.org/biss.pdf), an English professor whose father is a doctor, sets out a "literary pain scale":

> Like the advanced math of my distant past, determining the intensity of my own pain is a blind calculation. On my first attempt, I assigned the value of ten to a theoretical experience – burning alive. Then I tried to determine what percentage of the pain of burning alive I was feeling.
>
> I chose thirty percent—three. Which seemed, at the time, quite substantial.
>
> Three. Mail remains unopened. Thoughts are rarely followed to their conclusions. Sitting still becomes unbearable after one hour. Nausea sets in. Grasping at the pain does not bring relief. Quiet desperation descends.
>
> "Three is nothing," my father tells me now. "Three is go home and take two aspirin."

What hits you between the eyes about Eula Biss's pain scale is its own literary sophistication: explanation as poetry; explication as image. The tension between an "advanced" math and a "distant" path sets up the paragraph to act like a stretched piece of elastic. This is reinforced by "intensity". The quality of the experience is highlighted by the dismissal of quantification (pain scales) in "blind calculation". The most extreme pain is illustrated through a metaphor of extremity: "burning alive". Biss tunes us to worldly references: an increasing level of pain is "Mail remains unopened" (a lovely phrase for a terrible level of pain). Enactivism also tunes us to the world for reference. Every personal pain is relative to the suffering of a child buried in rubble in a conflict zone and dug up seven hours later.

Bahar Orang (2020: 77) again: "… this patient never / asked for the feeling of morning in any tablet or vial". How could we package "morning"? Yet already this worldly reference not only provides a felt emotional counter to the pharmacy's wake-up pill, but also a poetic counter, resonating in the mind as "mourning", and then you think of somebody waking up depressed and anxious or suicidal and "morning" takes on a different and scary character.

In the literature on the medical mind and clinical reasoning, there is little poetic forming of sensibility. The notion of an aesthetic dimension to how doctors think is elided in order to protect from criticism by literalists bounded by information land ("give me facts"). Surely medical thinking shaping clinical activity can be "poetic", or to be specific: subtle, graceful, rounded, elegant, beautiful, surprising, comforting, majestic, and even ecstatic? Can a diagnosis not tumble, rejoice, bend over backwards to please, fire an arrow into the unknown, impress with concision, bake to perfection, and manage the complex and ambiguous with diligence and grace? We believe that all of these conceptualisations are already at work in billions of lives.

The metaphors may be corny, but the point is that thinking in metaphors is fundamental here. Invention of new metaphors is medicine for medicine. Struggling to strip the colourful metaphoric framework into a more programmatic meta-metaphoric organisation around medicine-as-war and body-as-machine doesn't remove the metaphoric basis for our knowing, but it does consolidate and strengthen the odd cultural preference for biomedical primacy. If you read this as saying: "The authors say change some metaphors and we have a different medicine", then you are apprehending the utter simplicity of our general case. This book is a more complex investigation of the general case in the way that biomedicine is a vast investigation into the nooks and crannies of the biochemistries and biophysics of the body. Every epistemology worth its salt – we are deliberately using clichéd, dead metaphors in this paragraph ironically, in solidarity with medicine as war and body as machine – can be summarised in a few words.

What kind of thinking would allow us to create fields that can be sown to produce new metaphors? James Gibson's formative models of ecological affordance and the senses working as a system suggest that perception is not a passive process in which the world impinges on the senses and is then made sense of in the brain. Rather, as bodies move through worlds in time and space so the immediate environment shapes how the body will respond – enhanced through specific artefacts such as instruments that extend the senses. We are again bathing in beauty, but beauty (and the Bogeyman too) is also just around the corner. The curve on the road signals that we must slow the speed of the car we are driving, while a "blind" bend prepares us for sudden eventualities (the "blind" is in the bend first and in the mind second). The brain is ahead of the senses in anticipatory awareness and predictive processing, in a feedback loop with what the world affords, preparing the body's responses ("blind" bends offer a familiar trope). The senses act in complex co-ordination through adaptive expertise constantly pressing the body into innovation – a continuous series of small-scale experiments and subsequent adjustments guided by feedback loops. These cognitive experiments are simultaneously grounded in memory and anticipatory "lines of flight" (Deleuze and Guattari 2004a, 2004b).

A complex system is always at play, in which one's "self" is an attractor basin with a good degree of stability, but always adapting and flexible within a field of changing forces and presences. Of these, major attractor basins are other persons in our social world, and key artefacts such as languages, symbols, mobile phones, computers, ambulances, and diagnostic testing. These constitute "landscapes" and "fields" of affordances. The car-driving example can readily be extended to, say, a surgeon navigating a set of blood vessels and nerves, or a urologist performing a cystoscopy. In a field where the attractor basins are fluid or ill defined, there are high levels of uncertainty and crashes on the blind bend are possible as speeds in relation to topography are poorly judged.

Object-Oriented Ontology

Object-Oriented Ontology (often referred to as "OOO") is a contemporary philosophical movement that has been developed largely within circles of art theory and architecture (Harman 2018). A sister to Enactivism, but radically extending its reach to the world of objects and their intentionality, Object-Oriented Ontology adopts the radical stance that artefacts or things can be read as having the same ontological status as persons (a "flat" ontology), and that objects have "intentions" (as consequences) in the sense that they impinge on our lives in ways that both enhance and restrict existence.

The movement does not focus on epistemology (theory) but ontology (states of being) by placing appreciation before explanation. Its primary concern is then aesthetics, or how qualities might be explored. It is radically democratic, where all objects are given equal ontological status; poetic, where every object's being can be enhanced through close exploration; and non-reductive (objects are not known as essences but only as qualities emerging from relationships with other objects). Importantly then, this perspective is neither materialistic nor reductive – it does not want to know matter as a chemist might, cataloguing component parts, but rather what potential an object has for change and development as it engages with other objects. It does not reject that objects have "standing" qualities (zinc as an element: Zn) but is more interested in how these qualities change through interaction (solids to liquids; or oxidations; or how zinc looks as roofing material). Again, this is an aesthetic and not a pure materialistic view, where "expansion" of objects leads to an increase in their sensuality. This contrasts with material science, where potentially sensual objects are held in material form.

Poets specialise in Object-Oriented Ontology, in close description of objects as *ekphrasis*, modelled by Keats's "Ode on a Grecian Urn" that opens: "Thou still unravish'd bride of quietness, / Thou foster-child of silence and slow time". The closely observed urn is given character, just as forceps, blades, stethoscopes, pills, and MRI scanners can be given character. Why complain only about objectifying patients when we continue to treat objects mechanically where they have character, voices, styles, temperaments, and kickbacks? These habits are related.

Our cognition has been extended through computers and mobile phones; mobility through transport and prosthetics; medical judgement is supplemented or replaced by tests and scans; and our emotional lives are enhanced through shared semiotics (signs and symbols) such as architecture, furnishings, fashion, nationalism and its insignia, literature, and mass media. Medical semiotics is legion, and always in the process of change (traditions of white coats, stethoscopes, ward round protocols, specialty-specific languages, and so forth).

Somehow everything fell into place

All this talk about ecological or distributed cognition in diagnostic reasoning is all very well, but how does it play out in the clinic? We'll give you an example from experience. One of us (AB) developed a lateral collateral knee ligament strain surfing. Some weeks later, during the recovery period, he developed severe sciatic pain from the lower back down one leg. He went to a physiotherapist who suggested traction and a series of follow-up exercises. As she examined him, standing up, she put a full-size skeleton in front of him and behind that a poster showing the anatomy of ligament attachments in the areas of concern and another poster of the nervous system. She guided him through the anatomy with the skeleton so that he had a hands-on experience of how his own body was reacting, and talked him through her diagnosis of the origin of the sciatica as a result of compensatory movement for his original knee ligament injury. She matched this up against the muscular and nervous system anatomy pictured on the posters.

She then stood him in front of a full-length mirror and talked him through the whole picture of articulations, stresses and resultant symptoms; and then took a video of him walking up and down a hallway outside her treatment room and they analysed this together. It showed the level of compensation he was making for his original injury. This helped her too, in framing the best treatment regime. He had studied human anatomy many years ago and so plugged in readily to the information she was feeding him; but more, the information, presented as a gestalt or whole picture, became wisdom. She treated him with traction and gave him a series of exercises, as noted and he had one more consultation two weeks later. The sciatic pain was relieved as he adjusted his posture.

Easy to pick a success story perhaps (one of our critiques of Narrative Medicine's public relations), and this was a relatively uncomplicated clinical situation, but it illustrates the power of distributed cognition in practice. First, the physiotherapist instantly involves the patient in the diagnostic work. The "story" of symptom onset is quickly glossed. The meat of the consultation is the concretely poetic moment of practitioner, client and a range of artefacts (skeleton, posters, mirror, video) collapsed into a practiced form. There is a diagnostic field at work, and an Object-Oriented Ontology, where skeleton, posters, mirror, and video act as extended mind and as ecological affordances. Patient and physiotherapist were thinking outside the skull, collaboratively, embracing a field of material objects. This literally made a world of difference.

On recalling this occasion, what foregrounds is the hanging skeleton. An ancient (generic) shamanic ritual called "cleaning the skeleton" involves the shaman going into a trance and undergoing a journey to the otherworld of animal spirits, where he is helped by his familiars to "take" his skeleton out of his body bone by bone, "clean" or refresh the bones, and put them back, to renew the body from within (Bleakley 1999). The shaman is asked to name the main bones and their articulations. The lore says that the shaman is familiar with animal anatomy from hunting and with human anatomy from deaths in the community. The spirit journey is a way of refreshing anatomical knowledge, a kind of action poem. Our best equivalent here is anatomy classes in medical schools that still teach from cadaver dissection. Our connection here is with the Art of Memory as heuristic device.

We are reminded here also of Jennifer Richter's poignant poem "My Daughter Brings Home Bones" (https://www.poetryfoundation.org/poems/90104/my-daughter-brings-home-bones):

> and piles them on the driveway: femur, rib, jawbone with a few
> flat teeth attached, dozens of thin arced parts

The poem describes a mother letting go of her daughter to make her own way in life, as the daughter strides down the walkway in the drive made of the bones of her mother. Where "… Her line of bones / makes an arrow; sun lights them like a sign. She'll go …". The mother, now 40, remembers giving birth to the daughter, so that the daughter emerged: "… Gleaming, after living in my dark. Gleaming. So I can / always find her". The daughter is in, and of, the mother's bones; just as the animal familiar for the shaman is in, and of, his bones. The skeleton is placed in space. It has its history, of course, its narrative: one of ageing. But importantly it is an interior poem that both the shaman and Richter have brought out for display as an ecological gesture. The skeleton is part of the body's hidden mystery in life but, of course, joins the field of poetry at death. Meanwhile, it gleams. The physiotherapist made it gleam too, or the functional was made beautiful, efflorescent, as Richter's bones glow – anatomy as aesthetic medical education.

Sylvia Plath's Object-Oriented Ontology

Objects are ambiguous. They are at once inanimate and yet they speak and move. They extend our senses for example (spectacles, implants, prosthetics, pharmaceuticals, tools, computers, vehicles) and house us; meanwhile, doctors rely on objects such as low-tech bedside extensions (stethoscope, dermatoscope, pen and paper) and hi-tech apparatus (imaging equipment). As our experiences are widened, deepened, and sharpened (but also dulled and sometimes annulled) by objects, we have an ontological link to them. We experience objects, but more, we experience through them – they are essential media. Further, we are one among many objects at any one time in an environment to which we are subject. Objects form our subjectivities or experiences where they become artefacts – objects of use. We know whom we are in relation to the ways that we use, avoid, and consume objects.

Objects – we use the term in the same way as phenomenologists, to refer to phenomena generally – are also ambiguous and surprising. Sometimes surprisingly dull, but often infuriatingly animated (we might think of forces of nature such as winds, thunder and lightning storms and oceans as objects; computers open to malware that get glitches and crash). We like to pin objects and display them. Critics of medicine typically say that patients are objectified by biomedicine, as abstracted diseases or symptoms. Poets see puns in such occasions: objects objectified or rendered cold in painting are collectively called "still life". "We think that there is still life in the old boy", we say about an elderly relative, inadvertently rendering him as pinned, like a butterfly displayed, the Freudian slip showing that we want to see the old boy as still life (dead) just as we celebrate that there is still life in him. We also might object to the object that is in our way, objects as intrusions and obstructions as well as aids.

The etymology of "object" is interesting in this respect – from the Latin *ob* (in the way of) and *jacere* (to throw). This might imply that an object is a stumbling block to our smooth progress, or it might be that the object is the very thing we sling forward because that is our chosen trajectory. Either way, these would be good definitions of the uses for poetry. In Medieval Latin, the object becomes something "presented to the mind" and here we enter one of the main stumbling blocks for cognition. The "object" is not the mind itself, but something the mind contemplates, or makes through objectification. The mind is one object among many, objectified as the brain. There is then no identity between private self and objects in the world and we drift into Cartesian doubt that there is anything in the world at all. This is unnecessary lumber for Object-Oriented Ontology, which starts with the proposition again that we are one object *among* many and our world is one of learning how to negotiate meanings for objects. We think that poetry prefers it this way. It is par excellence the giver of life to the object world, the revealer of the object-ness of the object (the stoniness of the stone again; the stone known within a field of differences from other objects).

We have then referred throughout to one of the clearest overlaps between poetry and medicine – that of *ekphrasis*: detailed or vivid description, closely noticed; differences also closely felt and noted. For medicine, close noticing of symptom expression. For poetry, identification or deep description so that the reader notices these things too by proxy, in the idiosyncratic and often slantwise way that the poet might approach an object. We see that the pan has a lid, but exactly how does it look, or sit, and what does it do? Without this, we are in the world of objectification (the pan lid is x cm in diameter and made of copper, Cu). We need metaphors (the lid lifted reveals a stained and steam-spattered underbelly, the copper scuppered). How will you know the measure of Eula Biss's pain and the uselessness of 1–10 general scales without her scalding invention of the "maximum pain" metaphor as "burning alive"?

One of the central ambiguities created by poets through metaphor use is the projection of identity onto objects such that they become the speaking voice of the poet. This is more than symbolism, it is a state of being in which experience is defined by an object orientation rather than a subject-orientation, where metaphors are always embodied. This problematises the whole notion of "objectification" of patients, where making a patient an "object" in an object-oriented cosmos can be taken as both compliment and complement to a surrounding *umwelt* of objects. We are signalling connection, not isolation. Objectification becomes a means of contact, a meshing. Here, objectification is not a dehumanising but a placement. We know the patient by how she sits in relation to other key factors in her world. A diagnostic field emerges in which differences between symptom expressions (often revealed by testing) is the poetic field that the doctor navigates.

Again, poets are good at object orientation. Freud saw this as a mild neurosis, calling it "object fixation" – the transfer of libido onto objects. As noted earlier, post-Freudian object relations analysts such as Melanie Klein note that libido as a child is primarily centred on a favourite toy such as a doll or teddy bear, these days maybe a superhero figure or Pokémon cards. The object acts as a sounding board for rehearsing social communications, but is gradually replaced by actual interactions with people and the object dissolves in terms of its emotional function. Unresolved emotional ties to the object can reappear in fixations in adulthood where libido is transferred onto a desire to have and to hoard objects, or to objectify persons who are treated as collectors' items. Poets, in contrast, work out their object libido issues first by *ekphrasis* (deep object cleansing) and second, subsequent unhooking from the object of the poem itself as it circulates among readers and listeners.

We will illustrate Object-Oriented Ontology in action through a poetic example. Sylvia Plath's poem "Tale of a Tub" (https://plathpoetry.livejournal.com/) – written on February 20, 1956 – advertises such an ontology that ties worldly things and identity, where identity is formed as an affordance of the objects of the *umwelt*. In Plath's case this is an identity in crisis, depressive, and the *umwelt* is the small and stifling space of her bathroom and its object contents. "Take care it doesn't get too general" she wrote of the poem that detailed specifics of the objects around her in the tightest of spaces, the bathroom. Plath sublimates her mood in object-oriented art.

Ironically, Plath's poem is a take on Jonathan Swift's (1704) preachy *Tale of a Tub* – a glorious, bloated tub-thumping satire on English manners, the pomposity of the Church, and even the claims of medicine at his time. Plath's poem is the opposite of tub-thumping. It is melancholic and tub-bound.

Plath, contemplating limbo between life and death, draws on the apparatus of the bathroom as contemplative medium. It is essential poetry-as-placement. Again, the bath is already a place associated with reflection on mood, and a dark depressive current runs through the poem: "In this particular tub, two knees jut up / like icebergs ...", reversing the usual expectations that the bath is hot and a place for relaxation. Here, we are nervy, jumpy, and turning to ice. Frozen by fear. Plath becomes one object among many and is defined by them: the mirror being the most obvious; but also taps, the turning on and off of emotions. The last lines of the poem read,

> we shall board our imagined ship and wildly sail
> among sacred islands of the mad till death
> shatters the fabulous stars and makes us real.

Reading this, who could object to such sad beauty? Who could refuse to join this imagined "we" and form a community of suffering, being so moved, having most likely felt so at least once in the past? The object of the poem makes our shared suffering "real". When we read Plath, we often pause or outright stop, for we're with her on the ship, hushed by the voyage.

Plath starts by objectifying herself, turning her eye into a "photographic chamber". The *umwelt* of the bathroom provides a tight web of ecological object affordances: bare painted walls, electric light, chromium "nerves" of plumbing, lavatory mirror, ceiling, washbowl, towel, window, bathtub, water faucets. Each object can be seen to not "represent" Plath's persona, but "create" it:

> ... caught
> naked in the merely actual room,
> the stranger in the lavatory mirror
> puts on a public grin.

The mirror "scrupulously reflects the usual terror". And she cannot penetrate this persona, so practiced that it has become a perfect front: "when the ceiling / reveals no cracks that can be decoded". The persona is "disguising the constant horror / in a coat of many-colored fictions", where "we mask our past / in the green of eden, pretend future's shining fruit / can sprout from the navel of this present waste".

The bathroom towel steals her face: "dryly disclaims that fierce troll faces lurk / in its explicit folds". The window is "blind with steam" – there is no illumination for her dilemma. Indeed, Plath does not want the light to come in, but rather wants illumination of her darkness by the dark. But she cannot get to grips with her mood "which shrouds our prospects in ambiguous shadow". And here is the heart of the poem – the ambiguity laid bare. Again, Plath doesn't want to illuminate her stretch of sadness, but to engage productively with the darkness, for it is the dark that "shrouds our prospects in ambiguous shadow". Plath struggles with "putting on a face" and not being able to gain authenticity not by psychological introspection but by Object-Oriented Ontology, by a knowing through naming. She literally objectifies herself not by bringing out the glory in the objects – they are, in fact, dull, tawdry, and pedestrian – but by gathering the objects around her as fellow passengers on the ship that is her imagination.

She imagines the bathwater as a kind of acid that might strip away her persona to reveal a truth: "will pluck / fantastic flesh down to the honest bone". This kind of morbid dwelling has been going on for some time: "Twenty years ago, the familiar tub / bred an ample batch of omens". She wants out of this world, and perhaps fantasy will help, but the world is still there when you close your eyes: "the tub exists behind our back". The tub becomes a ship of suffering occupied by the suffering, transporting those who feel displaced to placement. Plath imagines death as that placement. And so the poem becomes a way of managing her sadness, but for us the sadness is transported to the objects around her. We see them affectively and not objectively.

Plath summarises: "Twenty years ago, the familiar tub / bred an ample batch of omens; but now / water faucets spawn no danger". The objects remain animated but now they are depressed, like her: "… when washbowl / maintains it has no more holy calling / than physical ablution …".

We are not calling here for animation of objects, but for object relations, and we ask whether or not medicine has such a relationship with its objects and instruments that moves beyond the instrumental, for this is its primary extension of cognition. Step one is then to embrace the object world. Step two is to notice it in detail. Both steps are essential for poetry and medicine.

Tisha Nemeth-Loomis (2012) sees Plath's poem as an exercise in Freudian object fixation, the attribution of libido to objects as a "visual embracing". The poet Ted Hughes, Plath's husband, had described her as an object hoarder. For object relations psychologists and psychiatrists Plath's fixation on objects would suggest that she has not resolved childhood issues about utilising objects (favourite toys for example) to work through human encounters issues. Fixation on objects as an adult such as hoarding suggests work to do on unhooking from libido invested in objects that should be returned to persons. We have ventured into classic post-Freudian territory, embracing Melanie Klein.

We will finish this section on Plath then with her unresolved object connection to her German father. Written in 1962 but not published until 1965 (posthumously, after Plath's suicide in early 1963), the confessional poem "Daddy" (https://www.poetryfoundation.org/poems/48999/daddy-56d22aafa45b2) was written just after Plath separated from Ted Hughes, who can be seen to have acted in the displaced role of Plath's overbearing and controlling father, the latter an entomologist specialising in the world of honey bees, an inveterate and apparently controlling observer. As Plath's father was an observer of insects, so Hughes was famously admired for his close observation of raw nature. Plath was only eight years old when her father died, but he left a significant imprint. She objectifies her father as a kind of punishment. For Sylvia the poet, the father was a

> black shoe
> In which I have lived like a foot
> For thirty years ...

Plath had been pinned by her father the entomologist and now she pins him in what must be the ur-poem of revenge. But it is clear from the poem that this is the scab over an unfulfilled love. For our part, we find poetry to be an effective psychiatric lens, a medical object of merit. But here we don't want to leave you the reader feeling punished by poetry, or, indeed, that poetry is psychoanalysis redux. The psychoanalytic is just one of many lenses. In the next chapter, we return to lyricism, praising lyrical poetry and promising a lyrical medicine.

References

Biss E. The Pain Scale. *Seneca Review*, 2007: 5–25. Retrieved from https://www. snreview.org/biss.pdf

Bleakley A. 1999. *The Animalizing Imagination: Totemism, Textuality and Ecocriticism.* London: Palgrave Macmillan.

Bleakley A. Broadening Conceptions of Learning in Medical Education: The Message from Teamworking. *Medical Education.* 2006; 40: 150–57.

Bleakley A. 2021a. *Medical Education, Politics and Social Justice: The Contradiction Cure.* Abingdon: Routledge.

Bleakley A. 2021b. Re-Visioning Clinical Reasoning, or Stepping Out from the Skull. *Medical Teacher.* 2021b; 43: 456–62.

Charon R. Narrative Medicine: A Model for Empathy, Reflection, Profession, and Trust. *Journal of the American Medical Association.* 2001; 286: 1897–1902.

Charon R, DasGupta S, Hermann N, et al. 2016. *The Principles and Practices of Narrative Medicine.* Oxford: Oxford University Press.

Clark A. 2016. *Surfing Uncertainty: Prediction, Action and the Embodied Mind.* Oxford: Oxford University Press.

Dalby A. 2006. *Rediscovering Homer: Inside the Origins of the Epic.* New York: WW Norton.

Deleuze G, Guattari F. 2004a. *A Thousand Plateaus.* London: Continuum.

Deleuze G, Guattari F. 2004b. *Anti-Oedipus.* London: Continuum.

Engeström Y. 2018. *Expertise in Transition: Expansive Learning in Medical Work.* Cambridge: Cambridge University Press.

Gibson JJ. 1979. *The Ecological Approach to Visual Perception.* Boston, MA: Houghton-Mifflin.

Hallyn F. 1987. *The Poetic Structure of the World: Copernicus and Kepler.* Princeton, NJ: Zone Books.

Harman G. 2018. *Object-Oriented Ontology: A New Theory of Everything.* London: Penguin Random House.

Hill G. 2019. *The Book of Baruch by the Gnostic Justin*. Oxford: Oxford University Press.

Hughes AM, Gregory ME, Joseph DL, et al. Saving Lives: A Meta-analysis of Team Training in Healthcare. *Journal of Applied Psychology*. 2016; 101: 1266–1304.

Neilson S. Pain as Metaphor: Metaphor and Medicine. *Medical Humanities*. 2016; 42: 3–10.

Nemeth-Loomis, T. The Beautiful Mundane: Plath's Object Transformations. *IUScholar Works Journal*. 2012; 5: 109–12.

Orang B. 2020. *Where Things Touch: A Meditation on Beauty*. Toronto: Book*Hug.

Padfield D. Perceptions of Pain Project. 2016, 2021. Retrieved from https://deborah-padfield.com/Perceptions-of-Pain

Rowlands M. 2003. *Externalism: Putting Mind and World Back Together again*. Chesham: Acumen.

Shapiro J. 2009. *The Inner World of Medical Students: Listening to Their Voices in Poetry*. Oxford: Radcliffe Publishing.

Sharma S. The Poetic Resonance. The Asian Age. May 20, 2020. Retrieved from https://www.pressreader.com/india/the-asian-age/20200520/282046214292961

Soldati G, Demi M, Demi L. Ultrasound Patterns of Pulmonary Edema. *Annals of Translational Medicine*. 2019; 7, Supplement 1, 516.

Sparrow T. 2014. *The End of Phenomenology: Metaphysics and the New Realism*. Edinburgh: Edinburgh University Press.

Stilwell P, Stilwell C, Sabo B, Harman K. Painful Metaphors: Enactivism and Art in Qualitative Research. *Medical Humanities*. 2020; E pub ahead of print.

Tucker WF, Lewis F. Culinary Curiosities – Resemblances between Common Skin Disorders and Food. *Journal of the American Academy of Dermatology*. 2004; 50: 40.

Varela F, Thompson E, Rosch E. 2017. *The Embodied Mind*, 2nd ed. Cambridge, MA: MIT Press.

West M, Eckert R, Collins B, Chowla R. 2017. *Caring to Change: How Compassionate Leadership Can Stimulate Innovation in Health Care*. London: The King's Fund. Retrieved from https://www.kingsfund.org.uk/sites/default/files/field/field_publication_file/Caring_to_change_Kings_Fund_May_2017.pdf

Wyer P, Charon R. 2011. Foreword. In: JP Meza, DS Passerman (eds.) *Integrating Narrative Medicine and Evidence-Based Medicine: The Everyday Social Practice of Healing*. London: Radcliffe Publishing, ix.

8 Celebrating lyric poetry, beauty, and medical moods

Celebrating lyric poetry

A lyrical medicine is poetry enacted. Here is an example from Abraham Verghese's (2009: 139) novel *Cutting for Stone* in which he describes a doctor at work:

> (Dr) Ghosh took the proffered hand and while supporting it he felt for the radial artery. The pulse was bounding at one hundred and twelve per minute. Ghosh's equivalent of perfect pitch was to be able to take the heart rate without a watch ... 'When did this start?' he heard himself say, taking in the swollen abdomen that was so incongruent on this lean, muscled man. 'Begin at the beginning ...' 'Yesterday morning. I was trying to ... move my bowels.' The patient looked embarrassed. 'And suddenly I had pain here,' he pointed to his lower abdomen. 'While you were sitting on the toilet?' 'Squatting yes. Within seconds I could feel swelling ... and tightening. It came on like a bolt of lightning.' The assonance caught Ghosh's ear. ... He asked the next question even though he knew the answer. There were times like this when the diagnosis was written on the patient's forehead. Or else they gave it away in their first sentence. Or it was announced in an odor before one even saw the patient.

The patient required an operation to sort out the obstructed bowel, to undo the twist. What interests us in Verghese's account (and, of course, is part of his reconstruction) is the insistent consonance (sitting, squatting, swelling, tightening, lightning) that is noted in the text. The language echoes the symptom. The episode is collapsed into space in two senses: the clinical poetics and the poetry of the bodily space as symptom. While there is a narrative element (what happened yesterday and what is happening today) this is secondary to the poetic field of activity, and the lyricism of the account.

"Lyric" derives from the ancient Greek *lyros* – referring to the lyre that was played as poetry was recited. The pre-Homeric Greek rhapsodists sung the epics, such as the *Iliad* and the *Odyssey*, before Homer wrote them down – so there was no longer a need to commit them to memory. As noted earlier, *Rhapsodos* – the word describing the ancient Greek singer – literally means

DOI: 10.4324/9781003194408-10

"a stitcher-together of songs" (Dalby 2006) referring to the balance between improvised performance and traditional, rule-bound memorised verse with strict metre or rhythm and recurring emblems and images as prompts, such as "wine dark sea". While the performer may be singing within an epic genre, there is evident beauty both within the epic tales and in his or her performance, as "embodied lyricism" or style (Marshall and Bleakley 2012). This also describes the well-rehearsed "songs" of hospital routines such as ward and teaching rounds that, nevertheless, require the singer (attending doctor or consultant) to think on her feet as she composes and decomposes "winged words" or metaphors (Ratzan 1992).

Once a quality within verse, lyric is now the major category of poetry (Greene 2012). The quality is referred to as "lyrical" (adverb) where the element is "lyric" (noun), and for consistency, we intend one or both when referring to "lyric poetry" throughout. In fact, lyric has been a dominant poetic form over the past 300 years, diverging from narrative forms such as the once dominant forms of the epic and tragic. Aristotle's *Poetics* ranked epic, tragic and comic poetry above dithyrambic (Dionysian, orgiastic, wildly enthusing) verse, and lyric poetry aligned with music. When the epic and tragic genres were once dominant, lyricism was yet evident within them. For example, Homer's (c800–c701 BCE) epics include sensitive and psychologically sophisticated descriptions of Achilles's wildly fluctuating moods, and his loyal, tender feeling for his companion Patroclus (in sharp contrast to his fierce disposition towards both the enemy and Agamemnon, his leader). More than a century after Homer, Sappho's (c630–c570 BCE) poetry is often taken as one of the earliest examples of pure lyrical expression. However, it is widely accepted that lyricism did not emerge as a fully formed genre and dominant style in poetry until the Romantic Movement from the late 18th century, championed, in particular, by Wordsworth, Coleridge, Keats, Byron, and Blake (ibid.).

Walt Whitman's 1855 "I Sing the Body Electric" is often taken as a primary illustration of confessional modern lyric verse with its direct, plain speaking and celebration of the physical caught in long, loose-limbed lines that so distressed traditionalists in his time. Especially poignant to us now, as we write these lines during another Covid lockdown with social distancing as the norm, Whitman (https://www.poetryfoundation.org/poems/45472/i-sing-the-body-electric) writes that he desires,

> To pass among them or touch any one, or rest my arm ever so lightly
> round his or her neck for a moment, what is this then?
> I do not ask any more delight, I swim in it as in a sea.
> There is something in staying close to men and women and looking on
> them, and in the contact and odor of them, that pleases the soul well.

Reductive and instrumental "clinical communication skills training" might ponder the educational value of reading and discussing Whitman in the context of a theme such as "embodied communication and ethical behaviour". After Covid, a tender medicine is surely required; but then, poetry is for all seasons and can inaugurate or be the subject of much discussion when paired with contemporary pedagogical subjects.

Immanuel Kant's 1784 essay "Answering the Question: What is Enlightenment?" is often taken as a watershed for the emergence of humanism and the legitimacy of a personal voice such as Whitman's. The Romantic Movement innovated by adding that such an expression of voice cannot be detached from the expression of feelings. Voice is not purely rational. It is not just what you think that matters but how thinking is shaped and enhanced by feelings as it is given depth, tone, character, expression, and form, thereby arriving at beauty. Where Frederick Turner (in Cowan 2012: 375) describes lyric as the "most important humanistic art form", a "lyrical medicine" can be seen to draw its forms and practices from lyric poetry as praxis seeped in care and intensity of engagement. A lyrical medicine and lyric poetry share these characteristics:

1   Character, achieved through approaching subjects "slantwise".
2   Intensity, depth and brevity with focus on particulars.
3   Epiphany or sudden insight.
4   Use of metaphors, with focus on invention and expansion.
5   Subjectivity and confession stressing emotion, mood and passion, or embrace of affect.
6   Tolerance of ambiguity embracing empathy.
7   Beauty (privileging quality over quantity, and form over function or the purely instrumental).
8   Orientation to here-and-now space and place rather than there-and-then time.

We will discuss each of these categories in more depth.

Character, achieved by approaching subjects "slantwise"

Lyricism is a method of choosing words "slantwise", and combinations of words and phrases laced with metaphor that are pregnant with possibilities, meaning-heavy and often surprising, confounding expectations. It was Emily Dickinson who advised poets to tell it "slant", as asides from the primary moment. Something poets do well (and prose writers too) is to capture the moments and issues around a central object, event or character and explore these in detail as a way of "slantly" illuminating the main event. This is common in haiku also. It is a key capability for medicine, as the twin exercise of a vigilant and paradoxical attention in diagnostic work.

Vigilant focus on what is going on (main event or frontstage) is paralleled by "fuzzy", distributed focus on what is "really" going on (untold or as yet unexpressed context, or backstage). Good diagnosticians sniff out the latter. We think that poetry does this exceptionally well too. The East Texan poet Betty Adcock (2008) pays homage to Dickinson in her collection *Slant-wise*: "where memory breathes its midge-cloud". Out of the side of her eye a recollection is garnered, against the grain of the main irritant, the midge cloud. The pervasive recollection becomes a paradoxical balm for the insistent midge cloud that demands vigilance.

Dickinson again exhorts us to "Tell all the truth but tell it slant", where "Success in Circuit lies" (circle around the issue, don't just burst in, head first, impatient) and then you may be rewarded with "The Truth's superb surprise" for "The Truth must dazzle gradually" (https://www.poetryfoundation.org/poems/56824/tell-all-the-truth-but-tell-it-slant-1263). This reminds us of the old saw that is the surgeon's irritation with the internist coming out in sarcasm: "don't just do something, stand there!" Rapid action is a main cog of surgery and emergency medicine, otherwise the internist wants to take her time, approaching the patient slantwise, gathering a sense of what is going on without the irritating midge cloud. The character of the diagnostic work is often a product of several alchemical operations: distilling, refining, sublimating, purifying, boiling down to dry essences, extracting the gold from the dross. Here, laboratory chemistry meets the chemistry created in the patient encounter. Character emerges from careful processing and not head-on encounter in non-emergency situations. Doctors might be advised: "don't wade in, but fade out; and let the patient do the talking".

In poetry, Dickinson uses form – slant-rhyme, unusual punctuation, and conceits – to shape the poem slantwise so that we get a reformed enjambment, a kind of web inevitably drawing the reader to the waiting spider at the web's centre. No matter how you try to read the poem, there is a truth or an epiphany at the centre of the web that you must encounter.

The Japanese haiku poet (Kobayashi) Issa (1763–1828), however, shows us how to write slantwise without the spider's pull, leaving us with a dilemma. This is the internist contemplating a complex case. Issa's technique is one of suspension of disbelief, an unfolding of dramatic ironies:

A world of dew,
And within every dewdrop
A world of struggle.

The gaze and the glance

Returning to Emily Dickinson's slantwise as both poetic and diagnostic diction, Michel Foucault (1976) in his masterwork on the historical conditions of possibility for the emergence of the "medical gaze", or the way that doctors do their clinical work, pins the birth of modern medicine down to two main issues – both architectural in their own ways. First, Foucault (ibid.) describes how "opening up a few corpses", or learning anatomy through dissection, educated a way of looking into the body that is literalised in dissection, post mortem examination and surgery, but acts as a metaphor for a characteristic way of looking (and then a way of being) that is the medical diagnostic gaze. The doctor looks at, and "into", the body as it expresses symptom, to metaphorically seek the source of the lesion. (In contrast, a cross-cultural point not exploited by Foucault, Chinese culture has a history of resisting the direct gaze [considered rude] for the – more subtle – sideways "glance"; where, coincidentally, dissection of corpses has been banned historically. François Jullien (2000) terms this way of looking poetically, as access-by-detour. We see below that Foucault has a parallel take on the glance).

Of course, the doctor is helped in cultivating this medical gaze by literal interior examination through auscultation, palpation, and percussion (Bleakley 2020), while this is extended later through more sophisticated testing and imaging such as MRI. But such techniques have been overlaid historically by a masculinised discourse of penetration rather than a feminised one of revelation (ibid.). The first architectural feature is then the interior of the body, mapped initially by Vesalius, managed clinically as both literal inspection and metaphorical map.

Second, the doctor is helped in executing the medical gaze by a secondary architectural feature, that of the "clinic": the white, antiseptic space that is the equivalent of the modernist white cube gallery space. Here, just as objects are "presented" in the gallery, the patient is objectified and presented in the clinical space as docile. For Foucault, the shift from examining patients in the privacy of their own home to examining them in the clinic allowed for a power differential to emerge in which the doctor dictates the conditions of exchange, or accrues capital (at the expense of the patient's labour).

Foucault (1976) also mentions that doctors both augment and prelude the direct, penetrating gaze with a slantwise "glance". This is an important point and so we illustrate this with a lengthy quote from a paper written by AB (Bleakley and Bligh 2009):

> We are aware that a close reading of *The Birth of the Clinic* in English is compromised by idiosyncratic translation. Sheridan (in Foucault, 1989, p. vii) who translated the first English edition (1973) offers a cautious note, where some of Foucault's "key terms" in French have "no normal equivalent" in English. The primary key term is *regard*, which Sheridan translates as "the unusual 'gaze'" in the text, but the much broader "medical perception" in the subtitle (as "a concession to the unprepared reader.") Commonly taken to mean a 'glance' (*coup d'oeil*), *regard* had been used by Sartre to describe a look that fully acknowledges the 'other', and means both to 'look' and the 'look in one's eyes.'
>
> In a key passage, Foucault (1989, pp. 120–121) discusses the emphasis placed upon an overall "fine sensibility" of diagnostic acumen, where a differentiation is made between 'gaze' and 'glance.' 'Glance' (Sheridan's translation) is described as a kind of rapid holistic grasp of the patient that the doctor makes in an instant look of recognition based on expertise.

This, paradoxically, Foucault ascribes to "touch." Foucault moves between looking, seeing, saying, and touching (as sensibility), and saying (as apprehension), in a description of diagnostic expertise. However, again the literal and the metaphorical are interchanged freely, particularly in the descriptor "touch" (which can easily be read as the doctor and patient being 'touched' by each other in a metaphorical sense of mutual respect). For example, "the glance is silent, *like* a finger pointing" (Foucault, 1989, p. 121, our emphasis) – an analogy not a literal palpation; and "The glance is of the non-verbal order of *contact*" (Foucault, 1989, p. 122).

This is further complicated by the contact being "ideal" and not literal, where it is described as "*striking.*" Later, this is described as the "kinship" of the "clinical eye" with a "new sense" that is "no longer the ear straining to catch a language, but the index finger palpating the depths." In the next sentence, Foucault (1989, p. 122) describes the "metaphor of 'touch'." The English language reader thus has to deal with an idiosyncratic translation of Foucault's already paradoxical language. This is further confounded by the meaning in French of a variety of gazes that 'strike' or are 'striking' thus giving sense to the notion of a gaze that 'penetrates' another's body or sees into its depths. The literal and the metaphorical are brought together in the *coup d'oeil* – the 'knock' or 'blow' of the gaze. To counter more empirical English language readings, we should read these translations of Foucault with a fine sensibility, following Foucault's (1989, p. 121) own description of the emerging artistry of the modern doctor in diagnostic technique as "taste," again aesthetically grounding an idea in a sense domain.

We are struck with the beauty of Sartre's observation of the glance as the "look" in the eye of somebody, the doctor perhaps, in a gesture of empathy, of identification with another's *pathos*; or even of longing or *pothos*. We read Foucault's "glance" as a summary exchange with the patient, one of first impressions but also one of communication "scene setting" – a brief negotiation of the meaning of the consultation. We see the glance as a more tender poetic gesture that sets the conditions for the gaze by initially softening the encounter. François Jullien (2000) again contends that Western inquiry is governed by impatience and haste, a need to know now, where Chinese philosophical tradition, embodied in Taoism, tarries and moves slowly, gathering moss. Within this tradition is a cognate element of communication and social exchange that is, as noted above, a "glancing off" another, rather than a direct gaze, considered to be impolite.

In our two examples below, from the poets Anthony Hecht and Rachel Long, we try to encapsulate the moods of gaze and glance under our general heading of *character*. Jonathan Post (2015) describes Anthony Hecht's ability to engage big themes through specifics in the appropriately titled *A Thickness of Particulars*. It also parallels the medical gaze as a "force" rather than a "presence" (a better descriptor for the glance) to borrow Wallace Stevens's terms (see Bleakley 2017a). As a Jewish American soldier during the Second World War, Hecht helped liberate Flossenbürg, a Nazi concentration camp. He addresses the vast horrors of the Holocaust through a single illustrative scene set outside a German wood "In which the two Jews are ordered to lie down / And be buried alive by the third, who is a Pole".

The Pole refuses the order, so the German soldiers make him dig a grave for himself at gunpoint, whereon he was ordered to change places with the Jews. Here, "The thick dirt mounted toward the quivering chin". Then, to compound the torture, he was dug out of the grave and immediately told to get in again, when he was shot in the belly (https://allpoetry.com/More-Light!-More-Light!). This huge and terrifying poisonous cloud of inhumanity, the Holocaust, is caught in a concentrated moment of inhumanity. How can we gaze at this? We must glance, hearts in mouth, stomachs churning.

In sharp contrast to Hecht's gravity, Rachel Long (2020) recalls a moment of levity and erotic pleasure on which we must exercise the long gaze. To glance would show manners, but to gaze is to confirm sensuality. Hecht condenses deep cruelty into one scene whereas Long collapses the opposite – human love – into one fleeting erotic episode she describes as her first experience of "being all-consumingly in love, holding your breath all the time (remember that?)". In "Hotel Art, Barcelona" (https://www.panmacmillan.com/blogs/literary/inspiring-poems-by-female-poets), the couple are on the balcony on the highest floor of a hotel:

> *Shhh.* You lift my dress. I shoulder-width my legs,
> Is love not this? – gripping a fence in the sky

The beauty of these lines is that the question ends, and then "gripping a fence in the sky" comes as a statement after a long pause instruction through hyphenation. It is just there, unquestioned, to be done. Passion brings experimentation and extra powers – the spirit is elevated. Medicine can learn from the sensual face of poetry because in essence the state of being we call "compassion" and its instrumental act of "empathy" are forces of eros, life forces.

Intensity, depth, and brevity with focus on particulars

Intensity is a *pharmakon*, a "healing poison" that can be as straightforward as putting the foot on the pedal, or as paradoxical as lifting off the beat as a jazz drummer does to create space: intense presence and absence. Here is how they exist together as qualities: mixed with pedal-down intensity are delicate tracings, light touches, and sudden but elegant turns in expression. Better poems remain balanced and do not run away with themselves, although the balance may be at cliff's edge. Lyric poetry strives for depth – of feeling and engagement with particulars. Surely good medicine demonstrates such intensity and depth of engagement?

In Issa's haiku above, the tender and delicate is turned into the tough through enantiodromia. Good medicine is both tough- and tender-minded, but often lacks a delicacy. We see a remarkable delicacy of touch (and honesty), however, in Bahar Orang, a young psychiatrist in training in Toronto, who has provided an essay for us in Chapter 14. Orang sees "beauty" as the aim of both medicine and poetry (http://open-book.ca/News/Read-an-Excerpt-from-Bahar-Orang-s-Where-Things-Touch-A-Meditation-on-Beauty). More, beauty is expressed through "the articulation of a / series of ruptures". These ruptures are often centred on relationships, but they also embrace what doctors find every day: literal ruptures of body and imaginal ruptures of psyche. This is a complement to Spinoza's idea of beauty as a series of folds, where truths reside within each fold but are hidden from view. In Sylvia Plath's "Tale of a Tub" considered in Chapter 7, Plath describes how her life is dried out, there is no longer any surprise, and each object in her bathroom is now a plain thing and no longer has voice or character. Of the towel, Plath says: "and the towel / dryly disclaims that fierce troll faces lurk / in its explicit folds". The disclaimer is that beauty no longer resides within. It has been squeezed out by mood.

Bahar Orang on intensity

Orang (2020) wants to puncture Spinoza's Fold and see what mosaic of fluids emerge. In *Where Things Touch: A Meditation on Beauty*, she confesses:

> I'm sitting in a psychiatry clinic, on my first rotation as a medical student. I wanted to start with psychiatry because the sight of blood still makes me uneasy.

It's pretty straightforward personal-confessional prose until the next line kicks in, bringing a deeply focussed meditation on the colour red that continues her self-analysis to include her reaction to the sight of blood:

> It's too much redness at once, a colour too arresting, too unambiguous, without intimation or forethought. I can't find the words, there are no words, really, for a red that symbolizes nothing, that is only the thing itself. Red for red's sake.

In such a quiet reflection, we are favourably reminded of Christopher Logue's louder re-working of Homer's *Iliad* where the stain of battle is "All Day Permanent Red", a bloodbath in the war between the Greeks and Trojans where wounding and deaths film the eyes and stain the earth (https://poetryarchive. org/poem/all-day-permanent-red-extract/). Blood for Orang is,

> too much redness at
> once

less a metaphorical concept than a spreading of a quality so that it permeates existence. Orang makes life be constituted of this essential quality. The enjambed line falls away to "once" to give extra emphasis and gravity to the word. "At once" (in the instant) and "just once" (not to be repeated) are fused in an inhalation of breath, a moment of queasy surprise. Our lives hang by this sudden spurt of colour. Orang says on watching surgery,

> I'm sputtering at the sight of blood—a rising in my belly
> for which there are few words ….

Again, she despairs that she "can't / find the words" for this sudden appearance. In fact, "there are no words". They are folded away. Symbolism must be suspended as superfluous, where "Red for red's sake" does not even attempt to capture the shades and varieties of red. Orang mines her sources well, such as "The Red Poppy" (https://poets.org/poem/red-poppy-0) of poet Louise Glück, a poem of 16 words that summarises perhaps the central work of poetry, that of raising affect:

> The great thing
> is not having
> a mind. Feelings:
> oh, I have those; they
> govern me

Orang moves on to make a comparison with the red of the flower's petals:

> Another red thing: poppies, *khash khash*. Poppies are not meant to be potted, they can never be kept by florists, they are wildflowers that resist any other kind of life. What happens to beauty when it's removed from its own dirt? If you pick a poppy, it withers within the hour

(*khash khash* is Urdu for "poppy" and "poppy seed", used in cooking). Here, we get a lesson in the difference between surgery and psychiatry: "How simple a practice, then, to let flower, let flower, smelling its own / earth". The poppy cannot be cut but must be allowed to bloom in its own being.

The poet bypasses the Western symbolism of the poppy – Armistice Day, the latter-day Opium Wars mirrored in the Taliban's coffers – for the thing-in-itself, the phenomenological appearance, back to red for red's sake. Permanent Red. But, here, the poppy is given a death sentence as beauty removed from its context and substrate. Beauty as an isolated idea is infertile, but the beautiful poppy's fertility is guaranteed by the soil that it inhabits. Beauty is in things and things may be severed one from the other, as the poppy is from its soil, or the conflict or climate crisis refugee is from her homeland. We must

> let flower, let flower, smelling its own
> earth

again an enjambed line – falling away into the earth, rooting with the poppy. This seems to be a metaphor for recovery. And then we get why poetry is so important to her medicine, as Orang moves on to discuss a patient with a supervising psychiatrist: "Borderline patients, he says, are afflicted with 'chronic / feelings of emptiness,' with 'unstable relationships,' / with 'a shifting sense of self'". They are folded away too, their intentions often invisible to themselves. And where they are divided, they need undivided attention (as does the poem).

The poem allows for a graphic or spatial representation of borderlines, and the "shifting sense of self" falls away into a new line. We follow it with our eye as we might feel the patient falling out of sightline and cognitive work and into a tangled bunch of feelings in our gut, garnering impressions of "emptiness", "unstable relationships" and "shifting sense of self", the latter driven home through both consonant and vowel alliterations. Orang continues her observation of the supervising psychiatrist: "It's strange to sift through his language" she says, observing that the psychiatrist sometimes speaks of borderline "people", sometimes of borderline "diagnosis" and sometimes of borderline "traits", so that "borderline" itself becomes a weasel word. We need to know more about "borders" – otherwise how "can we trace the borders that are dashed or wrecked, or know what's swelling at some seam?" The alliteration, outwardly like a hiss, hints at a birth of beauty rather than a bursting forth of suffering (although pathos, of course, can be beautiful). Primarily, there is intensity at work in the lyric. The intensity is the seam itself, zipped, holding back what is as yet unsaid. We are in the presence of a strange repression of forces that want to question lines drawn around "identity", borders imposed on authenticity.

And so poetry, crossing the line, inhabits the clinical report or the case study by representing the complexity of the patient at his or her borders that have been somehow broached to express symptom: "dashed", "wrecked" or "swelling at some seam". Meanwhile, a ghost hangs behind the enterprise of the poem as a milky red presence of borders, poppies, and wars. Unsettled and unseated by blood, Orang gets back in the saddle, resettled, to restore identity to borderline patients, forced migrants from the stability of normality or a settled psyche. The illness does not reside with the patient but with the abstract notion of "borders" imposed, a symptom of what Deleuze and Guattari (2004a, 2004b) refer to as a "territorialising" imperative that pathologises the nomadic impulse. You might like to turn to Bahar Orang's essay on "abolition medicine" and Palestine solidarity at the beginning of Chapter 14 to flesh out the de-territorialising gambit. We like the fact that Orang can set the soft edges of poppies against the hard edges of separatist politics; of course, as we insist throughout this book, clinical medicine's soft edges must sit with biomedicine's harder outlines without attempting to resolve the contradiction. Indeed, the contradiction acts as resource and opportunity.

Peter Redgrove on intensity

Following the mytheme of hard and soft edges co-existing, few poets have written around this theme with the sustained intensity of the late Peter Redgrove (2012), whose *Collected Poems* (over 40 years) runs to nearly 500 pages, maintaining a remarkable consistency. This borderline position stems from Redgrove's melding of a background in academic natural sciences with symbolist poetry. We take Redgrove's body of work as a remarkable advertisement for the power of lyric poetry – of celebrating the imagination and the flows of affect.

For example, in "The Cave" Redgrove takes the big theme of the natural cycle of life and death and focusses it on the interior of a rotting apple. The mouldering fruit, held in his hand, is a "winged apple" containing the promise of rebirth – where Redgrove told AB that these kinds of images, recurring in his poetry, are flashbacks to his periods of mental illness where he felt like he was rotting out. Poetry rebuilt his confidence. In the same poem, Redgrove sets out his own version of existential authenticity. This also stood as his version of the goal of psychotherapy, where mental illness equated with an alienation from the natural world. How to connect back to an authentic life through identification with nature? Do not glorify nature or idealise it, but notice its pathologies.

Drawing on the same poem, Redgrove describes an audience as if watching a play where some unknown force strips their clothes from them, a metaphor of unmasking or calling out the "frontstage" personae. They sit, naked and helpless, watching "… their talking clothes, their / Eloquent masks and attitudes …" fly away. "The handless, headless, hollow clothes", meanwhile, "… pull themselves through each other's textures" and "… lie in heaps like leaves" while the audience sits naked and vulnerable, where Redgrove compares them with the apple seeds introduced early in the poem, again awaiting planting and rebirth (see Redgrove 2012: 227). The poet then embraces the biggest of existential questions and concentrates these in the smallest of nature's particulars, the seed.

Crushing pain

Such intense compression as Redgrove captures characterises not only lyric poetry but also a lyrical medicine – key not only to the time-pressured medical encounter but also to the circulation of knowledge where "head space" is at a premium for busy clinicians. As the patient's presentation is translated into a "case", and where the latter may become, say, a presentation on a Ground Round, so brevity and concision are prized in both medical work and medical education. These are again the compressed, well-rehearsed "songs" of the medical teaching rounds (Marshall and Bleakley 2012). However, where poets encourage wonder, scrutiny, thinking against the grain, ambiguity and complexity, medicine generally uses compressing technical language to reduce ambiguity: "Mr Smith is a sixty-year-old man who came to A&E with crushing, central chest pain, which radiated down the left arm and up into the neck. There has been no previous episode. His ECG showed ST elevation …". Yet at the heart of this brief description there is a powerful metaphor at work: "crushing" chest pain; overused, yes – but striking, nevertheless, in physical presence. The metaphor works because the word "crushing" in the embodied context in which it is used forces us to test the veracity of the description.

A "crushing" pain implies an insistent force over a period of time. Crushing a flower in our hand doesn't at all get at the intensity of the crushing pain, while the experience of a crushing chest pain can feel like an outward motion pressing on the ribs rather than an inward pressure on the heart, or pressure from within the heart. Lyric poetry's compression, often a soft crushing, is again best advertised in the haiku, with a regular structure of three unrhymed short lines of (usually) five, seven, and five syllables. The 17th-century Japanese haiku master Matsuo Basho writes:

> Autumn moonlight–
> A worm digs silently
> Into the chestnut

In his early poem "Marriage" (1916), William Carlos Williams might be seen as the American master of the adapted haiku:

> So different, this man
> And this woman:
> A stream flowing
> In a field.

Which is the stream and which the field, the man or the woman, one permanently active, the other resting? Here are two very different kinds of patients, perhaps presenting with the same physical or psychological symptoms. How will the doctor engage the characters that Williams encapsulates in just four brief lines? Williams's metaphoric descriptors of the difference between the man and woman, one a field, the other a stream flowing, reminds us of how important it is for doctors to be conversant with general and idiosyncratic metaphor use. The "crushing, central chest pain" in the report above is a typical, generalised medical metaphor. We have indicated that it can be differentiated. Patients may specifically experience "stabbing", "burning", or "like a belt tightening across my chest" (Albarran 2002): see how haiku lines, by virtue of an essentialised context, reflect the quality and intensity of their experience of chest pain with sensory and emotive components.

Williams's poem is haiku+, the surplus being the final line that snatches us out of haiku territory (the image of "a stream flowing" would be a natural haiku ending) and into Olson territory of the field of composition. The line's introduction puts us into the territory of medicine's major dilemma – that the linearity of biomedicine (reduction to information) sits with the complexity of clinical medicine (the introduction of the human factor and uncertainty), or the general case and the specific instance. Placing the stream literally in the field gives us a dividing line: in Williams's poem the difference between men and women equally apportioned. In the haiku, the hanging stream, unplaced, takes on the mantle of the "difference" between men and women, a lovely image (if reinforcing a stereotype).

Epiphany or sudden insight

Among poets, Wordsworth called it "spots of time", Coleridge "phantasy", Shelley "moment", Browning "infinite moment" and "good minute", Yeats "great moment", Eliot "timeless moment", Pound "image", Wallace Stevens "moment of awakening", Heaney "revelation", and Redgrove "hole-in-the-day" (as noted previously, a pun on "holiday" as away from the daily grind in a moment of revelation and relaxation), while among critics and novelists Pater called it "pulsations" and "pauses in time", Henry James "sublime instants", Conrad "moment of vision", and Virginia Woolf "frozen moment".

These terms all refer to "epiphany", derived from the Greek *epiphaneia* meaning the sudden appearance or revelation of a god. To the list above we might add Sigmund Freud's clunky "parapraxis", typically instrumentally weighty, as an unthinking gesture that reveals a hidden or unconscious motive. We prefer the conversational metaphor "Freudian slip" for its own parapraxis, where "slip" has several meanings. In analysis, an epiphany occurs as an insight following the revelation of an unconscious desire. But, also as the revelation of the universal through the particular, a key feature of poetry, parapraxes are themselves evidence of a shared unconscious life. The archetype shadows the idiosyncratic.

Abraham Verghese (2013) uses epiphanies constantly as tropes in his writing, reflecting his clinical work. Epiphanies – sudden insights – act as pivot points in a narrative that changes the nature of both the patient and doctor's experiences. He gives an example of such epiphanies drawing on John Berger's (1967) *A Fortunate Man* – a literary ethnography of an English country doctor John Sassall:

> An unhappy patient comes to the doctor to offer him an illness in the hope that this part of him, at least — the illness — may be recognizable. His proper self he believes to be unknowable. In the light of the world he is nobody. By his own lights, the world is nothing. Clearly, the task of the doctor is to recognize the man. If the man can begin to feel recognized, then such recognition may well include aspects of his character which he has not yet recognized himself. The hopeless nature of his unhappiness will have been changed; he may even have the chance of being happy (ibid.: unpaginated).

Although Verghese casts them as such, these are again not necessarily moments in a narrative arc:

> Most of people's daily activities do not involve story. But the moment someone shows up to see a physician in his office," he observed, "there is inherent drama, because most of us in this room will get the news that our lives will be shortened, or affected, or changed in some fashion in a doctor's office. "I remind my students that there's always story, there's always drama, when a patient comes to hospital or the doctor's office. Even if it's routine for you, it's not at all routine for the patient." Listening well to a patient's story … can produce an epiphany (an "ah hah" moment), when he suddenly sees things in a different light (ibid.: unpaginated).

Such epiphanic "ah hahs" are also like an unfolding poem, deeply concentrated, specific. These epiphanies may be muted, as a reflection of circumstance such as a matter of fact transformed into a matter of tact. Berger (1967: 60) recounts Sassall's home visit to a couple where the husband had informed the doctor that his wife was "bleeding from down below":

> … the wife was lying on the ottoman. Her stockings were rolled down and her dress up. 'She' was a man. He examined her. The trouble was severe piles. Neither he nor the husband nor she referred to the sexual organs that should not have been there.

James Joyce might be taken as commentary on Freud's method, at once satirical and learned, where epiphany is the cornerstone of his work. Joyce designed text so dense, allusive, alliterative and punning that epiphanies became the equivalent of punctuation, allowing pause for the harried reader after the shock or pleasure of the insight. In Joyce, characters now stand in for gods, and it is through their appearances and utterances that epiphanic moments occur. In *Ulysses,* Deasy asks Stephen Daedalus "what is God?" to which Stephen replies "That is God … a shout in the street". Molly Bloom echoes this in the final chapter with her cry of "yes", where the epiphany is the orgasm, the "little death". Death, of course, is Chief Epiphany and poets linger much on this, as do doctors, of course, where the medical epiphany is death's enantiodromia, the saving of life – medicine's chief concern. We might deflect attention away from the heroic and epic tags often used to narrate intensive medical work towards the epiphanic: the first blink from a Covid-19 patient who has been on life support for days or weeks.

Emily Dickinson wrote an untitled poem whose opening line runs, "I heard a Fly buzz – when I died" (https://www.poetryfoundation.org/poems/45703/i-heard-a-fly-buzz-when-i-died-591). This is an epiphanic moment, a strange shock. Better, the poem's penultimate line runs, "And then the Windows failed". The light leaves. The reader is now grappling with the death herself. Conventional readings take "the Windows" to mean the eyes of the dying person. But what if we take the word literally and not as symbol? It is a sudden jolt to the system that the windows in the room fail, as light no longer enters.

Epiphany is also the revelation of beauty, often sudden and deeply moving. Poetry designs epiphanic moments at the level of form. Indeed, there is an argument that all poetry is necessarily epiphanic (as is all medicine, discussed below). Recall that Wallace Stevens called epiphanies "moments of awakening". Epiphanies range from lightning flashes to pleasurable knowing. Either way, they are sudden and suddenly sharpen the senses. We feel and see beyond our usual capacities. This might be pleasurable surprise (the presence of beauty) or violent shock (the interpellation of awe).

If a moment of cognition is everyday, then surely it is not epiphanic? Yet medicine might be thought of as the singular practice of cultivating "ordinary epiphanies" where medical habits are by their nature extraordinary. In adaptive expertise, the reasoning process of experienced doctors, the primary method of diagnosis is Type 1 reasoning, clinical gestalt, or pattern recognition as set out in the previous chapter. Abraham Verghese (1999) characterises this as "the blink of an eye diagnosis". To those outside medicine, this can look miraculous, but it has a simple explanation, a logic, that we explained in the previous chapter. Doctors mainly do not "know" how or why they make instant diagnoses, because by definition pattern recognition is a tacit or unconscious event, it is black-boxed.

Where the cognitive psychologist stands in for the unconscious life of the doctor, as illustrated in the previous chapter, so this is augmented by the life of diagnostic instruments and objects. Here is a recent example from experience. A family member of AB suffered a knee injury surfing and consulted an experienced orthopaedic surgeon who specialises in sports injuries. At consultation, the surgeon noted that the knee could not be straightened on downward compression in a prone position. And from the description of the accident and exploration of how the person was experiencing a range of symptoms, a definite diagnosis was made of a "bucket handle" tear of the knee meniscus (cartilage). This would require urgent arthroscopic investigation and surgery, either removing (worse-case scenario) or repairing (best-case scenario) the cartilage, the latter often a challenging procedure. A date for theatre was booked. As a matter of protocol, an MRI scan was arranged. When the scan images came back, the surgeon saw that the meniscus was undamaged – the problem was a tear in a medial collateral ligament that would repair on its own, hastened by physiotherapy, tailored exercise, and careful management.

The epiphanic moment is advertised as of two kinds: an "ordinary epiphany" in the pattern recognition diagnosis (that turned out to be a misdiagnosis); and the epiphany linked with the arrival of the scan results that showed not only that the initial diagnosis was wrong but also why it was wrong. In this case, the "unconscious" revelation is the MRI scan (scanners and other equipment act as a collective unconscious for medicine: generating, storing, and retrieving images).

Poetry too has ordinary and extraordinary epiphanies. All poetry is epiphanic in an ordinary way by its nature – the strange compression of words and the arduous exercises of arranging them according to forms and structures, choices of rhythms and slantwise approaches to subjects and objects: all of this is extraordinary in a prosaic world. But poetry also excels in the extraordinary epiphanic in which the god does speak, the image confounds, or the idea electrifies. By definition, the epiphany cannot be pre-ordered but is a fortunate product of the poem. Epiphanies then depend on serendipities or fortunate coincidences. Medicine surely moves in this way too, despite its claim to be grounded in the logic of biomedicine. The science is the main explanatory basis for symptom (not all symptoms, as psychiatrists know too well, although since the 19th century the profession seeks brain-based explanations and regulated chemical interventions), but doctor-patient encounters are exploratory prior to explanations. It is in the exploration, and the appreciation prior to explanation, that epiphanies may occur.

Again, there is a structural symmetry between the use of epiphany in poetry and medicine. The poet arranges language such that revelations may occur in the reader's mind or shift of affect; the doctor draws on the structures of clinical reasoning that we detailed in a previous chapter as the basis for diagnostic insight, as "ordinary epiphany". Revelations also occur where a differential diagnosis suddenly resolves itself.

Epiphanic knowledge and enjambment: stepping out with poetry in mind (mind the gap)

Noted pathography theorist Anne Hunsaker Hawkins (1994) suggests that a key value of poetry (in medicine) is that it offers, in her phrase, an "epiphanic knowledge" – sudden or immediate insights, revelations or realisations out of time, nonrational images, and horizons that cannot as yet be articulated but bear importance. Narrative and tragedies (the latter yielding, in her phrase again, "passional knowledge" or the deepening of emotional connections) do not necessarily afford such insights.

George Saunders (2021) claims that "escalation" is key to story may illuminate meanings, and possible outcomes, of tension between the narrative and poetic imaginations. Yet patients and doctors do not necessarily engage with escalation (an echo of hierarchies, now much challenged in a democratic medicine). The "slipping" and "sliding" that doctors may do around the emergence of cues and clues, as a form of sensemaking, draws on what poetics detail as "enjambment", referred to across chapters. Enjambment is formally described as "incomplete syntax at the end of a line; the meaning runs over from one poetic line to the next, without terminal punctuation" (Greene 2012: 435–36). This involves line breaks as sudden sideways slippage to gain a new footing as this opens a new perspective. This in turn reflects the patient's own mind and imagination as it slips and slides around the appearance of worrying symptoms. The patient does not find herself in an unfolding story, but in a state of fluid confusion, worry and uncertainty.

Here, any attempt at escalation results in slippage away to a new level that resists increasing narrative tension, to produce a new line of inquiry. Enjambment takes the reader to the edge of a cliff as the following line picks up at the cliff fall. This is the opposite of an end-stopped line. It is more a mini version of one tectonic plate sliding over another. The surface result may be an earthquake. Poets use this technique regularly. (Indeed, many have been criticised for overuse.) As an example, Shakespeare's sonnet 116 has an opening line:

> Let me not to the marriage of true minds
> Admit impediments

The sudden cliff edge at the comforting marriage of two minds brings a contradiction. As we fall off the end of the line, the new line presents an uncomfortable conundrum: "Admit impediments", where the author promises in the previous line not to do ("Let me not") exactly what he might do. The enjambment suggests that impediments may, indeed, be admitted, so watch out. This serves to heighten tension like the Shakespeare example above. The doctor and patient may wish for the marriage of minds in reaching a plateau of understanding and an ironing out of tensions and worry on the patient's side, but the consultation must "admit impediments": unknowns, let's see what develops, I'll refer you to a specialist, let's wait until the test results come back, give it some time, I'm not sure how this will unfold.

George Young, a retired doctor, writes about a patient with Alzheimer's who suddenly breaks the "night silence" on a locked ward (https://www.acpjournals.org/doi/10.7326/0003-4819-137-5_Part_1-200209030-00016):

> Tell me the night silence
> on the locked Alzheimer's ward is broken
> by a yell from room 206.

The doctor on call moves into action to find the man "… standing / in the middle of that room, naked, / his freckled face a clenched fist, / urine and feces running / down his legs". But this is not a medical call. The man used to be a boxer, he has a "flattened / nose and crumpled ears" but now he is reduced to a man at loss. As the doctor arrives, already a carer or a nurse,

> … twelve years on the job,
> working her second shift because
> someone's car won't start,
> comes with a pan
> of warm water, a sponge and a towel

and cleans him up:

> … her hand reaches out

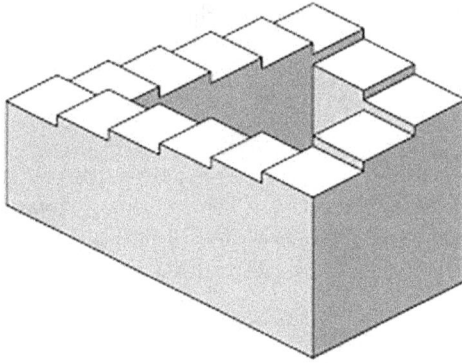

Figure 8.1 The "Penrose Staircase".

to flick down his wild flame of hair.
Now tell me again
why you don't believe in angels.

The epiphany is complete. Both doctor and patient are enjambed, falling to the level of spectator. The patient, the old boxer, slips in memory. The nurse or carer's loving presence upstages the doctor and he slips away, in admiration (Demarco 2020).

Enjambment is the opposite of George Saunders's "escalation". It is a kind of slipping in and out of grace, but it is a way to create beauty. Indeed, it is better to think of enjambment as a kind of anti-escalation best illustrated by the visual illusion of the never-ending "Penrose Staircase" first created by Oscar Reutersvärd in 1937 (Figure 8.1). We will leave this section and enjamb into the next with these images in the reader's mind, with the important reminder that enjambment in poetry does work that prose cannot do at the level of form.

Metaphors as vehicles of expression

Deployment of metaphor – both use and abuse – is a main characteristic of lyric poetry and of medicine (especially in the talk of the consultation). A metaphor expresses one thing in terms of another and in the process promises an enrichment of appreciation and meaning. Emily Dickinson's "Tell all the truth but tell it slant", introduced earlier in this chapter, uses "slant" as a metaphor for "telling something truthfully"; as if to tell the truth required a method of indirection, that a direct method would not include the full apprehension. We expect "direct" for truth, but Dickinson invites a slantwise view of truth by asking us to "tell it slant". Dickinson sees "Success in Circuit lines" – the "roundabout truth", because direct Truth and the whole Truth may be "Too bright for our infirm Delight", where

> The Truth must dazzle gradually
> Or every man be blind –.

More, Dickinson describes "The Truth's superb surprise / As Lightning ... ", exhorting that it must be "eased" but hinting that it is worth taking the risk to face it direct. A "superb surprise / As Lightning" is both metaphor and another epiphany. And then Dickinson adds a conundrum:

> The Truth's superb surprise
> As Lightning to the Children eased
> With explanation kind

means that "The Truth must dazzle gradually / Or every man be blind – ", except that because of lack of punctuation, we don't know as reader if the truth is a superb surprise as lightning to the children (i.e. the inno-cent can take it), or the lightning of truth must be "eased" for the chil-dren "With explanation kind". Dickinson sets us a brilliant moral puzzle. It is one of direct concern for doctors breaking bad news. (The poem is still in copyright. Access at: https://www.poetryfoundation.org/poems/56824/tell-all-the-truth-but-tell-it-slant-1263).

We have already noted that production of new metaphors in medicine is necessary to productively guide and check instrumental technological frames and forces that shape medical practice. However, we can give plenty of living examples of practice-enriching metaphor use in medicine. For example, to conceptualise healthcare organisation and medical education in terms of ex-pressions of complexity requires the use of metaphors both to enrich thinking and to bridge conceptual frames.

In discussing how a medical school's pedagogical work may be best evalu-ated, Jorm and Roberts (2018: 401) draw on what they term "sensemaking", or holistic grasp of complex interacting patterns and features. They found that a "powerful means of sensemaking is through the use of metaphor" as "the organization as a neuron situated within a complex neural network – to make sense of medical school evaluation". They call this "the medical school as neuron metaphor". This is an "organic metaphor rather than a mechanical one". and is very much defined by its connections. Importantly, it signifies complex system rather than linear connection.

Thus, brain science is mobilised to explore a pedagogic and organisational issue – that of how to best educate doctors. But the authors attempt to ex-press the science poetically, drawing on metaphor. Further, the metaphor itself is organic (neuron), rather than a tired industrial or machine metaphor (body as machine, organisation as production line). The authors rather trip themselves up where "we used a modified program logic model" (straying into the territory of linear engineering), but this is quickly resolved where "inputs and outputs were nonlinear". Importantly, the model has face validity for biomedically oriented medical educators and affords a step towards better understanding of the central role that metaphor use has in clinical practice.

This is then the opposite of reduction of behaviour to brain function as brain functions are expanded to encompass the metaphorical. Nevertheless, we recognise that "neuron" here as metaphor for medical school could readily be nudged out for "switch" or "wire", putting us back to square one (one of our tired metaphors, at breaking point). We will describe the use of metaphor throughout and so won't waste any more time here. If you want to cut to the chase, see the work of Laurence Kirmeyer (1992) and our own work (Neilson 2016, 2019a; Bleakley 2017b).

Subjectivity and confession – stressing emotion, mood and passion, or embrace of affect

Anne Sexton's poems are confessional, straight to the point: "At night, alone, I marry the bed" she says of masturbating ("The Ballad of the Lonely Masturbator": https://www.poetryfoundation.org/poems/42574/the-ballad-of-the-lonely-masturbator). Emily Dickinson, in contrast, takes us by surprise (epiphany) by transferring mood from the world (context) to person. This mirrors current ecological reasoning models of medical diagnostic work as described earlier. We have already met Dickinson's disconcerting opening line: "I heard a Fly buzz - when I died". The dying person's emotions are bleached out or stripped out and transferred to the irritating fly.

In contrast to Sexton's and Dickinson's bleaker visions, we previously met Rachel Long's warm, confessional eroticism in "Hotel Art, Barcelona" where she describes her first experience of "being all-consumingly in love, holding your breath all the time (remember that?)". The epiphany arrives with the suddenness of the passion and its place – on the balcony on the highest floor of a hotel. Long asks the reader to hush in the presence of the scene. We are voyeurs (we make no apology for repeating the quote here):

> *Shhh.* You lift my dress. I shoulder-width my legs,
> Is love not this? – gripping a fence in the sky.

The metaphor is unusual but apt. The epiphany is in the realisation of falling in love, but also in the moment a promised orgasm. The confession is embracing. The mood and affect are explicit.

Wordsworth defined lyrical verse as "the spontaneous overflow of powerful feelings", and famously as "emotion recollected in tranquillity". The lyric form became associated in particular with the subjective voice or the expression of the personal. In recent times, this has transformed into expression of identity, where the personal is located as national, ethnic, disabled, political and gendered; and dis-located as migrant, political refugee or sex-trafficked woman (advertising modern slavery). Turner (2012: 359) notes that: "The distinguishing mark of lyric as against any other kind of poetry is the intense presence of the self of the poet". Well, each age and style has its own version of subjectivity and identity, but yes, lyric poetry coincides with the invention of "self knowing" in the modern sense of psychological insight or making of a private identity. This intensity can be icy, judgemental, or expressly cynical, but it is more often embracing. Turner (2012: 167) notes of the poet "the world" he or she "describes is marinated with the poet's feelings and intentions". Hegel described the main interest of lyrical poetry simply as "mood". Selfhood and intensity of feeling are intimately entangled.

Where the poetic imagination flowers because of this, medicine has trouble with such entanglement. The identity of the doctor in training is carefully cultivated as one in which the suspension of emotional states is central to the success of the clinical consultation and of working professionally with other doctors and healthcare workers. The lyric poet adopts a different stance – not one of unreflective catharsis, but of speaking through the emotions wisely. Poetry here, then, can educate the medical mind and body, where Turner (ibid.: 168) suggests that through the praxis of affect: "lyric takes the most direct, searching and immediate path to the mystery of selfhood". It is an arc that does not have to encompass a story but reflects rather a composite of critical incidents. In many cases, contra Turner's description, lyric poetry does not act as if the self is a mystery, but rather engages the audience to join the poet in exploring how selves are differently engaged by mysteries in the world. Wallace Stevens (1951: 93) stresses the importance of lyric poetry's interest in the peculiar and the particular as "reality in its most individual aspect".

Lyric poetry has broken away in modern times from collective rules, such as formal metre, to focus instead on idiosyncratic expression – intonation, phrasing, stutter, pause, silence, emotional expression, lilt, insecurity, grasping the moment, dispensing sureties, and so forth – from the emotionally annihilatory and tentative (for example, Sylvia Plath) to the unsentimental and blissfully confident black comedic (for example, Frederick Seidel). But confessional poetry does not necessarily offer balm to writer or reader. Famously a cynic, but one of the best of modern poets, Geoffrey Hill described poetry as "The crassest form of self-harm, that I have long practiced". Then why do it? The answer is simple. *Because it presses you, because it beseeches, implores and entreats; and not doing it leads to symptom* (p.s. doing it also leads to symptom!) For example, as noted earlier, Peter Redgrove once told AB that poetry literally saved his life. (See SN's "Poetry Will Save Your Life" (2019) for an ironic take on this phenomenon in the medical context).

Let us return to the issue of how unprepared doctors may be for dealing with emotional flux or catharsis in their selves and in their patients (who naturally present with anxiety). Lyric poetry specialises in quality of engagement with affect, whereas conventional medical education sets out not to put medical students in touch with their feelings, but to educate for a particularly stringent separation of the professional self from the emotional self (Bleakley

2020). There are good reasons for this. If a medical student is to face suffering, disease and death, she must maintain a professional distance between these expressions of persons (as patients) and how this touches her emotionally. The latter, it is argued, must be controlled rather than expressed, suspended rather than cultivated. This is exacerbated through medical students learning how to objectify their patients as diseases rather than persons. This keeps potentially disruptive emotional invasions at arm's length. Emotions can infect medical judgement and professional relationships.

This is the opposite of what a psychotherapist learns in her education, such as the range and possibilities of catharsis, just as a musician learns expression through tone, melody and interpretation. The difference with her education and that of the medical student is that she learns how to "manage" emotions and catharsis, or the release of emotions, rather than to repress them or keep them at a distance. She discovers that cathartic experiences yield insights that cannot be obtained rationally. There is a sophisticated educational approach at play here. Affect release or catharsis requires parallel "free attention" to be at play so that one is not drowned by the cathartic episode. She gains expertise in emotional flux.

Philosophers such as Richard Rorty and Martha Nussbaum collapse emotion and feeling such as compassion and pity into one state as a ground for moral and political value judgements. Psychologists, however, have long distinguished emotions from feelings on the basis of location. Emotions are grounded in bodily forms and their metaphorical offshoots (gut wrenching, sickening, heartening), where feelings are grounded in the conscious working through of these bodily states (catharsis). The best unit of analysis for emotions is bodily site (literal or metaphorical), where the best unit of analysis for feelings is behavioural expression (catharsis). John Heron (2001) makes a useful distinction between emotion and feeling. Emotion is raw and direct, where feeling is more cultivated as the apprehension and education of emotional life through psychological reflection and insight. Here, we don't drown in our tears or "lose it" in our anger; we don't impulsively act out erotic charge. Catharsis is not simply venting feelings (from belly laughter to howling with grief, and from the quiet smile of satisfaction to a lingering sadness) but gaining subsequent insight through aware release. Doctors have chosen a stressful occupation, but it strikes us as contributory that the stress should be exacerbated in their education rather than drawn on as a resource. Poetry engages this resource.

We can see this slantwise in the work of William Carlos Williams. In the poem "A Cold Front" (1939) (https://www.poetryfoundation.org/poetrymagazine/browse?contentId=22429), Williams describes a house call to a woman "with a dead face" and,

> seven foster children
> and a new baby of her own in
> spite of that.

The enjambed line suddenly falling away from "in" to "spite" speaks volumes about how Williams grasps the essence of the woman's conflict. She doesn't want any more children and asks Williams for abortion pills. The father(s) of the children are notably absent from the poem. Williams describes her as like a cat in the treetops "on a limb too tired to go higher // from its tormentors" while in the background "the baby chortles in its spit". Then there is a tender moment: "a dull flush / almost of beauty to the woman's face", the face that had previously been "dead". His heart goes out to her: "In a case like this I know / quick action is the main thing". No wonder the poem is entitled "A Cold Front" because the woman can do no other than to put on a cold front. She is beaten by life, frozen out from exhaustion, apprehension and fear. Here, Williams's decisions as doctor and poet are aligned, where the poetic imagination and the medical mind are bedmates. The heart as much as the mind engages the patient, but more, also writes the prescription. The episode speaks of cathartic-engagement-to-come, a horizon of feeling. The woman has shut off and grown cold. Williams warms to her situation. Having decided to engage in "quick action" there is no doubt that the woman will thaw and break down.

Medical students are shaped by traditions that privilege factual biomedical knowledge, but this is now balanced by approaches to ethics, communication and professionalism that stress the importance of the single, unique patient and her lifeworld. Further, where closed, linear models of science explore isolated body systems and demand reduction of ambiguity, open adaptive and complex systems thinking invites high tolerance for ambiguity. Here, we think rather in terms of a patient's "embodiment" in a context rather than just "the body" as abstraction. These approaches are now being adopted in a new wave of medical education (Bleakley, Bligh and Browne 2011; Bleakley 2014).

Despite these positive shifts in medical education, their very nature exposes an enduring and serious flaw – again that of a lack of attention to medical students' and junior doctors' emotional or feeling states culminating in poor understanding of, and working with, catharsis. Unlike psychotherapists, doctors are not educated in the main to understand and work with the movement between potentially swamping catharsis (release of emotions) and free attention (the ability to reflect on emotion as it happens); through fear of being swamped by feeling states, emotional lability is then denied, repressed, distorted, and rationalised (Heron 1977). Poorly managed emotional states, rather than their educated (and not raw) expression, can lead to accumulative stress and breakdown.

Medicine (outside of psychiatry) has failed to fully address the emotional vicissitudes of the inter-subjective abject – what a patient's suffering means in interpersonal terms. Illness inherently disturbs identities, creating scenes and territories of "abjection", or what is most feared, disliked or terrible (Kristeva 1982). Doctors and patients must occupy this space simultaneously in mutual understanding of the emotional movement that is catharsis. This requires intensive dialogue and the parallel exercise of a dialogic imagination (Bakhtin 1981). There is a particular art form that specialises in occupying this space "without any irritable reaching after fact & reason" as John Keats defined "negative capability" and that, again, is poetry. The power of the poet is to not simply tolerate ambiguity in states of desire and feeling, but to cultivate this as specialty and to give it forms of expression. Poetry is essentially cathartic. Lyric poetry is the ideal medium through which tangled episodes of care embracing emotional flux and cathartic possibilities can be illuminated.

Tolerance of ambiguity embracing empathy

Like metaphors, tolerance of ambiguity is central to both the poetic imagination and the medical mind at work, and is discussed in depth in later chapters, so we will not tarry here. We close this section with a metaphor involving ambiguity. We do not think that the intimate relationships between the poetic imagination, drawing on lyric, and the medical mind as it works particularly in imaginative and engaging consultations and subsequent diagnoses, can be understood fully without applying complexity theory as an informing framework. The doctor and the poem both act as attractors, pulling effects into being rather than directly causing them. They are the lights towards which the moth is inevitably drawn. The patient visits the doctor and the reader visits the poem because they may benefit; effects are then pulled into being as a result of this attraction. As the doctor diagnoses and the poem exerts an attractor effect, lives are changed mainly for the better. Medicine can act as an attractor for poetry, and poetry as an attractor for medicine. The mutual exchange can be life changing. Attractors again pull effects into being rather than cause them.

Beauty or form (qualities)

Because beauty is in many ways the point of poetry, we're going to linger with this one a while. This section will complicate beauty as aporetic, for when we shake out beauty some darkness falls, partly as the sublime (comprehensively dealt with by the Romantics) and partly beauty's "surplus" as penumbra or mood (dealt with by the deconstructionists).

But we begin briefly with beauty as epiphany (the appearance of Aphrodite in Greek myth) and as self-negation (Narcissus falling in love with his own image). Archetypal Psychology (Hillman 1975) deals with these themes as they offer a background to clinical work in psychotherapies, medicine and healthcare. We can take the major archetypal theme that the soul or imagination (whatever nourishes the person as extra-personal) is buoyed by epiphanies, and we return to our claim that medicine is, dutifully, epiphanic in its devotion to the traditions of Greek Asclepius (Latin Aesculapius), the god of medicine. The god had one rod entwined with a single snake. The traditional (historical) symbolism for healing is almost certainly the epiphanic moment of the snake shedding its skin and growing a new one, taken as the moment of healing and turning a corner to recovery for the patient.

We are reminded here of Williams's encounter with the destitute mother who is about to be brought into beauty's light by the doctor's heartfelt pity. Williams notices "a dull flush / almost of beauty to the woman's face" where previously she had been frightened and "cold" like a cat needing to be rescued. An epiphany of Aphrodite is described in myth as immanence in the world of sense – both a sensibility and sensitivity – the core of a relationship-centred medicine that favours Homeric heartfelt "pity" over the modern instrumental term "empathy" (Marshall and Bleakley 2012). This is at the core of Bahar Orang's poetry that we discuss a little more below, where her main themes are manifestation and occlusion of beauty within an aesthetic medicine. The shadow side to this is embodied in Narcissus, as the negation of humility. Modern medicine, a stereotyped surgery in particular, has often displayed a hubristic and narcissistic bent that strays from beauty because objects and practices are reduced to their raw instrumental forms, and repeated as mirror images (the object is never developed sensually). It takes poetry to develop the sensual qualities of objects. Psychology has therapeutic antidotes for this habit of reductionism to mirror image. We don't necessarily recommend using poetry as therapy, but we do like the idea that poetry provides the alternative mirrors of epiphany and the hall of mirrors of qualities (size of mirror is secondary).

Bahar Orang's (2020) *Where Things Touch: A Meditation on Beauty* calls "beauty" (the concept) an "aporia", an internal contradiction that cannot be resolved. Again, let's leave that work for canny philosophers such as Crispin Sartwell, discussed below. Orang continues "And then there is your beauty". We like the use of the mirror of the Other to cancel narcissistic gazing. When it comes to specifics such as the flames and cold embers of passions gained and lost, the poet can step in. Beauty in intimacy is transferred quietly to the intimacy of attending at a birth:

> The OB guides my hand inside our open patient so
> that that my palm is pressed against uterus: smooth,
> warm, alive.

Then, "she releases the baby from its shelter // ... – ugly sweet, / and writhing". Orang looks into the eyes of the newborn "... who, it seems to me, must be queer as / sunlight seeking every empty space ...". Oddly, the mother is bracketed out, only addressed in the third person ("our open patient", "this woman") but the baby, simultaneously "ugly sweet", is greeted with an open honesty in first gasp, a moment of surprise ("strange bundle"), and then an overwhelming intimacy:

> Good morning
> first morning, sweet babe. I have books heavier than
> you.

… here we are – basking in the afterwardness of the
day's events, like two sparrows studying the forest,
picking broken branches after a storm.

Beauty works here by multiple transpositions, meaning: the transfer of affect
entirely from mother to newborn as if Orang had become the mother herself; the transfer of scene from delivery room to imagined forest; the transfer of weather from storm to calm; and of affect from the uncertainties of
"first gasp" and "surprise" to a "basking", even making that strange choice
of term "afterwardness" seem familiar. "Afterwardness" (*nachträglichkeit*) was
first coined by Freud to explain the moment of insight a patient has into
the realisation of how early trauma affects current psychological life and its
symptoms. It describes a kind of "catching up" on events. The baby's birth
is already a trauma but Orang allows her and the baby to "bask" in its after-
math. Poetry has become this baby's cradle and, perhaps, the poet's analytic
couch.

The Iranian-born, UK-based poet Mimi Khalvati (2019) entitled her series
of sonnets "Afterwardness" – to describe recollections recovered that make
deep impacts on personality. An 11-year-old boy from Aleppo develops a
"thousand yard stare" in the face of bombing. But "through the long tunnel
of that gaze" the boy recalls, "a yard, a pond and pine trees that surround …"
as a counter to his trauma. The gaze of Williams's frozen-by-fear patient too
was a "thousand yard stare", a gaze through a "tunnel" until Williams helped
mitigate future trauma a little by providing a prescription for an abortion pill.
Freud's "afterwardness" must be extended from prescription to prediction,
prognosis, the full arc of the medical encounter. Khalvati writes of poetry
as the work of gestation in which the subsequent birth is always a surprise"
"Poetry startled me awake last night" with "Stray lines, excited to be up so
late". And on beauty, Khalvati is gnomic: "Everything seems too beautiful to
grasp. I don't know what to feel, other than yearning".

We can get at beauty in medicine by the back door – by saying what a
beautiful, lyrical medicine is not. A lyrical medicine embraces the aesthetic,
or sensitises, where an instrumental medicine can an-aesthetise or dull. A lyrical medicine engages the elegant, inspiring, imaginative, animated, digni-
fied, graceful, sensitive, distinctive, passionate and expressive. In contrast, an
instrumental medicine interested in function rather than form, and in quantities rather than qualities, may be uninspired, flat, unimaginative, ungracious,
clumsy, insensitive, tiresome, numbing, restricted and even ugly. But, while
medicine has embraced ethics, it has little time for aesthetics, preferring again
what can be more easily applied. But what is left behind on the road to easy,
competence-based instrumentalisation?

For those inculcated in the rites of biomedicine, the word "beauty" still
niggles, loaded as it is with Romantic notions of "high art". We appreciate
the symmetry of such a resistance with the kind of critique that might come
from a more progressive political quarter which would charge that "beauty"
is intimately connected with class structures and power, as Jacques Rancière's
(2013) extensive work on the historical engagement of aesthetics with politics

shows. The philosopher Crispin Sartwell (2006) addresses this complex issue of beauty through cross-cultural comparison, looking at six "names" of beauty from six cultures that educate us to tolerate differing perspectives on how we gauge "quality". An overview hardly does justice to Sartwell's ideas and his elegant prose, but we hope readers will follow up the reference.

Sartwell reminds us that defining our terms is important. In English, *beauty* characteristically encompasses an object of longing or desire and is often ascribed to physical appearance and character. In Hebrew, *Yapha* describes glow, bloom or efflorescence: beauty as growth and expression. In Sanskrit, *Sundara* describes beauty as holiness, a spiritual state of ecstasy, or transcendent identity. In Greek, *To Kalon* describes an ideal, or an idea of perfection, the model of beauty that Romantics claimed, where beauty equates to truth. In contrast, in Japanese *Wabi-Sabi* describes necessary imperfection, the beauty of the designed or accidental flaw in objects. In personal character this is humility, and in relationships beauty is cultivated as shyness embodied in the sensual and erotic glance. In Navajo, *Hozho* describes health and harmony as a way of life, an aesthetic of balance rather than character, where beauty is all embracing and all consuming. Without invoking beauty, a blanket, a gesture, a friendship, the preparation of a medicinal herb, or a ceremony is lifeless, empty of meaning. Beauty then is marked differently across cultures where all expressions, says Sartwell, should be embraced.

Lisa Samuels (1997: 1) defines Beauty in terms of a process of scaffolding of ideas, where: "Beauty wedges into the artistic space a structure for continuously imagining what we do not know". We might gloss this, or rephrase it, as continuously imagining what we cannot know. Beauty is as explicit as it is implicit. It is bold and exclamatory as it is under erasure (~~beauty~~) or a condition of surplus (unexplained and inexplicable beauty, as awe). Rather than interpellation into an ideology of "narrative knowing", could doctors in consultations with patients, with each other and with other healthcare professionals, not "wedge" into that same "artistic space" that invents in the absence of knowing? In other words, the conjuring of Beauty is surely the poetic imagination at work. Here, what is important is what we do not as yet know, a horizon of understanding or a "supplement", to borrow from Jacques Derrida (1967). Here, we are back also to surplus – what we do not and cannot know about beauty that, nevertheless, impresses itself on as yearning, or desire. Beauty too is a Black Box that our habits exclude or keep at arm's length.

Samuels (1997: 1) continues, "Beauty is therefore endlessly talk-inspiring, predictive rather than descriptive, dynamic rather than settled, infinitely serious and useful". Note an important about-face: beauty is predictive and open, just as it is pragmatic and useful. Beauty does not just inspire, it "works", is labour. Stephanie Burt (2019) suggests that the best way to get your head and heart around poetry and its wide remit and stylistic concerns, is to compare it to music and its genres, styles, and range. Poetry can be classical, jazz, crooning, folk and country, show, pop, electronic, hip-hop, or grime. Poetic lyricism is born in ancient Greek song focussed on the vicissitudes of feelings.

Wallace Stevens described music as "feeling" rather than "sound". In the same vein, while a doctor-patient encounter obviously embraces technical knowledge and insight, its overriding feature is surely one of affect. The patient's emotional response overrides immediate understanding of the diagnosis, and the sensitive doctor's engagement with the patient depends on attunement and response to this emotional flux.

For Samuels (1997), poetry as relationship between writer and reader can be defined as "subjective interestedness". This also defines the patient-doctor engagement. Samuels continues: "Interestedness requires sympathy, so poetic beauty might be defined as the result of subjective sympathy: paying enough attention to a poem for it to teach us how to read it and (crucially) feeling that it fulfils the terms it lays out. ... This is not to say that all poems are beautiful".

That last warning is important. Poems need not do anything at all, but some can strike terror into the heart of their readers just as they can leave them cold. Let us linger on Samuels's description above and translate it into the clinical encounter. The doctor must display "subjective interestedness" requiring "sympathy". An encounter with a patient demands attention to "lyricism, word attention, sound dissonance, even of a faltering which is part of the poem's point" (ibid.), or the patient speaking through a first-hand account of symptoms. We recognise neither poetry nor medicine as panacea, but we do claim that in either field, one does have to take care (of patient, colleagues, and self).

Orientation to here-and-now space and place rather than there-and-then time

Our final category returns us to poetry's primary concern with space and place as opposed to narrative's primary concern with time. We are reminded again of Bakhtin's neologism "chronotope" that collapses time and space into a single instant, but are suspicious that this drives away the particular qualities of "place" sans time: the exact moment of death and the withdrawal of light in Emily Dickinson's poem; the living space of the woman with the frozen stare and the "cold front" in Williams's poem; the balcony of the hotel room in Rachel Long's poem; Anne Sexton's momentary and masturbatory marriage to her bed; Peter Redgrove's interior of the apple; Bahar Orang's account of a birth as "sunlight seeking every empty space", and so forth, all "fields".

Doctors will see a beauty in symptom and in configurations of diagnoses that patients might take as insulting where the content is illness and suffering, but this is the nature of medical curiosity that feeds on the beauties of illnesses as it seeks remedies in other beauties. Medicine is again aesthetic work, making sense of form. Importantly, the clinical encounter may not be best explored as a narrative gaze even where it deals with spatial scene rather than temporal unfolding of plot. Such scenes may be functional – an instrumental frame (focussing purely on symptom presentation) rather than a positioning of observations (focussing on the context for symptom). Here, doctors need to cultivate *a sense of interiority* rather than superiority (translating the patient's story into medical capital), and focus on place and space rather than temporality – to enter their patients' psychosomatic houses as guests, and strike up inquisitive conversations about the expressions and meanings of their symptoms.

In the safety of the doctor's clinic, a house call can still be made in psychological space. This medical imaginary is not on the conventional undergraduate curriculum. Its primary text is Gaston Bachelard's (1964) *The Poetics of Space*, a phenomenology of small or tight spaces – cupboards, corridors and so forth. This offers a counter to anatomy texts that merely map the body's interior space with articulating parallel human experiences of inhabiting, studying or treating those spaces. Lisa Samuels (above) describes "an aesthetics of intensity", an apt descriptor for a medicine of qualities that revolves around tight spaces – a collapsed lung, a furred artery, an overcrowded operating theatre, an Intensive Care Unit during the height of Covid, the shelves of a pharmacy.

John Burnside (2019) calls 20th-century lyric poetry "the music of time". But we think it is better called the music of place. Ed Casey (2013) notes that in Western philosophy, interest in time engulfed interest in space, while interest in space engulfed interest in place. As noted, lyric poetry specialises in intensity or concentrated moments, and is characterised by being indifferent to time or its (re)constructed unfolding arc. We are in step with Bainard Cowan (2012: 2) who says that time is the "enemy" of, and "threat" to, lyricism. "Lyric", says Cowan (ibid.: 5), celebrates "the place where human nature encounters immortality". Immortality is the moment in place, the gasp, and the recovery of sight.

Cowan goes further than heroic medicine when arguing that immortality is the apex of beauty as enduring resplendence of the world, the paused moment that is exquisitely and intensively examined, articulated, dissected, deeply sensed and emotively engaged. In conclusion, let us pause medicine for a moment and ask whether the qualities of great poetry can be borrowed by traditional medicine. In the best of poetry, time stands still and, in the moment, the words knock your socks off. Chugging along in the clinics, hectically, frantically and antically attempting to batten down everyone's hatches in the most reductive of checklist styles, let's pause that medicine, our medicine, has now stopped, completely, and there is just space to look at and perceive. How strange it is that you can see humans here. What they are doing seems to matter less than where they are, and how they are there. This is a beautiful kind of medicine that needs to steal the socks of the run-off-its-feet kind.

References

Adcock B. 2008. *Slantwise: Poems*. Baton Rouge, LA: LSU Press.
Albarran J. The Language of Chest Pain. *Nursing Times*. 2002; 98: 38.

Bachelard G. 1964. *The Poetics of Space.* New York: Orion Press.

Bakhtin M. 1981. *The Dialogic Imagination Four Essays.* Austin: University of Texas Press.

Berger J. 2016/1967. *A Fortunate Man: The Story of a Country Doctor.* Edinburgh: Canongate.

Bleakley A. 2014. *Patient-Centred Medicine in Transition: The Heart of the Matter.* Dordrecht: Springer.

Bleakley A. 2017a. *Thinking with Metaphors in Medicine: The State of the Art.* Abingdon: Routledge.

Bleakley A. Force and Presence in the World of Medicine. *Healthcare.* 2017b; 53: 58.

Bleakley A. 2020. *Educating Doctors' Senses through the Medical Humanities: "How Do I Look?".* Abingdon: Routledge.

Bleakley A, Bligh J. Who Can Resist Foucault? *The Journal of Medicine and Philosophy.* 2009; 34: 368–83.

Bleakley A, Bligh J, Browne J. 2011. *Medical Education for the Future: Identity, Power and Location.* Dordrecht: Springer.

Burnside J. 2019. *The Music of Time: Poetry in the Twentieth Century.* London: Profile Books.

Burt S. 2019. *Don't Read Poetry.* New York: Basic Books.

Casey E. 2013. *The Fate of Place: A Philosophical History.* Oakland: University of California Press.

Cowan B. (ed.) 2012. *The Prospect of Lyric.* Dallas, TX: Dallas Institute.

Dalby A. 2006. *Rediscovering Homer: Inside the Origins of the Epic.* New York: WW Norton.

Deleuze G, Guattari F. 2004a. *A Thousand Plateaus.* London: Continuum.

Deleuze G, Guattari F. 2004b. *Anti-Oedipus.* London: Continuum.

Demarco S. 2020. Doctor-Poets Search for the Right Words to Help Patients Heal. Los Angeles Times, March 11. Retrieved from https://www.latimes.com/science/story/2020-03-11/column-one-doctor-poets).

Derrida J. 1967. *Of Grammatology.* Baltimore, MD: Johns Hopkins University Press.

Foucault M. 1976. *The Birth of the Clinic: An Archaeology of Medical Perception.* London: Routledge.

Greene R. (Ed.) 2012. *The Princeton Encyclopaedia of Poetry & Poetics,* 4th ed. Princeton, NJ: Princeton University Press.

Hawkins AH. Literature, Medical Ethics, and "Epiphanic Knowledge." *Journal of Clinical Ethics.* 1994; 5: 286.

Heron J. 1977. *Catharsis in Human Development.* Guildford: University of Surrey. Retrieved from http://www.human-inquiry.com/catharsi.htm

Heron J. 2001. *Helping the Client – A Creative Practical Guide,* 5th ed. London: Sage.

Hillman J. 1975. *Re-Visioning Psychology.* New York: Harper and Row.

Jorm C, Roberts C. Using Complexity Theory to Guide Medical School Evaluations. *Academic Medicine.* 2018; 93: 399–405.

Jullien F. 2000. *Detour and Access: Strategies of Meaning in China and Greece.* New York: Zone Books.

Khalvati M. 2019. *Afterwardness.* Manchester: Carcanet.

Kirmeyer LJ. The Body's Insistence on Meaning: Metaphor as Presentation and Representation in Illness Experience. *Medical Anthropology Quarterly.* 1992; 6: 323–46.

Kristeva J. 1982. *Powers of Horror: An Essay on Abjection.* New York: Columbia University Press.

Long R. 2020. *My Darling from the Lions.* London: Picador.

Marshall R, Bleakley A. 2012. *Rejuvenating Medical Education: Seeking Help from Homer.* Newcastle-Upon-Tyne: Cambridge Scholars.

Neilson S. Pain as Metaphor: Metaphor and Medicine. *Medical Humanities.* 2016; 42: 3–10.

Neilson S. 2019a. The Practice of Metaphor. In: A Bleakley (ed.) *The Routledge Companion to the Medical Humanities.* Abingdon: Routledge, 144–54.

Neilson S. Poetry Will Save Your Life. *Canadian Family Physician.* 2019b; 65: 820–22.

Orang B. 2020. *Where Things Touch: A Meditation on Beauty.* Toronto: Book*Hug.

Post J. 2015. *A Thickness of Particulars: The Poetry of Anthony Hecht.* Oxford: Oxford University Press.

Rancière J. 2013. *The Politics of Aesthetics.* London: Bloomsbury Academic.

Ratzan RM. Winged Words and Chief Complaints: Medical Case Histories and the Parry-Lord Oral-Formulaic Tradition. *Literature and Medicine.* 1992; 11: 94–114.

Redgrove P. 2012. *Collected Poems.* London: Cape.

Samuels L. Introduction to Poetry and the Problem of Beauty. *Modern Language Studies.* 1997; 27: 1–7.

Sartwell C. 2006. *Six Names of Beauty.* New York: Routledge.

Saunders G. 2021. *A Swim in a Pond in the Rain: In Which Four Russians Give a Master Class on Writing, Reading, and Life.* London: Bloomsbury.

Stevens W. 1951. *The Necessary Angel: Essays on Reality and the Imagination.* London: Faber & Faber.

Turner F. 2012: Lyric and the Self. In: B Cowan (ed.) *The Prospect of Lyric.* Dallas, TX: Dallas Institute, 359–77.

Verghese A. 1999. *The Tennis Partner.* New York: HarperCollins.

Verghese A. 2009. *Cutting for Stone.* London: Chatto & Windus.

Verghese A. Medicine, Literature and the Power of Epiphany. UCLA Center for India and South Asia. November 12, 2013. Retrieved from https://www.international.ucla.edu/southasia/article/134973

9 Poeticising with a medical imagination

What medicine can do for poetry

Where reductive biomedicine is information not wisdom, and where it fails to feed poetry

Poetry about medicine is called *iatroversalia*. We have a concern that such medicine-sourced work may only offer poetry scraps and not a decent meal, placing poetry in the position of having to make up for medicine's deficit. An example can be gleaned from John Keats in the role of surgeon trainee describing the heart in purely reduced, descriptive terms as having four cavities (the informational eye) – "4 Cavaties surrounded by muscular fibres" (Ghosh 2017: 35), yet when writing about love and the heart, abstracted from medicine (https://www.poetryfoundation.org/poems/50375/this-living-hand-now-warm-and-capable) Keats says,

> This living hand, now warm and capable
> Of earnest grasping, would, if it were cold
> And in the icy silence of the tomb,
> So haunt thy days and chill thy dreaming nights
> That thou would wish thine own heart dry of blood
> So in my veins red life might stream again,
> And thou be conscience-calm'd—see here it is—
> I hold it towards you.

This fragment was one of Keats's last pieces of writing before his death. From our perspective, here is a transfusion/donor metaphor: "you would drain your heart dry for me" he seems to say to his lover or friend, on his death-bed suffering from tuberculosis. Our use of it here is to illustrate that Keats could not effectively join medicine and poetry, where he had to ditch the former for the latter. Poetry pressed harder than medicine. Of course, they are damn hard to get into conversation where anatomy wants to drain away the better heart metaphors, reducing it to pump, machine or information (but we must remind ourselves of technical descriptors that remain poetic and invoke pathos, such as "hole in the heart"). Here, we are back to the core of Object-Oriented Ontology (Harman 2018): the heart benefits (develops,

DOI: 10.4324/9781003194408-11

is made more sensuous) where it is put into relationship with another object that brings out its beauty (love, passion). This, of course, is how metaphors work. One thing is compared to another such that a larger than life, more sensuous image is formed: "The heart has its reasons which reason knows nothing of ... We know the truth not only by the reason, but by the heart" (Blaise Pascal).

Keats is saying that he wants to nourish a relationship through transfusion of love. What we want to do in this chapter is look at how medicine can nourish and shape poetry through reciprocal love, or shared passion. Some poets, doctors among them, love medicine in this way, of course; but, where medicine does not reciprocate, we suspect that they are often milking a dry cow in the main, eking out nourishment for poetry more in hope than expectation.

We draw on T.S. Eliot's distinction between "information" and "wisdom" to develop our argument that we need an adventurous wise medicine, rather than a reductive one that seeks to remain within the safe boundary of information. In 'Choruses from "the Rock"' (https://www.poetrynook.com/poem/choruses-%C3%B4%C3%A7%C2%A3the-rock%C3%B4%C3%A7%C3%B8) (a poem within a play), T.S. Eliot says,

> Where is the wisdom we have lost in knowledge?
> Where is the knowledge we have lost in information?

Recall from Chapter 7 that this is how an Object-Oriented Ontology works: Information is the object-in-itself. Once paired with its enhancing partner knowledge, there is an aesthetic transformation. Information grows wings and aspires to wisdom. Objects flower in relation one to the other. The stone reveals its stoniness.

This may seem obvious to the reader – who would not want an enhanced and rich medicine that is not purely informational, as biomedicine? More, who would welcome a similar pedagogic reductionism in medical education (to training, skills, and competences)? Yet medical education can be seen to regularly draw on almost anti-poetic strategies of educating for insensibility and insensitivity by closing down students' feeling states, deflecting catharsis and refusing lability of emotional life. Students are asked rather to maintain a frontstage "professionalism" in which repression or sublimation of feeling is central (Bleakley 2020). This produces a culture in which many doctors have difficulty in approaching their work therapeutically or psychologically, again in dealing with affect through catharsis and insight. An outcome of such psychological naivety – doctors unable to turn a psychotherapeutic lens on their own work – is high rates of anxiety and burnout (Peterkin and Bleakley 2016).

Poetry welcomes and feeds a more sophisticated approach to the lability and expression of feeling and the shaping of subsequent insights from catharsis. We suggest that to think and feel this way in the consultation, a

diagnostic-affective approach of close noticing, is already engaging and feeding the poetic imagination, taking the weight of responsibility for the "art"
of medicine off poetry's shoulders as compensatory feed-in.

Medicine expanded to a lyrical form can provide a transfusion for poetry,
saying, "look this is how we do our job and expand our culture; is this not
substance for your art and medicine, and for your maintenance of health?" The
object of medicine tied to the object of poetry creates an object-orientation
of aesthetic possibilities, one feeding the other, again. Poetry's body can then
be nourished and expanded by drawing on a developed medicine, rather than
an impoverished variety where, again, poetry is constantly compromised and
stretched by having to act as a supplement to, emotional voice for, or alternative to the medical imagination. Poetry is more than an "equal partner";
poetry is the dominant partner. Not recognising this fact is why there is so
much tired or burned-out poetry in medical/health humanities circles: it is
bearing an unnecessary weight of responsibility for maintaining the vigour
of medicine itself.

Here is a poem by a medical student (anonymised), refreshingly honest,
if unimaginative, in its title: "I demand you consider us humans: A medical
student poem" (2017, from the KevinMD website: https://www.kevinmd.
com/blog/2017/01/demand-consider-us-humans-medical-student-poem.
html). From dozens that we might have picked out, this was our first hit. It
advertises our point.

> Slave, I am not
> Servant, I may be
>
> Arrogant, I am not
> Ignorant, I may be
>
> Un-engaged, I am not
> However, Quiet, I may be.
>
> Your coat is long, mine short
> Your knowledge mile deep, mine mile wide
> You have seen 100 patients this week, I have seen 10
> You trained for 10 years, this is my first
>
> If I look scared, it's because I am
> If I seem intimidated, I indeed am
> If I appear confused, I in fact am
> If I show up tired and exhausted, I really am
>
> I accept my role as a student
> I am satisfied with it
> I wake up at 4 a.m. every morning

I put a smile on my face

I worry about my patients
I want to invest in their care
I do not wish their misery to be wasted
I want to learn from their suffering

I only ask,
You accept your role as an educator
You take pride in the opportunity to shape young minds
You understand you are enriching future doctors
You realize we will treat you, your children, and your grandchildren
You invest in turning us into clinicians, not technicians
You encourage us to engage our minds, and think critically

Finally, I demand
You know that I am a person
You respect us as team members
You consider us humans
You treat us with respect

We understand the sentiment where this is an apologia. It is unclear if the poem is simply generally descriptive of the relatively powerless being of the student, or if it points to a specific oppressor. We also understand that the poem is a cathartic or personal-confessional opportunity. Our primary question is: if the student were making a diagnosis, or offering some biomedical insight while presenting a case, would the technical latitude that is allowed for this poem be extended to his or her medicine? We think not. There are poetic elements for sure, for it is too easy to pick a completely egregious case, just as that is true for any "bad case" of art. We choose a poor example, not a disastrous one. In the poem, a relational field is made, and there a rhythm is established in the opening stanzas, but it is quickly lost. The poem is technically inept and frankly dull as it abandons its opening premise of contrast, becoming a unidirectional complaint that floats lazy abstraction rather than doing the work of imagery. This is a reflective narrative cut up into lines with stilted diction, an absence of adjectival zest, and a lack of awareness of the necessity of metaphor.

The poem lacks imagination. How could it aesthetically resolve its conflict other than through its direct statement? Worse, the poem comes disguised as liberator, but acts as assassin of language. We are aware that we, acting in the role of critics, are mirroring the critical eye of the senior doctor, the very object of the poem's attention. But the poem was put in the public domain, and we are the public, reading the poem (critically) as poem and not as student's logbook.

Medicine has fed into this first year medical student's poem as an object aching for aesthetic treatment (the student's passion is for an engaged medicine), but the poetry-object is not aesthetically formed and so cannot provide the means of expansion for the first object. It may strike readers as gauche for some supposed authority to say, "This is a bad poem", but we revel in the act for it is one not done enough in public medical humanities spaces. There is no good that can come from poetry branded as such when it is published in this form. Poetry that is dead will accomplish nothing other than perpetuate poetry's invalidation in medical culture. In this respect we eye the many medical humanities journals that publish poems no better, and often worse, than the one we've reprinted here.

We want medicine, in doing its own thing properly – and we would accept a competent poetry only, as a standard of poetic care – to provide a readymade substrate for poetic invention. This student, lumbered with informational medicine, has no platform with which to expand that object and so is a fish out of water, flapping. To feed poetry, rather than rely on poetry's charity, medicine must move its base from Eliot's "information" to "wisdom". Poetry is fed up with trying to make art solely from medicine's "information", but it also can't make art from medicine's information if poems like these are not recognised as – shall we be Charonian here? – lacking in "poetic competence".

If we return to Eliot's questions, "Where is the wisdom we have lost in knowledge? / Where is the knowledge we have lost in information?", this should offer caution against reduction in both medicine and poetry to paucity of form. If our direction of travel is from poetry to medicine, we may be able to lift medicine as object into aesthetic worth if our poetry is good enough. This student's was not, and that is unfortunate, because tutoring in the discipline may have given a kick-start to a better, revised poem with the same strong intentions. If our direction of travel is from medicine to poetry, we do not want the lumber of an informational medicine. So what is a cultured medicine that can readily feed poetry? This is medical education's challenge – to educate, and not train, doctors who are wisdom carriers, who have outgrown competence and nourish capability or the unfolding of potential: lyrical doctors. So first, what medicine can do for poetry is be more attentive to the use of poetry in medicine by calling for a better standard of work. Read good doctor-poets – we provide plenty of examples in this book.

Chapped hands sift greasy suds: the domestic interior of community medicine

We urge you to read poets too who stand in for healthcare workers, by making "general case" interventions about issues such as poverty and deprivation (major causes of ill-health). Elise Partridge – in "Domestic Interior: Child Watching Mother" – offers a domestic scene that can be read as poet in the guise of family doctor or social worker (https://howapoemmoves. wordpress.com/2016/10/27/domestic-interior-child-watching-mother-by-elise-partridge/). The poem leapfrogs a biomedical diagnosis moving from information through knowledge to wisdom. Partridge cannily uses an observant child as if making a physical examination (as a good family therapist would), scrutinising the body and emotional leakage of her mother, whose

> Chapped hands sift greasy suds.
> She can't make rent. Quietly,
> she's crying again.

Then, "Vessels tip in the rack" just as the mother's emotions tip. Through the eyes of the child: "Each night I watch her eyes / to make sure they keep drying". The mother is likened to the plates in the rack – all she needs is a rinse, but the child knows better. Partridge uses alliteration (on the "a" and the "s") – "Chapped hands sift greasy suds" – to underscore the wear and tear that domestic chores can bring. The woman's stress is echoed in the poem's word stresses. The words are chapped through their work of stress.

Repetition hammers home the symptom: "She can't make rent / ... she's crying again". The poem's hook is a big metaphor to deepen the everyday to a mystery: "Vessels tip in the rack" – they must drain. So she drains and is drained, every night: "... I watch her eyes / to make sure they keep drying". There is some recovery. The vessels do dry. The mother dries out and then the tears start over. The child watches her mother with increasing worry. They're both trapped it seems. While the vessels dry out, the income has dried up: "She can't make rent". "Rent", of course, has a double meaning, not just what she pays but also a tearing or a making of a space through which she might escape or some illumination enters. The associations echo, where "tears" as crying imply a tear, rent, or rip in her being and life.

We can hear dissenting voices muttering, "how can poems about domestic interiors and the life of a hard-pressed single mother help us to teach medical students or do our jobs better as doctors?" Well, instrumentally speaking (yes, sometimes we do this), shifting our gaze from the hospital setting to health inequities and inequalities in the community is a necessary step for medical education and medicine as a whole to make (Bleakley 2021); preventative medicine must be a priority. The wisdom to be found here is that there is more in medicine than a symptomatology of illness, but rather a context of suffering.

Via Partridge, we have gone to poetry to illuminate a medical dilemma – not enough attention is paid to community care at a time when resources are oriented towards hospitalism, yet our major pressing health issues are grounded in social inequity and inequality (summed up beautifully in the image "Vessels tip in the rack" that has multiple resonance – we'd love to see this kind of language in the social worker's report). But we have only used the poem as mirror. We come back to a wisdom-based (in this case community wisdom) medicine feeding into an eager poetry that fattens on its issues. As such, we have symbiosis between medicine and poetry. What is happening in Partridge's piece is what we'd wish for the untutored bard of KevinMD above.

In the same passage where T.S. Eliot asks his famous paired questions – we hear them in our minds like scissors cutting – he also summarises the difference between the busy and scattered diagnostic minds of novices and the focussed minds of experts as a kind of Zen awareness, where novices may have both "knowledge of motion, but not of stillness" and "Knowledge of speech, but not of silence". Poets, resonating with Eliot, know only too well that finding the still point at the centre of the storm, fully inside the experience, yields satisfying poetry as the re-telling of incident in specifics. Look at the quiet stillness in Partridge's poem above: therein is the place from which to ponder the morality of the situation. We read into the stillness of this poem a medical silence, a dawning realisation that the future of medicine is one in which resources are shifted to community-based practices addressing structural issues, away from the "whiz-bang" medicine of hospital treatment (ibid.). As medicine grabs this bull by the horn, it may contribute to a poetry expressing social conscience and examining strategies for change. What Partridge does too is set off associations in the reader's mind: "vessels"=vassals, "rack"=wrack. The mother is on the rack and wracked, subordinated. Once we irrigate the poem it flowers into different meanings, of course.

Irrigating an otherwise arid EBM to see if it flowers

Medicine can irritate, or bring to expression, the critical facet of poetry and lyricism – just as the resting snake, constantly provoked, will strike out, maybe gobble its prey and thus expand its voice. Medicine can bring poetry out in a rash, but this is good. (A rash of poor poetry stimulated by medicine is not so good, and all too common as noted above). While we argue above that a rich, imaginative, expressive, lyrical medicine (Eliot's "wisdom") will feed an always-hungry body of poetry, there is an argument that poetry also waits to be provoked by the limitations of dry medicine. We follow the line of archetypal psychology that symptoms are not there just to be eradicated, but first must speak their lines or have voice (appreciation before explanation). Dialogue with symptoms (except, of course, acute, life-threatening, or dismally insistent) is prior to their fervent and heroic eradication (Hillman 1975).

Evidence-Based Medicine (EBM), considered as panacea, provides such an iatrogenic symptom, often eating away at the honest practices of dedicated doctors, constantly putting them on the rack that is the tension between the general case (population studies) and the individual patient (idiosyncratic presentation). We again follow the advice of archetypal psychology by asking the symptom what it wants, rather than trying to eradicate it (for EBM this is an impossibility in any case). One of us (SN) shows how a lyrical poetic eye can be used as a critical perspective to, ironically, expand the province of EBM rather than shrink it through humiliation as other critics have (Neilson 2021a, 2021b). Neilson wants to irrigate the arid EBM and see if it can flower. He exposes the limits to EBM from the point of view of its application to a family medicine context as "a data-rich lurch into the sideways". His compensatory position and means of expansion is "(T)hrough the lyric essay technique of juxtaposition and by employing lived experience in the narration". As the most primal form of medical reductionism, EBM feeds into the poetic imagination in this way so it is cooked, and emerges not as reject or waste matter but as substrate for medical practice that needs improvement through lyrical attention and reformulation. Again, we are feeding the body of medicine into poetry as a means for expansion.

We wonder if anybody has written a poem critically addressing EBM, or bringing its deficiencies home to roost? In the process of searching, we did come across the acronym POEMs – for "Patient-Oriented Evidence That Matters". The *American Family Physician* has published its top POEMs for the past three years (https://www.aafp.org/journals/afp/content/top-poems.html). We are amused that POEMs and medicine should meet this way, under the EBM banner and where poems have to disguise themselves so heavily! Beware – if you Google "poems and medicine" you might find yourself in this EBM thicket too. We wonder what an "Evidence Based Poetry" (EBP) might look like, where the "proof" of the poem is in its wisdom and not just its knowledge and information. One key aspect of such wisdom is creative metaphor generation.

Generating new metaphors

Metaphors can be coined in single words in relation to other words, that flower as ideas and images. Returning to Elise Partridge's sad domestic interior (that we take as a metaphor for poverty), see how single words multiply up meanings and associations by transfer: rent (as unaffordable payment and a tear), tear (as sadness and a hole in one's life), tip (as tipping over or emotional instability, and as gathering rubbish), rack (as drying out and as emotionally wracked), drain (as a place for drying things out literally and emotionally), and drying (literally with the mother's and daughter's plates, and becoming desiccate). She has so much on her plate. The domestic interior is a house of many associations (metonymic chains) and multiple meanings (metaphoric echoes) hinging on such a small store of words that collectively paint a picture of misery and breaking point. These multiplying image potentials are the evidence of poetry and an inevitable product of intense collapse of ideas, images and descriptors into a field of form. Singular metaphors generate pluralities.

Contra EBM, medicine can also bear gifts that feed into poetry such as the invention of new metaphors. Abraham Verghese (TEDMED Video: https://scopeblog.stanford.edu/2015/04/07/a-grand-romp-through-medicine-and-metaphor-with-abraham-verghese/) bemoans the lack of invention of metaphor in contemporary medicine as it has become more commodified and reductive or instrumental. The Covid pandemic has brought this home where doctors have had to resort to virtual consultations with their patients. Nicholas Pimlott (2020), a Canadian family physician, claims: "An in-person examination gives the physician a sense of true craftsmanship and inspires confidence in the patient". Pimlott extends the notion of medical craft using fly-fishing as an analogy:

> Catching a fish is like making a diagnosis – the skilled fly-fisher must have consummate skills in "history taking" (reading the water, understanding when the seasonal mayfly hatches are on and fish are feeding on them) and "physical examination" (powers of observation as to where fish lie, fly casting skills, and hooking, playing, landing and releasing the fish with care).

The point being that the craft of medicine and fly-fishing are both hands-on in essence. Virtual medicine, no matter how practical, is a distortion of the craft. Pimlott cites Verghese's worries about the decline of the physical examination.

In our contradictory, paradoxical fashion (the spirit of poetry, the rebellion against the rebellion) we suggest below that technology-driven medicine can, in fact, generate new metaphors and imagistic ways of thinking. Technological science can be poetic. From the point of view of the development of diagnostic languages as metaphoric and poetic, we can temper Verghese's and Pimlott's claims above. For example, here is Soldati and colleagues' (2019) description of ultrasound patterns of pulmonary oedema that we might see as poetic abduction informing diagnosis:

> A characteristic ultrasound picture of the hyperdense, non-consolidated superficial lung is sonographic interstitial syndrome (SIS): the presence of multiple focal, patched or diffuse vertical artifacts (B-lines) fanning out from the lung-wall interface. White lung, characterized by a granular and mostly white texture which starts at the pleura line and ends at the bottom of the screen, is also an aspect of SIS for some authors.

The metaphors, embracing technical descriptors, are striking: "hyperdense", "sonographic", "patched artefacts", and "white lung". Others are familiar, such as "interstitial" and "fanning out". Medicine then can offer poetry a metaphor horde after all. Developments in imaging – where ultrasound is at the low-tech end – offer one of medicine's most important scientific advances. Making the body transparent (there's a long-standing metaphor) through imaging (Dijk 2005) need not reduce the body to the status of Eliot's mere "information", it can also offer "wisdom", for imaging is already a kind of poetics masquerading as information and technical-rational reductive 'hands-off' medicine. In Chapter 6, we saw how a radiologist uses

Minimalist diction ("the undercut edges") and draws on metaphors ("apple core") to make a crisp (and brisk) diagnosis.

As new technologies develop in medicine and surgery, we return to their role in the generation of new metaphors thus again feeding poetry from within the body of medicine. For example, from an ethnographic study, the science anthropologist Rachel Prentice (2013: 188) describes teaching scenarios in surgical education, including the inventive "fieldwork" of looking at videotapes of minimally invasive shoulder arthroscopies. Prentice describes the focussed anatomical view as "like looking through a porthole at a red and white undersea floor with white tendrils undulating in the current". Further, "(T)he view made me mildly seasick". Will the surgical imagination match this or even conceive that it is entering poetic territory? Thinking metaphorically, Prentice herself turns anatomy into landscape painting and arthroscopy into undersea exploration.

In Prentice's study, Anna the surgeon says, "This is his humeral head and there's just a lot of arthritis, a lot of fibrillation" (as formation of fibres). She identifies "messy white tissue descending into the image frame as the rotator cuff tear". Anna then describes the tissue as "falling in our face" (ibid.: 191), an embodied metaphor, tissue as morbid snowflakes or interior air pollution. (A metaphor because the tissue is not literally falling in anyone's face – it is on camera, and actually a nuisance for the surgeon as it temporarily blocks her view. But it signals that the surgeon, in keyhole surgery mode, is morphing her perception from distanced observer to active participant.) Metaphors of space (Bachelard 1964) are key to this engagement of the observer – the enactive and the embodied, so different from the emotional disengagement and an-aesthetising, or de-sensitising, that traditional medical education has encouraged among students as we have regularly argued (Bleakley 2020). The sensuous metaphor, weather-like, brings patient to surgeon as a poetic bridge. More, the science of imaging has facilitated an aesthetic moment of beauty where the science image is expressive and gripping. The technology is no longer the problem as potentially reductive, but acts rather as facilitator of imagination. Biomedicine's tech baubles are thus reclaimed for humane care.

As a principle, technical descriptors in medicine and surgery (such as the "naming of parts" of surgical kits) are withdrawn into a utility mindset and their poetic value is squeezed dry. But reverse this process, and allow surgical equipment an ontology or existence (following Object-Oriented Ontology), a voice; and think of these instruments as extensions of the human senses. Then the utility perspective is dissolved by an aesthetics of "speaking" instruments, as a web of poetic possibilities emerges: grasping forceps, skin hooks, needle holders, tapered needle, locking forceps, rake retractor, and so forth. To make the stone stonier, the poetic imagination encourages not thinking about the instruments listed above, but rather thinking with them: precisely how the forceps "grasp" for example.

Two cultures, or one culture in two minds?

We will continue with the theme of medicine feeding poetry by widening this to the modern cultural dilemma of arts and sciences nourishing, rather than eating, each other. In our era, it is not easy for science and the arts/humanities to converse and entwine. The Spanish poet and philosopher Maria Zambrano (Zambrano 2008; Burnside 2019), however, argued that the poetic imagination and scientific mind form a whole psyche, where, "In poetry we directly encounter the concrete, individual human. ... Poetry is encounter, mastery, discovery through grace". Science and art, says Zambrano, possess an elective affinity in which one is deficient without the other. Following this imperative, medical science and art can be re-aligned, but this would require a significant overhaul of science teaching at medical school, disengaging it from instrumentalism. Fixated on compensating for science's perceived lack, the medical humanities have totally failed to engage with the idea that science can be intrinsically beautiful and imaginative, and this needs to be drawn out.

For example, Hume, Mulemi, and Sadock (2018) point to the difficulties of trying to integrate humanities into a medicine curriculum in Kenya, South Africa, and Tanzania, where medicine is strongly bounded as biomedical territory:

> We argue overall for the great potential of humanities in the health 'space' – as well as the need for improved dialogue between the disciplines to bring a diverse community of knowledge to bear on our understandings of experiences of health. And we suggest the need for a robust awareness of our own positions in relation to medicine, as humanities scholars, as well as a patient persistence on both sides of the humanities–health science equation to create a broader and ultimately more effective research system.

But maybe the issue cannot be forced as the round plug of the humanities approaches the square hole of biomedical science. Rather, think laterally, defamiliarise, expand the object of biomedicine by bringing the aesthetic object of the humanities to touch on it lightly, not to attempt to colonise it or march in critically. Look for the humanity and artistry already evident in biomedicine (we have given many examples here): the metaphors, the rich vocabulary that at times is poetic ("white lung", "hyperdense", "fibrillation", "rotator cuff tear"), the "geography" of human anatomy – the precise word, as metaphor, that Foucault (1976) uses to describe the rise of Western anatomical knowledge through cadaver dissection. As noted above, think with the object rather than just about it.

Science is very good at excluding the wrong words in its precision, formulaic methods and object descriptions. However, this can lead to desiccation, so that the work of poetry is needed as supportive aesthetic object, staining the object of science with its presence, not its insistence or intrusions. The work of poetry is summed up by Zambrano in the embodied metaphor of the kiss, as "A // pearl that goes from mouth to mouth" ("Lengua": https://www.wordswithoutborders.org/article/lengua-mara-zambrano). "Lengua" means "language", but also "the lingo of the tongue". So Zambrano sensualises language by imaging persons speaking into each other's mouths through kissing and tonguing, as they pass pearls. Pearls of wisdom maybe, but also pearls made from the grit of conversation and love. However, surely the orthopaedic surgeon above creates pearls through abrasion and cleaning of the joint as she imagines this both literally (the mechanics must be right) and metaphorically (one must love the work – it must be aesthetically satisfying). Actually, when the mechanics are right, so are the aesthetics (and vice versa). This is the first rule of Minimalism (Chayka 2020): clean surfaces, accurate joins and repetition of satisfying forms.

For both Anna the surgeon and Zambrano the poet, issues of power are necessarily implied in their work. Anna has a technical authority bound by an ethical code to do the best work on behalf of her patient. Zambrano's poetry and prose embody a philosophical commitment to a socialist and feminist imperative of equality (she was a politically engaged revolutionary in Spain prior to the Spanish Civil War and the reign of terror of Franco). We can think of biomedical science passing through the filter of poetry and being radicalised in the process, but really our vision here is not that poetry colonises science but instead that science meets poetry on the road and is expanded by the friendship.

The sensual diction of the consultation: a carnal hermeneutics

Rafael Campo (1997: 166–67), one of the most celebrated of contemporary physician poets, suggests that "formal poetry" (adhering to rules of metre, pulse, and structure) presents "the beating contents of the body at peace" and "the gentle ebb and flow of breathing, or sobbing". Where "[p]oetry is a pulsing, organized imagining of what once was, or is to be", it is also a "distillation of the process of living itself". Campo uses straightforward Keatsian comparisons: the source domain of knowing the body from medicine/surgery maps on to the target domain of the embodied metaphor. Yasir Al-Jumaili (2020: unpaginated) provides a comprehensive list of Keats's body metaphors:

> "morbid fancy", "fancy-sick", "brain-sick", "sick hearted", "heart-sickness", "sick eyelids", "sick pride", "sickly imagination", "bosom pain", "mind in pain", "pained heart", "scarlet pain", "balmy pain, "heaving in pain", "heart-ache", "eyelids ache", "aches in loneliness", "full of ache", "fever", "feverous hectic", "feverous boiling gurge", "fevered parchings",

"eye all pale", "pale of cheeks", "pale cheeks", "thy cheek is pale", "pale limbs", "pale mouthed", "pale faces", "pale forehead", "pale were the lips", "drowsy numbness", "drowsy hour", "drowsy noons", "drowsy gloom", "drowsy wing" and, "drowsy chimes".

Drawing on a 19th-century analysis by two surgeons teaching at Guy's hospital while Keats was a student, Jumaili (ibid.) further provides an illustration of a medical definition of "fever" used in Keats's time:

Increased frequency of pulse, - preternatural heat, preceded by sensation of cold, -feeling of languor, lassitude, and general uneasiness:-pain of head, back, and limbs:-memory and judgement confused and indistinct; - senses of taste, smell, touch, &c. altered or impaired:- want of appetite, - defect of saliva, - thirst;- discolouration of the tongue; -respiration frequent and anxious:- changes in the urine (Babington and Curry 1811: 2).

Keats translated this via poetic imagination in his poem "Hyperion" as,

This passion lifted him upon his feet,
And made his hands to struggle in the air,
His Druid locks to shake and ooze with sweat,
His eyes to fever out, his voice to cease.

The descriptive tone of the medical, as symptom description, is transformed into an animated encounter with the patient himself. In four lines we are intimate with his suffering and its sensual nature: feet, hands, (hair)locks, eyes, voice gives us a body scan; while the lifting to the feet, the struggling hands, the shaking locks, the oozing skin, the fevered eyes, and the loss of voice fill in the particulars. Underneath this frenzy, a regular iambic pentameter beat shows that the body is still stable within the episode. But this is the body of a god – Saturn, or Chronos, the Lord of Melancholy and of Time, who struggles to understand his loss of power (that Keats represents as being gripped by a fever). And so we all identify with his suffering, live in his penumbra, know that time affords healing. Keats reminds us that suffering is both all-too-human and otherworldly simultaneously. Fever takes us out of ourselves and into realms at the lip of death.

Poetry is fed also by the violence and dread of symptom or pathology: a racing heart of anxiety, a crushing chest pain, the singular crash of depression, a skin erupting with acne that will surely scar for life and leaves a teenager with deep embarrassment, a relentless blinding headache, a relationship torn asunder, a lump discovered in the breast. A seed of cancer, a rogue cell, expands sideways and territorialises, so the body is "riddled". The riddle to the patient is "why me?" Poetry is both body at peace, body at war; although poetry includes them, it is also far more than these familiar medical metametaphors. Poetry takes mortal suffering (for example) as the singular case (this blinding headache) and places it among the gods, the archetypes, the disease formulations, the public sphere, as the general case. In this way we identify symptom as a shared concern and then democratise medicine.

We continue with our theme of medicine feeding into poetry not to expand poetry's remit – for example as a therapeutic device – but to allow poetry to do its work of reciprocal nourishment, again through metaphor invention, expansion and renewal; through formal processes such as the handling of enjambment (line slippage in poetry, slippages in clinical encounters in medicine); and through infusion of lyricism in otherwise tough-minded, rational work. Above all, as we keep insisting, while poetry emphasises the importance of *ekphrasis* – vivid description – medicine can teach poetry about close noticing, the first step in physical examination; and the first step in a carnal hermeneutics (Kearney and Treanor 2015), or a knowing of the body (as interpretation) through the body. All the time we are bouncing between idiosyncratic presentation and general cases and their rationales (such as EBM).

Patient presentations bounce off the drumhead of the listening doctor, play on the eye, and resonate against her skin in physical examination. The senses are always intimately engaged: Bahar Orang's (2020: 72) "detailed ekphrasis, description as / analysis". Poetry too engages the senses and educates for deeper sensibility. A sensibility for sound educated by poetry can reclaim the sonic elements of a clinical encounter. Homer teaches us that poetry is first sound on a field (battle cries, death throes in the *Iliad*; lamentations (as longings for homecoming) in the *Odyssey*. Poetry is not, of course, confined to aural epiphanic imagery but is felt, or embodied, through metre and rhythm, assonance and dissonance, and – sometimes bruising – emphasis, as a "tactile poetics" (Jackson 2015). Sarah Jackson (ibid.) describes the many associations between text and tact, using the poet Anne Michaels ("Into Arrival": https://allyourprettywords.tumblr.com/post/35252972260/into-arrival-anne-michaels) to introduce the relationship between skin and language, with "each word of skin / a decision".

The through-line here is twofold. First, not that poetry is literally tactile (which it can be in raising "felt sense"), but rather that tactility is poetry. Hands touch and skins exchange wisdom, not just information. In Elise Partridge's poem considered earlier, the mother's "Chapped hands sift greasy suds" and "can't make rent", or can't make a hole in the situation to escape; while again "tear" brings us back to the mother's tears at the sink that the child hopes will dry up, just as the mother is doing the drying up – a round reverie – while the mother and child engage glances but do not touch. A Freudian reading of "can't make rent" suggests self-harming ideation that is frustrated or suspended – making cuts. Of course, this is what the mother wants – for the landlord to make cuts, to lower the rent, adding to the metaphor store described earlier. A metonymic chain is promised. Or, the poem has wings.

The orthopod Anna touches her patient's shoulder joint remotely but through metaphor ("messy white tissue … falling in our face"). Zambrano has us touch through an imagined series of French kisses that do not pass information but pass pearls of wisdom from mouth to mouth. Orang's title *Where Things Touch: A Meditation on Beauty* is self-explanatory. Permissive touch is beauty. Saturn's infectious touch in Keats turns us all to fevered melancholics as archetypal force. All this is for an appreciation of the source domain after the metaphoric work of the target domain – in other words, the poetry must make us look at the world again with renewed vigour, fresh senses, unusual perspectives. And medicine can take us to that edge of a New World.

A fire inside

Let's take an extended example of how medicine feeds into poetry by igniting metaphors that then feed back to the medicine with enhanced intensity, for a consequent defamiliarisation of habitual practice. Laurence Kirmayer (2000) analyses a patient's interview with a psychiatrist where the 23-year-old woman explains that she has recurring burning sensations in her chest and abdomen. She uses the metaphor: "a fire inside" to describe these sensations. Exhaustive examinations and exploratory procedures revealed no somatic issues, no gastrointestinal or cardiac cause, yet the symptoms persist. Her doctors suggest it is psychosomatic, what they refer to metaphorically as a case of "nerves", necessitating the referral. He elicits talk from the patient about a recent relationship where she says that she was in love, but the relationship went sour because the man was excessively controlling, possibly abusive. She agrees with the psychiatrist that there is more than a lingering passion here that was cut short, and that she has not had the opportunity to release, and gain insight from, repressed feelings – an equal mix of love and anger for the man. Could this be the "fire inside"?

The psychiatrist, however, turns the conversation towards the woman's mother and sees that here is unfinished business between the mother and daughter (the Object Relations reflex). He steers her towards framing this as being trapped by a maternal web that she needs to free herself from to gain a sense of independence. She seems to be in agreement with this, but it deflects from the unfinished issues with her failed love affair that have left her "angry" and she resorts to the familiar metaphor of her emotions being "bottled up inside". She still seems to seek a somatic explanation rather than a psychological one for her symptoms, and while the psychiatrist concludes this initial consultation with an invitation to make a second appointment with him, the woman fails to do this.

Kirmayer uses this frustrated consultation to challenge the notion that the medical encounter should be framed in narrative terms. He sees a failed narrative here on the part of the patient (who still harboured the belief that her symptoms were somatic) and a forced narrative on the part of the psychiatrist (who attempted to fit the patient into a classic psychoanalytic frame of unresolved mother-daughter psychological conflict, where the daughter needed to break free of a perceived suffocating but probably well-meaning mother).

Having introduced the overarching metaphor of "nerves" – a stand-in for "psychosomatic" – into the analysis, Kirmayer (ibid.: 171) does not attempt to address the poetic work of this source (and nascent) metaphor. While he talks of "poetic evocation through bursts of figural language", this is not developed. Actually, it feels more like the young woman is about to burst, and certainly about to burst into tears. Strangely, towards the end of the consultation, as the psychiatrist seems to be steering her away from returning to the GI doctors for a further opinion, she says that there are other physical issues: "Internal bleeding, and hemorrhage" (ibid.: 165). The psychiatrist does not follow this up, even as a coded message. Perhaps she is talking about menstrual distress for example (Shuttle and Redgrove 1978), or is this a metaphor for the deep wounding that the relationship has caused? Is her major psychological symptom her inability to break free of literalism? The source metaphor of "nerves" conferred by the doctors has now mutated into a target metaphor of "internal bleeding and hemorrhage" offered by the patient – the metaphor that we imagine as extensive deep wounding from her rupture of the relationship.

She's maybe not nervy; rather the loss of her lover is experienced as a tearing away leaving a wound that bleeds profusely. Whatever the diagnosis, poetry is being drawn into the occasion by medicine's (psychiatry's) complexities. Poetry is not a therapy here, but embodied as the psychological rupture experienced as phantom pain, for metaphors are writ large on and within the body, where a carnal hermeneutics serves to examine and interpret or give meaning to such expressions. And they speak. Psychiatry, of course, is the twin use of the literal pharmacy and the poetry pharmacy, where minds make symptoms out of metaphors and metaphors make meaning out of symptoms.

The patient seems to want to play the sick role as she musters resistance to that role, mystifying her doctors. Kirmayer's account leaves the reader hanging with the unresolved dilemma of the two failed narratives. "Nerves" may be an inappropriate metaphor for the context, as it morphs into "blood loss". Indeed, the patient maybe thinks that the GI doctors have a nerve to keep palming her off (they are perfectly justified in doing so as they have seemingly exhausted all diagnostic testing avenues). A closer description may be that the woman is in limbo. Perhaps she fears self-responsibility by leaving decisions in the hands of experts (biomedical certainty), but also fears the authority of others as potential trap (her abusive boyfriend and emotionally suffocating mother are her models of authority). Actually, we know so little about this woman that all of this is conjecture, but let us play out the fantasy nevertheless. We are left with the impression of a double bind at work where the abusive ex-lover raises blood, but she also haemorrhages in his absence, losing life force. She wants her lover back, but not on his terms and knows that is impossible.

In a rather more severe psychological state, but possibly offering a lesson for our young woman patient here, in *Macbeth* (5, iii: 45–50) Shakespeare describes how Macbeth turns to his physician, seemingly in the throes of a severe case of "nerves", to demand a material cure for a psychological ailment:

> Canst thou not minister to a mind diseased,
> Pluck from the memory a rooted sorrow,
> Raze out the written troubles of the brain,
> And with some sweet oblivious antidote
> Cleanse the stuff'd bosom of that perilous stuff
> Which weighs upon the heart?

The sorrow squeezes the heart, promising rupture. The physician, an early master of patient-centred therapy, replies, "the patient must minister to himself". Returning to T.S. Eliot's distinction between information and wisdom, the doctor offers Hippocratic wisdom. We do not take Hippocratic medicine literally, but rather as aphoristic, and less diagnostic but more prognostic. To the young woman suffering from "nerves" we might suspend the seemingly fruitless diagnostic quest to ask not "what is wrong?" but rather "what are you going to do now?" We are loath to say that her narrative must be re-written. We prefer that her poetic field, clearly soiled, be renewed.

For the case described by Kirmayer, "nerves" is also too encompassing a metaphor; to make a biomedical equivalent, this as if a doctor says she must do "tests" to identify illness. But what tests? A biopsy? An X-ray? An angiogram? Our metaphors should be as attuned to patient symptomatology as we are supposed to be patient-centred in practice. We want to know precisely what her symptoms are like and how they change according to circumstance and mood. We want a keen diagnostic "listening eye" and "watching ear" to catalogue when and how symptoms appear in language – again, Orang's (2020: 72) "detailed ekphrasis, description as / analysis". We can be "metaphor-centred" and still care for patients. Indeed, metaphor as object in conjunction with patient as object likely transforms both.

But let's be specific, as poets like to be. As far as her self-reported "fire inside" is concerned, does she burn, itch, or smoulder? Is this, metaphorically, a "bloody nuisance"? And is she bilious, sickening, or sticky? We need a contemporary and biomedically sharp medicine, yes, but we need to bring back a little of what he have lost, the metaphorically rich medieval and early modern language of the humours, also an Elizabethan- and Jacobean-Shakespearean poetic language of psychological flux; and a Keatsian set of what rhetoricians now call "god-terms" but that we understand as abstractions, big forces, archetypes, or general cases. Again, many believe that a reductive biomedicine's ascendancy is a product of once productive metaphors draining away, leaving a burning, an itching or yearning for their recovery and for generous new inventions. The field must be re-invented, the plot thickened not in a narrative sense but in a horticultural move.

Robert McCrum (2016) notes how Shakespeare turned an adjective into a verb ("thick my blood" in *The Winter's Tale*); a pronoun into a noun ("the cruellest she alive" in *Twelfth Night*); and a noun into a verb ("He childed as I fathered" in *King Lear*). Perhaps some similar turn of language can help the young woman above, so that descriptors and qualifiers are turned into activities. Maybe alter the pejorative label "nerves" and convert it into an agency metaphor, asking: does she have the nerve to change circumstance? Is the "fire inside" and her "haemorrhaging of feelings" being frustrated by the psychiatrists' inabilities to facilitate catharsis leading to insight?

We speculate, we don't know; we are raising the spectre of poetry that in our book is the best facilitator of affect we have. How the doctors can help the young woman with "nerves" is surely not to be reduced to either bodily gastrointestinal findings or the psychodynamics of maternal love and loss, but is an archetypal question of this woman finding her daimon, her passions, or what drives her. This is work of the soul or imagination, where Shakespeare and Keats are established guides, although we can think of a host of contemporary voices who also do this work, such as Dionne Brand (2018). These are questions of prognosis or fate and they are determined by wisdom or lack of it, and not by information – as milk dry in the cat's saucer.

Danielle Ofri's offering

As of yet, we have not completely lost poetry to information. We write this ironically, we confess. Poetry can't be completely lost; poetry can't be lost in any quantity. We imagine that it aches for the love and touch of medicine, and there are few who believe in this connection more passionately than poet-doctor Danielle Ofri (2008: 110–11) who has long been a champion of incorporating poetry into medical rounds, where,

> Poetry is all about metaphor, and the great poets force us to think deeply when interpreting their metaphors. Challenging patients do the same. ... To successfully help those who come to us in need, we must interpret their metaphors, or they will hunt for other physicians with more nuanced understanding.

Ofri usefully switches our interest – enjambs, to make a metaphor – from the narrative gaze to metaphoric utterance. Artists, including poets, she suggests, avoid the direct and obvious gaze. Rather, they learn to see, as it were, out of the corner of their eyes (glance) and listen with an inner ear (insight). These are metaphors for a more subtle and sensitive approach to patient encounters, collapsing predictable narrative sensibility into a more concentrated unpredictable poetic imagination. Here, through a medical humanities-infused medical education, Ofri says we can "help our students become far better physicians if we learn a bit from the poets". Students, of course, do not have glance and insight as experts do, but practice educates for these qualities. Can practice be improved where diagnostic reasoning is aligned with the poetic imagination? And as those doctors improve their practices poetically so their practice of medicine will come to satisfy poetry's needs (to attract writers and readers interested in craft as well as raw expression). Doctor-poets might meet for (en)jam(bment) sessions.

Ofri, among others, recommends directly engaging not only medical students with poems but also poems with patients. William Sieghart (2017, 2019), in two volumes of *The Poetry Pharmacy*, gives an account of his long-standing and successful project to bring poems to individuals as therapeutic interventions through the media, libraries, and festivals. Different from patients writing poetry, Sieghart selects particular poems to be read to laypersons publicly or in private, for a range of (technically "undiagnosed") psychological conditions such as generalised anxiety, compulsions, obsessions, depression, insecurity, convalescence, bereavement, crippling shyness, loss of a child, and fear of death. From his face-to-face "pharmacy" encounters, he claims success, or at least satisfaction – although the reader is never sure about lasting effects, and sceptics will always ask for evidence of "success".

More importantly, people are introduced to poems they may never have previously read or heard of. Discovery can be epiphanic. Sieghart provides an unacknowledged service to psychiatry by providing an alternative *Diagnostic and Statistical Manual* (DSM) of mental health symptoms, poems both advertising conditions and providing insights into them. Sieghart errs on the side of poems giving pleasure (no bad thing in itself), but a better measure of "success" may be the ways in which poems upset expectations and engender uncertainty. Ofri (2006) gives an example of meeting a patient at Bellevue Hospital in New York who "displayed all the cardinal signs of a chronic Bellevue Hospital alcoholic: cantankerous mood, matted, stringy hair, stirring halitosis, a W.C. Fields nose, and bone-rattling tremors of the fingers and tongue".

She gets us off to a good start. Ofri is a good writer: alliteration, sharp observation, and embodied metaphors ("stirring halitosis", "bone-rattling tremors"). But how will her medicine entice, embrace, and bring into service a poem? Well, the first thing is to gain the trust of the patient who has "maladies of the bottle". This dishevelled character was faced with the ritual of the ward round comprising: "one attending physician, two residents, four interns, and six medical students—bunched around his bed, all attired in crisp white coats and equally crisp attitudes". How will lank and crisp be matched up? Ofri reaches for Jack Coulehan's "I'm Gonna Slap Those Doctors" (https://utmedhumanities.wordpress.com/2014/10/13/im-gonna-slap-those-doctors-jack-coulehan/):

> they write me off as a boozer
> and snow me with drugs. Like I'm gonna

go wild and green bugs are gonna
crawl on me and I'm gonna tear out
their goddamn precious IV".

The patient smiles and brightens up, relating to the moral of the poem as it criticises high-minded attitudes from doctors; a connection was made, trust was engendered. A medicine was administered.

Sieghart and Ofri are doing the same thing in different ways: introducing novice readers to poems. But Ofri's approach is a little more hot and instantaneous. Sieghart is not sure how the poetry will travel. Both are fervent believers in the medium eaten raw. Such use of poetry as *supplement* to medicine, and as potential therapeutic intervention, is now well established and widely discussed in arts and health and medical/healthcare humanities circles.

While recognising and applauding the value of such approaches, this book however takes a different tack, as readers will by now be aware. Here, the focus is on the process of the birthing of poetry (as opposed to any other creative act), or *the ferment of the poetic imagination*, and the meaningful overlaps between this poetic imagination and the work of clinical reasoning and associated care carried out by seasoned doctors as the core of their everyday work. If such overlap is found to be meaningful, the sceptic's "so what?" might be considerably tempered as we then find the education of the poetic imagination to be at the heart of a medical education.

This provides a strong rationale for the inclusion of a certain kind of medical humanities within medicine curricula, one shaped by the poetic imagination, focussed on metaphor production. In this chapter we have demonstrated that this is not a one-way traffic as poetry applied to medical practice to supplement it, beef it up, or to add finesse. Rather, the metaphor-inventing, wisdom-rich practice of democratic medicine is reflected back by poetry in a re-doubling of effort and intensity. Object relations are encouraged. Metaphors are deepened, enjambments are negotiated, *ekphrasis* is sharper, tolerance of ambiguity is increased, contradictions are seen as opportunities; and the reality of slippage and failure is matched by deepening of critical reflexivity. Too much of a load? Well, we warned that poetry's job is compression and often heavy lifting; but Ofri shows how this can be achieved with grace and a light touch.

Cat's milk needs topping up

The working of the poetic imagination is then, paradoxically, a mesh of "unseeing", or of withdrawal of sclerotic patterns of seeing such as habits and ruts, or blinkered traditions. This *via negativa* brings us back to T.S. Eliot's plea for knowledge of stillness rather than motion, and silence rather than speech. Some may take the alignment of the medical mind and poetic imagination as an interesting diversion from the day-to-day realities of clinical work. Their response may be, "Get real!" To some extent they are right – the argument in this book is an experiment, a proposal, a hypothesis, maybe just conjecture as an abductive conceit. But we have faith that it is worth rehearsing. Years of engagement with trying to convince sceptics of the value of the medical humanities (such as use of poetry) through often half-baked empirical research has left us a little counter-jaded. Sometimes, the proof is in the pudding. Wallace Stevens claimed that poetry is "an unofficial view of being". In an age where biomedicine has taken on the role of the official view of being, perhaps poetry and medicine are, indeed, two sides of the same bodily coin, both highly conversant with human suffering or the far reaches of the flesh and the off-kilter mind. Here, once more, as Wallace Stevens says, "Cat's milk is dry in the saucer". How shall we top up the saucer?

References

Al-Jumaili YA. Metaphors of Fever in the Poetry of John Keats: A Cognitive Approach. *Cogent Arts and Humanities.* 2020; 78(1). Retrieved from https://doi.org/1 0.1080/23311983.2020.1793445

Bachelard G. 1964. *The Poetics of Space.* New York: Orion Press.

Bleakley A. 2020. *Educating Doctors' Senses through the Medical Humanities: "How Do I Look?".* Abingdon: Routledge.

Bleakley A. 2021. *Medical Education, Politics and Social Justice: The Contradiction Cure.* Abingdon: Routledge.

Brand D. 2018. *The Blue Clerk: Ars Poetica in 59 Versos.* Durham, NC: Duke University Press.

Burnside J. 2019. *The Music of Time: Poetry in the Twentieth Century.* London: Profile Books.

Campo R. 1997. *The Poetry of Healing: A Doctor's Education in Empathy, Identity, and Desire.* New York: WW Norton & Co.

Chayka K. 2020. *The Longing for Less: Living with Minimalism.* New York: Bloomsbury.

Foucault M. 1976. *The Birth of the Clinic: An Archaeology of Medical Perception.* London: Routledge.

Ghosh H. 2017. John Keats's "Guy's Hospital" Poetry. In: N Roe (ed.) *John Keats and the Medical Imagination.* Cham: Palgrave Macmillan, 21–42.

Harman G. 2018. *Object-Oriented Ontology: A New Theory of Everything.* London: Penguin Random House.

Hillman J. 1975. *Re-Visioning Psychology.* New York: Harper and Row.

Hume VJ, Mulemi BA, Sadock M. Biomedicine and the Humanities: Growing Pains. *Medical Humanities.* 2018; 44: 230–38.

Jackson S. 2015. *Tactile Poetics: Touch and Contemporary Writing.* Edinburgh: Edinburgh University Press.

Kearney R, Treanor B (eds). 2015. *Carnal Hermeneutics.* New York: Fordham University Press.

Kirmayer LJ. 2000. Broken Narratives: Clinical Encounters and the Poetics of Illness Experience. In: C Mattingly, LC Garro (eds.) *Narrative and the Cultural Construction of Illness and Healing.* Berkeley: University of California Press, 153–80.

McCrum R. 'Perfect mind': On Shakespeare and the Brain. *Brain.* 2016; 139: 3310–13.

Neilson S. Nonevidence-Based Lyric Essay on Evidence-Based Medicine, Part I: What We Talk about When We Talk about Paradigms. *Journal of Evaluation in Clinical Practice*. 2021; 27: 578–83.

Neilson S. Nonevidence-Based Lyric Essay on Evidence-Based Medicine, Part II: Continuing Status Quo Maintenance Education. *Journal of Evaluation in Clinical Practice*. 2021; 27: 584–91.

Ofri D. 2006. The Poetry Ward: A Doctor Dispenses Poems to Patients and Medical Students. Poetry Foundation. Retrieved from https://www.poetryfoundation.org/articles/68616/the-poetry-ward

Ofri D. The Muse on the Medical Wards. *The Lancet*. 2008; 371: 110–11.

Orang B. 2020. *Where Things Touch: A Meditation on Beauty*. Toronto: Book*Hug.

Peterkin A, Bleakley A. 2016. *Staying Human During the Foundation Programme and Beyond: How to Thrive after Medical School*. Baton Rouge, LA: CRC Press.

Prentice R. 2013. *Bodies in Formation: An Ethnography of Anatomy and Surgery Education*. Durham, NC: Duke University Press.

Shuttle P, Redgrove P. 1978. *The Wise Wound: Menstruation and Everywoman*. London: Marion Boyars.

Sieghart W. 2017. *The Poetry Pharmacy: Tried-and-True Prescriptions for the Heart, Mind and Soul*. London: Particular Books.

Sieghart W. 2019. *The Poetry Pharmacy Returns: More Prescriptions for Courage, Healing and Hope*. London: Particular Books.

Soldati G, Demi M, Demi LD. Ultrasound Patterns of Pulmonary Edema. *Annals of Translational Medicine*. 2019; 7(Suppl 1): S16. Retrieved from https://atm.ame-groups.com/article/view/23881/html

Van Dijk J. 2005. *The Transparent Body: A Cultural Analysis of Medical Imaging*. Seattle: University of Washington Press.

Zambrano M. 2008/1939. Philosophy and Poetry. Text imprint Mexico City, Fondo de Cultura Económica. Retrieved from http://webshells.com/spantrans/Zambrano.htm

10 Diagnosing with the poetic imagination

What poetry can do for medicine

Medicine breathing the airs of poetry

It is vitally important to recognise the power of story, as much a democratising force through traditional folk tale and contemporary soap operas (Rancière 2013) as provocative art in the hands of novelists. But we will continue to bring poetry out from the shadow of clinical narratives, wringing out the last drops of our critique. Jeff Encke (undated) recognises that "Pedagogical applications of poetry in medicine are relatively nascent, lurking in the shadows of narrative theory". This is reinforced by Michael Theune's (undated) blog "Structure and Surprise: Engaging Poetic Turns" where he suggests,

> many readers come to poetry thinking that it, like the other literature with which they're acquainted, tells stories. Such thinking, of course, is misleading—it's not clear such thinking would help anyone really encounter and engage many poems. Certainly, lots of poems make use of narrative elements, but lots of poems, even poems thought to be generally "accessible," don't. Readers need to be presented with a different paradigm for how poems "work," for what it is that poems "do."

Again, Cecile Alduy (undated) further asks how we might challenge the dominance of narrative frames, where this is unproductive:

> to find ways to 'release the grip' of the narrative impulse which permeates the way we think about ourselves (and) the world … (where) some of the most fundamental of human experiences … are stripped down from their intensity, beauty, horror, and maybe their truth, when we try to make sense of them by forcing them into a narrative box.

Alduy notes, importantly, that *narratives may mis-shape our practices*, a point conveniently overlooked by narrativists in medicine and medical education. For example Alduy questions the value in medicine of "redemptive, 'meaning at the end of the story' kind of narratives … (that) rely on a teleological worldview", seeing consultations as more open-ended, messy and unpredictable.

DOI: 10.4324/9781003194408-12

Of course, while medical practices such as diagnostic work have purposes, their enactment can be messy, not at all redemptive but rather full of blind alleys and blind spots, open to error.

Lyric poetry, in particular, has developed to embrace concentrated accounts of singular sensory experience that describe objects and events by re-inscribing them. An example from medicine might be: a dermatologist looks closely at a melanoma asking the patient "how long have you had this?" as a temporal aspect to diagnosis and prognosis, but is more interested in spatial location and topography such as colour, prominence, and irregular borders. The dermatologist is perhaps thinking more about such spatial location and self-display than temporal plot (although the latter is important such as in the phase development in thickness and extent of a melanoma). The doctor is focussed primarily on immediacy of visual cues.

Paul Valéry's (1934) parody of the intense search that poets make to come up with the right words in the right place actually parallels the finest of sense-based diagnostics in medical expertise: "a word that is feminine, disyllabic, includes P or E, ends in a mute syllable, and is a synonym for break or disintegration, and not learned, not rare" (in Nowottny 1965: 2). Lyric poets draw on five chief qualities – sound, voice, metaphor, symbols and images, and ambiguity (sometimes as a conscious contradiction). Expert doctors also draw on these qualities, as,

> 'Let me listen with the stethoscope' (sound).
> 'I have some bad news, I'm afraid' (voice).
> 'There's something fishy going on with your gut' (metaphor and metonymy – fishing line can be made from gut).
> 'There's a question mark over the test results' (symbolism).
> 'It looks like a carcinoma, but let's not rule out a melanoma' (ambiguity and enjambment or sudden line breaks – the sudden slippage from carcinoma to the more threatening melanoma).

Alduy (undated) suggests that

> A poem is a gentle, ingenious device to make us stop, force us to be present, and present only to what is there, as it is, one word after the other, one line after the other, not rushing anywhere, and certainly not rushing to "the" meaning. Poems are anti-ideologies (or should be). They are instances of resistance to our own impatience, our tendency to simplify, our pragmatism, our constant efforts to be "efficient" and our unfaltering neediness, this need to cling on the belief that there should be a meaning at the end of the day, at the end of our lives, or at the end of history. I like to believe that poems work against interpretation (if interpretation is understood as the translation of a complex, alive system into a more legible, consumable dish), that they are agents of resistance.

We agree with Alduy that poems are "agents of resistance" in several senses. Alduy asks us to consider that the poem acts to resist haste, working against poet's bad habits, and that they are "anti-ideologies". Well, poetry can also educate for direct political resistance to oppression. Given the political fuse that a poem can offer, poems are not necessarily "gentle" devices, although they are "ingenious". The middle section of Alduy's meditation on poetry could certainly be taken as helpful advice on medical diagnostic work that avoids impatience, simplification, pragmatism, efficiency, and "meanings". Alduy echoes Susan Sontag's familiar rhetoric to move "against interpretation" by placing witnessing and close noticing before analysis. Surely medical diagnosis is interpretation, but initially its birth is in appreciation. But also, we want medicine to be politically aware, a liberatory practice (Bleakley 2021).

Jeff Encke (undated) further suggests that poetry can be placed in dialectical conversation with tragedy and epic narrative forms, so common in medicine as patients suffer life-changing and life-threatening illnesses. Poetry is then not subsumed in a narrative worldview, but informs and shapes narrative. It is in poetic instants that epiphanies may occur. Tragedy, suggests Encke, "marks the articulation" of a conflict between the lyrical poetic "embodied moments of crisis" as symptom is experienced, and the tragic genre marking the articulation of felt bodily conflict "as it encounters narrative language". The conversation between the partly unknowable but pressing concerns of symptoms and their expression in story as a sensemaking (diagnosis for example) leads to a synthesis in the form of the epic genre as "socially-accepted outcome".

This is the expression of diagnosis in the public domain. Encke then suggests, "Perhaps by understanding this progression from a pre-articulated state of truth to one of social acceptance, physicians would be more attuned to what epiphanic moments mean – to themselves and to their patients – and how to leverage them in the improvement of care-giving" (ibid.). We precipitated out epic poetry in our book because we feel it has a differential amount of lyric therein, dependent on the practitioner; but we appreciate Encke's delicate appreciation of genre, how different kinds of poetry might be particularly applicable, dependent on the clinical situation.

Poetry then stands as an affective and epiphanic knowing internally illuminated by metaphor, a "latent" knowledge that can be triangulated "with stories and propositions" (in the genres of tragedy and epic). The poetic imagination offers "a sudden recognition, cast in the form of a fully embodied impression" that is "knowledge not immediately present in narratives" or "hardly reducible to narrative form", Encke suggests. In summary, "Readers of poetry have the most demanding of listening tasks: like physicians, they must observe with uncommon empathy the gestures and silences of the poem – listen carefully to its breathing and monitor its pulse" (ibid.). But they are not just readers of the body and world; rather, they are activists within it, as our following section shows.

Hello to the soil of the fields. Welcome roots

What can poetry offer medicine? Sometimes it is a poke in the eye, a wake-up call, or a counterweight to an historical burden. From 1981, Anne Sexton gets straight to the point and raises the finger, and it is body-political, gendered: don't mess with my uterus! In "In Celebration of My Uterus" (https://www.poetryfoundation.org/poems/42573/in-celebration-of-my-uterus), Sexton uses a rhetorical ploy: my uterus is the ground ("Hello to the soil of the fields") to a future being who is rooting in me ("Welcome roots"). As the title attests, the poem bravely stands up to the dominant patriarchal medicine of her time:

> They wanted to cut you out
> but they will not. They said you were immeasurably empty
> but you are not.

We don't have the clinical details and Sexton may have been getting good advice, but the manner in which the advice was given (this is 40 years ago) may have been unwelcome. The uterus becomes a wider symbol for women's rights, linked back to the power of reproduction and growth, and as a container of women's knowledge identified with the generative earth itself:

> Hello, spirit. Hello, cup
> Fasten, cover. Cover that does contain.
> Hello to the soil of the fields.
> Welcome, roots.

There is a Biblical ring to this, and a kind of field song call-and-response. Not a story, but a revelation of connected objects, feelings, and meanings. This is an archaic pre-story, a metaphoric weave, where Sexton resists being inserted into a masculine medical story. The unfortunate back-story – a narrative of the poet's life retroactively informing the reading of the poem – is that Sexton had two children, but suffered severe postpartum depression leading to suicidal ideation. After periods of institutionalisation she took her life by car fume asphyxiation at age 46.

Because of her own harrowing mental health experiences associated with postpartum depression, Sexton stood for women's reproductive rights. Oh, drat: we see that we are now succumbing to "Queen or King Narrative's" biocritical imperatives, spinning a biographical story about Sexton, but we recall that her confessional poem itself stands outside – or prior to – story. Its power rests with articulating and amplifying the reality of a woman's deepest feelings towards her womb as this represents the collective womb that is maternal earth. This is repeated along a chain of metaphors standing for the womb, including a "cup" that can be covered, and "earth" that can be rooted. Metonymy and metaphor are then unusually and cleverly linked.

Sexton repeats mythology. In this double umbilical rooting is myth-making of a poetic and not a narrative kind. (You might ask how two male authors can speak on this matter – our main defence is that we have teachers like Anne Sexton.)

The poem is structured around powerful embodied images and metaphors. There is a list – indeed, a provocative and profane litany – of at once both specific and generic women that Sexton wants to celebrate:

> one is tying the cord of a calf in Arizona,
> one is straddling a cello in Russia.
>
> One is wiping the ass of her child.

The anaphoric strategy in each of these lines suggests that we could readily sing them, as a hoedown. For its part, the uterus itself is "singing like a school girl" and is "not torn". The use of "torn" here is ambiguous, possibly meaning that it is not damaged, but that it is somehow conflicted too – and in this case, it could certainly be conflicted capital. Sexton's body, and the bodies of women more generally, were caught between the territorialising impulses of the medical establishment and the primary ownership of the child-become-woman who has grown up with her uterus intact and now finds that it provides shelter for the embryo that roots, flowers and fruits.

Imagine the consultation between the gynaecologist and Sexton where a (we imagine) male doctor is speaking technically, while for Sexton: "Everyone in me is a bird. / I am beating all my wings". We've all had that intense fluttering; we've handled birds that have been caught in the house, or in a greenhouse, and we feel their elevated heartbeats and the attempted fluttering of their wings and we hold them briefly. "You are singing like a school girl", says Sexton of her uterus. Who says that of her womb but a poet? Sexton gives women a role equality: "Let me study the cardiovascular tissue, / Let me examine the angular distance of meteors"; and then, "let me suck on the stems of flowers // let me sing / … / for the kissing". The patient as poet speaks back to the doctor in extraordinary terms. Through poetry, Sexton asks for credibility for her expertise as woman.

With an obvious appeal to both medicine and surgery, Sexton's carefully crafted poem speaks of both torment and beauty. It would be pointless, even destructive, to try to force the poem into a time-based narrative medicine mould. Chronological hermeneutics, based say on Sexton's life history, are ill matched for analysis. The uterus, as cup and chalice, might be mythologised and historicised, but the poet here speaks of gendered space (subject to patriarchal territorialising) and gender-contested place (subject to rightful feminist reclamation). Sexton speaks rather of intensities of embodiment: the womb in the body and the prospect of the baby in the womb, the soil resting on the field and the roots bedding in the soil (as metaphors for the body). Of course, there can be poetic description in narrative, and there is a genre called narrative poetry, but we must declare a warning: where narrative becomes an instrument of medicine, poetry's value is compromised at best and entirely lost at worse as we have argued at length.

To squash, abstract, or otherwise abuse metaphor is to produce an illness in language for which poetry remains the best cure, if we were to resort to instrumentalisation ourselves. For example, illuminating mechanical medicine's deficiencies (such as its often crass use of tired metaphors of war and machinery) are liberational acts. A poem such as Sexton's above is spiritually, politically and materially important as a guide for a "close" lyrical medicine – close noticing, sensitive, deeply engaged, affective and moving the soul or imagination. It is again primary work of reclamation of place.

We will continue throughout this book to examine the work of doctors in relation to the perspectives of patients by "thinking otherwise" about medicine (defamiliarising ourselves to its familiar or underwhelming habitual practices) through the lens of poetry. Here is an example from the doctor and poet Dannie Abse, who, in "Anniversary" (https://www.poetryfoundation. org/poetrymagazine/browse?contentId=26744), says,

> The tree grows down from a bird,
> the strong grass pulls up the earth
> to a hill ….

See how Abse uses enjambment to make us fall away just as we are about to be pulled up the hill. This series of reversal of expected perspectives is what artists do well, as making strange. Where Sexton draws on the metaphor of soil and rooting to explore the sacred *topos* of the womb and its feminist implications, so Abse makes us think about rooting as a reversal of expectations. We are tumbled into another perspective. Abse makes us climb first to engage with downward rooting.

We see a similarity in anaesthetics where for example, in administering an epidural, the anaesthetist must be able to judge when to relax pressure – lifting off – on the syringe plunger as well as when to depress the plunger. This is signalled by sensitivity to differing textures of human tissue as the needle passes through five distinct layers: skin, subcutaneous fat, supraspinous ligament, interspinous ligament, and ligamentum flavum. The needle enters the epidural space and must be stopped in case it penetrates the dural sheath. The anaesthetist then enjambs through the layers with extreme caution, pressing, lifting off, pressing, lifting off (Raj et al. 2013).

Poets, of course, offer different kinds of injections. Here, we concentrate on how poets handle needle point perspectives to inject qualities into the work. Poets write in highly concentrated forms focussed on bringing feeling to the reader through extensive use of close description (intensity, sensibility, and sensitivity – terms that will be fully explored a little more before book's end), as well as metaphor and image. They do this through formal structures. Sexton uses the well-worn beat of iambic pentameter, throws in a nice alliteration ("cord of a calf") and uses repetition of "one is" to characterise singularity-in-multiplicity: "one is tying the cord of a calf in Arizona, / one is straddling a cello in Russia. // One is wiping the ass of her child".

Can you feel the needling going on? The "one is" works like the drummer lifting off the beat in jazz, creating a slight pause as the rest of the line or phrase kicks in. On the downbeat, as the drummer hits the snare, so Sexton strikes a muscular home run: (One is) "tying", (one is) "straddling", (one is) "wiping". There is, respectively, assertion of agency, sexual innuendo and celebration of motherhood: a mini feminist manifesto. To succumb to the biocritical impulse for a moment, always a narrativising one, we point out that Sexton's poem probably had to be such: she lived (1928–74) through the classic period of subjugation of women as "homemakers" in post–Second World War America, as well as the 1960s revolutionary political upheavals.

We are conscious that doctors and healthcare workers reading this, intrigued perhaps by how poetry and medicine might feed one another, are still saying, "I don't quite get it yet". Hang in there we say, there's plenty to be done yet. We keep providing illustrative examples and at some point we hope to reach most readers' tipping points.

While the study of medicine through narrative lenses is pervasive in the fields of medical education (including medical/health humanities and ethics), we recognise that it impacts on only a small slice of jobbing physicians. Throughout this book we refer to generic "medicine" and "doctors" or "physicians" quite aware that the majority have little interest in either narrative or poetry, or the relationship of medicine to literature and creative writing. Translating poetry's rebellious style into spirit, we say: it is this lack of interest – a powerful, resolute one – that is the problem. It is not poetry's problem. As William Carlos Williams (https://poets.org/poem/asphodel-greeny-flower-excerpt) has stated in the poem "Asphodel, That Greeny Flower", and this has often been repeated in standard narrative medicine seminars on poetry: "You can't get the news from poems, but men die miserably every day for lack of what is found there". This is as instrumentalist as we get: you want a cure for burnout? There isn't one. But you can read poetry and see what happens. We think that other things are going on with poetry and medicine.

Knocking at the door

A burning issue conveniently ducked by narrative medicine is that of "fiction" itself. A story is necessarily a representation of events. And the kind of story that narrative medicine deals with almost exclusively is the social realist kind. This cuts out a lot of fictional genres such as magic realism, science fiction, and its cousin "near future" (Don DeLillo, William Gibson). Related to this is the question: is the social realist story to be believed? This is particularly germane in an era of "post truth" and "alternative facts". The following question then arises: what are we to believe of the patient's "story"? This matters if, in the classic scenario, a patient is asked how much alcohol they drink during the week. It is a running joke among doctors that the answer should be treated with a pinch of salt.

For the sociologist Erving Goffman (1959), for example, these questions are moot, because everybody lives daily through creative fictions. The philosopher Hans Vaihinger (1911) wrote a book called *The Philosophy of 'As If'*, that suggested people live by emotionally driven values "as if" these were truths. Students of theatre have long described life as an enactment of roles that are "scripted" and can lead to feelings of inauthenticity. Jean-Paul Sartre (1956) made this the centrepiece of his existential philosophy, where we can choose to live inauthentic lives, behind ascribed roles and masks, or step out from these to claim authenticity. Goffman is one inheritor of these ideas, describing human interactions as "management of impressions" within a "dramaturgical" model. But for Goffman "authenticity" and "inauthenticity" are moot points where life is staged, a drama, and we play our (scripted) parts; and sometimes wander off script. Such scripted roles are embedded in "total institutions" such as hospitals.

Our pivot, or organising idea, for this chapter is then Goffman's (1959) dramaturgical frontstage/backstage metaphor. His anthropological fieldwork recognised and articulated what seems obvious, but by definition, of course, remains unarticulated: that our habitual patterns of social exchange are strongly coded and rehearsed (performance, scripts, manners). Behind the frontstage is unrehearsed material laden with affect as the "backstage". This differs from Freud's unconscious where repressed material is unknown, or out of consciousness by definition. With Goffman, backstage tactics are conscious but "unrehearsed". "Forgetting your lines" for example may not be repression or sublimation but a conscious tactic of deception or an act of self-sacrificial humility to avoid embarrassing another.

A woman visits friends where the walk up to the cottage door is long enough for the friends to see her coming through the window, while they quickly rehearse a greeting and terms for her visit that can be negotiated. Meanwhile, the approaching woman, now with her eyes looking down, is rehearsing her greeting and what she would like to say to those in the house. On meeting, there is formal eye contact, an invitation to enter the house, and the promise of tea and biscuits. The conversation unfolds with movement between frontstage (mannered, well-rehearsed) performance and backstage (running commentary, leaked semiotics, and nonverbal acts such as impromptu gestures; waiting in the wings and unspoken rehearsals to self as witness). Of course, gesture and what is outwardly said sometimes mismatch. Goffman (ibid.) again calls this interaction "impression management". Backstage emotional lava sources may just erupt hot, upstaging cold or lukewarm frontstage niceties. And so forth. Goffman is re-casting Freudian orthodoxy with sociology rather than psychology as the unit of analysis, and drama as the main metaphorical frame. But we recognise nascent poetry especially in the backstage brewings.

In a previous chapter, we anatomised the frontstage/backstage aspects of doctors' clinical reasoning processes, where "illness scripts" informed by biomedical knowledge are a central aspect of what is stored tacitly in the basement of doctors' minds (backstage) to be drawn on to inform frontstage reasoning. The poet too has a set of shaping practices (diction) once learned as a novice but then dropping into a space of tacit knowing as expertise develops. Here, we inquire at the level of interpersonal activity and the habits of roles to make sense of reasoning in action. This must include the wider sphere of how to build a therapeutic relationship.

The family doctor welcomes a patient in a consultation. She has less than 15 minutes to see the patient and research suggests she will interrupt the patient within 11 seconds of seeing her. Both doctor and patient have well-rehearsed frontstage manners (the doctor's are called "professionalism"). We can only guess at what matters backstage. Our method of inquiry is what Paul Ricoeur (2008) called a "hermeneutics of suspicion". Taking Nietzsche, Marx, and Freud as models, Ricoeur develops a literary method of reading texts for what they might say, or what remains unsaid. For Sartre, suspicion extends to the challenging of inauthenticity for authentic self-presentation. But for Goffman, there is no such value judgement applied to backstage activity. It is "merely" (but importantly) rehearsal. The poetry brewing here may remain unrecognised as such, and fails to emerge frontstage, or is overshadowed by the narrative tic.

We say that poetry is not there as an instrumental vehicle to improve medical practice (patient care) through medical/health humanities as pedagogy; rather, poetry is there to be nourished, explicated, and refined as a central task of medical education, shuttling between backstage and frontstage. Once the poetry is evident (and evidenced), we can approach Emily Dickinson's advice that saying things "straight" can sometimes be overwhelming. We need rather to approach the world slantwise with poetry in mind. Poetry is explicitly unnatural yet strives to make sense of the natural world with alarming intensity. We will try to make more sense of medicine through the nonsense of the poetic imagination that is, above all, sensuous.

Marriages between poetry and medicine: let us not admit impediments?

Forced, convenience, servile, lavender, political, shotgun, arranged, reality TV stunt, sham – these might be the kinds of real or metaphorical marriages discussed if you were to ask many doctors about a supposed close relationship between poetry and medicine. Simple bafflement would surely be a common response. Another is suspicion, for in our experience poetry and medicine are often thought of as opposed in meaning and intention. We welcome suspicion because it indicates that there is something worthwhile to be suspicious about: the possible validity of poetry. Yet we believe that the poetic imagination and the medical mind actually offer a marriage akin to Goethe's "elective affinity" – an attraction of seemingly different forces destined to share a common aim – and this book is not only the natural result of that belief but also a rebel yell of recruitment to poetry's side.

A graduate in English and French Literature before studying medicine, Allan Peterkin (2018: 4) observes that for doctors, "Diagnosis is actually an antinarrative act: it takes a wealth of details (the kind literature celebrates) and distills it into one or two words to be acted upon. Reading, similarly, becomes a sped-up instrumental, pragmatic act". At first sight, this observation is easy to agree with. As discussed in previous chapters, considering a so-called antinarrative act as a symptom of reductive biomedicine is the signal gesture of narrative medicine. And we agree: by challenging, tempering, and refining the objective scientific impulse, a literary sensibility turns the habitual "antinarrative act" of diagnosis into something richer and more investigative. However, there is more work to be done here.

Let us talk of a general tendency in the medical/health humanities to project a self-valorising biomedical "boogeymanism", a phenomenon that narrative medicine knows well. To project this idea better, we have invoked a version of Shakespeare's theatre and bring it in conversation with medicine for again the standard diagnostic act engages a tacit store of symbols and rules enacted through explicit *performance* as a scripted drama: the consultation as dramaturgy, or *poetry that is staged* (mirroring too the public reading of poetry). By invoking "dramaturgy" we use a term that takes into account the total context of the performance.

To conceive of diagnostic work solely as instrumental and stripped down – Peterkin's "antinarrative" distillation of the patient's presentation – is, we feel, an (albeit useful) oversimplification of what is actually a complex, messy, and aesthetic story happening backstage or tacitly. It is not enough to just shift the "antinarrative" act of functional diagnosis to a more considered grasp of the wider story; we – as previous chapters testify – encourage moving beyond story, testing its reach and limits, by conceiving of medical diagnostic work as poetic labour (cognitive, emotional and physical). More, the capital developed by such labour is not held solely by medicine but is redistributed across all stakeholders, patients in particular. We also – as loyal rebels – point out that the "signature technique" of narrative medicine can flatten story into data as efficiently as biomedicine reduces the body into data, often reinvesting this data in the business mill of Narrative Medicine[TM] as educational capital to be sold on at profit.

Perhaps our narrativist colleagues have treated the language of biomedicine unfairly? As Caliban says of Prospero's island in Shakespeare's *The Tempest*: "The clouds methought would open and show riches / Ready to drop upon me, that when I waked / I cried to dream again" (Act 3, Scene 2). Just as Prospero's island invites projections of either desolate wasteland or isle of riches, so science receives projections, many of which are biased. Let's look backstage, where projections can be conceived of as injections. "Backstage", recalling Goffman, is not only a metaphor for both formal and informal social interaction – as performed and rehearsed – but also refers to the backstage of cognition, again echoing a "cognitive unconscious" or "tacit knowing". Here, perhaps, rests existential authenticity. The ghostly play of purer intentions remains in the shadow of the muscular frontstage drama of ghastly proportions.

Where frontstage and backstage engage in conversation rests "adaptive expertise", as physicians become expert by "stitching together medicine and art" to draw on Roger Kneebone's (2020) craft metaphor. What a doctor "knows" (cognition) has to be explicitly performed (activity and affect), but the paradox here is that the expert doctor does not know what she knows. In other words, practice has become largely habitual, polished and automatic, as expertise. We love the fact that poetry, as inspiration, is largely in the backstory; if poetry were more obviously on stage, then it wouldn't be itself, it would be a commodity for narrativification and traditional medical education, made palatable and packaged as such.

However, the verse that is the language of the clinical encounter has to be composed, compacted and polished to be efficient. This is no bad thing – maybe the stripped-back, brief interpretive act on the part of the doctor can be rescued from the standard view that assumes the poor biomedical drone is performing a reductive functionalism. We believe that even the most devout biomedical acolyte operates within the aesthetic of Minimalism. We wish to impress on readers that the language of medicine might, in some mouths, be "cold" and "clinical" but that it very much possesses a style, and recognition of that style can be achieved when thinking of language as a poet does. Within that style is limitless beauty, and it is in this sense we challenge the narrativists to appreciate that which they casually discard as biomedical. For example, in her co-authored text Rita Charon (Charon et al. 2016: 1) opens, "Narrative medicine … emerged to challenge a reductionist, fragmented medicine", a vast generalisation that sweeps all productive and holistic (everyday) medical language and metaphor under the carpet, such as "grape-like vesicles", "sudden flashes and floaters", and "thunderclap headache".

In the opening paragraphs to Charon's (2006: 3) first text on Narrative Medicine, she says, "A scientifically competent medicine alone cannot help a patient grapple with the loss of health and find meaning in illness and dying": the same sentiment as her grumble above. We agree, but not for the reasons Charon puts forward. The patient's life is not necessarily improved because of the interpellation of Narrative Medicine, but more likely because of the love and support they feel from their family and friends. They are probably very grateful for the biomedical intervention of, say surgery, a drug therapy, or a course of physiotherapy. Narrativism, to be fair, is a minor intervention in comparison to coming home to a beloved pet dog, a local street community of helpful neighbours, or, most importantly, a national political decision to increase the pay of community nurses, or expand mental healthcare volunteer work through extensive grants. In a moment, we will bring forth the work of William Carlos Williams to assail the casual ascribing of coldness to what we view as often a beautiful, engaging style.

Some medical educators have sought, through the medical/health humanities, to educate a poetic imagination to bring emotional colour and imaginative flair to the medical mind (when poetry is even thought of at all, we should add). This is again based on the stereotype that the medical mind typically lacks a poetic imagination or stands in opposition to it. Isn't this just the flip side of the "antinarrative act" as applied to poetry, a recruitment of poetry to do narrative work? We explode the binaristic constructions of narrativists as advertised in the Charon quotes above (where Narrative Medicine is invoked to address a lack) by asking these questions: What if a poetic imagination already inhabits the structures and practices of diagnostic and prognostic clinical reasoning but doesn't readily show its face, or is largely a backstage, or tacit, underground and distributed activity? And what if the medical mind has a set of ground rules that echo formal poetic concerns such as genre, diction, rhythm, sensibility, style, and imaginative capacity as these represent feeling states? The poetic mind again may be in the wings, awaiting an entrance, while the frontstage drama has become over-rehearsed and over-identified with narrative concerns. We have already answered these questions formally in our chapters 6 and 7 on the architecture of diagnostic reasoning, but here we provide a gloss.

This chapter condenses two orthodoxies that we have set ourselves to challenge in this book. These orthodoxies are:

1 The compensatory position.

Medical thinking and the poetic imagination are naturally opposed rather than intensively and extensively entangled or implicated. Arts and health interventions bring these poles into an often forced or artificial conversation to compensate for the dominance of "objective" readings of symptoms over "subjective" life histories of patients. We say "artificial" because such arts-based interventions often do not actually lead to the production of decent art. And we say this defiantly, on poetry's behalf. We blame Keats, who told us to tell the truth so long ago as an act of beauty.

2 The narrative dominance position.

We have already set out how narrative medicine has been configured as the major compensatory force for reductive biomedicine. Our Part 1 shows how narrative has eaten lyric poetry whole. Narrative and poetic approaches can and should work side by side. Here we foreground the work of poetry.

We will, borrowing a philosophical tactic from Martin Heidegger, make a "Clearing" – an illuminating, a positioning, or perspective-taking – so that we can more readily see and feel the productive overlaps and entanglements between the poetic imagination and the medical mind. This will expose a treasure that artists call a "readymade". By putting the outwardly functional hat stand, bottle rack, bicycle wheel or snow shovel into an art gallery setting, Marcel Duchamp forced us to reconsider such functional objects aesthetically, revealing qualities that we perhaps had not noticed before, where the instrumental suddenly exudes beauty (recall "skin hooks" and other surgical instruments, rescued from instrumental reductions). We then re-site medicine in the "gallery" so that we can remind ourselves of its inherent beauty or see it refreshed. This is a double recognition, where not only are the objects of medicine re-sited (or recited through poetic diction), but also the frame, the field, of medicine – the clinic – is re-sited, à la Duchamp, as gallery. This is, again, the work of defamiliarisation.

We will rehearse this poetic reciting again, because it is central to our argument. Michel Foucault (1976) did the footwork for us by tracking the "birth of the clinic" as the origin of modern medicine in a space whose supra-function was the generation of power (of medicine overlaying other approaches to health and illness). This was a political gesture. We are now saying that the clinic must be re-birthed, or undone and re-invented, as an aesthetic gesture. Our vehicle for this work is poetry. We ask that we bring poetry into the clinic drawing on Duchamp's technique of shifting everyday or mundane objects – in our case the objects of medicine – and relocating them, or placing them. The clinic then becomes gallery, a placing of the aesthetic, and a call for medicine as poetry.

Back to *iatroversalio:* splicing medicine and poetry

We have seen how narrativism has been appropriated by the medical/health humanities to bring balm to patients buffeted by nakedly instrumental, bruising medicine. This is the accepted narrative. In this book however we stand for alter-narratives. We think there is plenty in naked medicine to admire and we have provided a lens for that: Minimalism. We ask that medicine consciously apply itself to the Minimalist ethic through study of its principles, particularly: "reduction in form does not mean reduction in complexity". But narrativism for us, for all the reasons already given, cannot do what poetry does. We know from our experience in the medical/health humanities that poetry is perceived as the most radical positioning away from biomedicine that one can achieve. We have partly addressed this perception by aligning poetry with medicine's clinical reasoning process. Poetry and medicine can breathe together, in synchrony. We continue by revisiting the notion of *iatroversalia* – poetry inspired by medicine, and invert it to describe medicine inspired by poetry.

Here, we must be clear again, we are not so interested in poetry being used to better doctors' wellbeing – a therapeutic function; or in poetry being used instrumentally to "improve" medicine ("a controlled trial shows that medical interventions informed by poetry had better clinical outcomes than the same intervention without the poetry" etc. Remember, poetry is *essentially* useless. But we are not interested in essentialism either. We are interested in poetry doing aesthetic labour: bringing beauty, form, quality, intensity, and so forth, to a life lived (and to the reverse, that lives lived feed back into the body of poetry to develop its form and qualities). The heart of this is the coining of new and more heart-stopping metaphors that turn mere events into experiences; and its effect is on style of medical practice as a medicine of qualities.

In medical judgements, patients' hopes, fears, recoveries, uncertainties, and suffering are at stake. We must make every effort to understand such judgements and hone them. This also addresses what the Spanish doctor-poet Pascual Iniesta (1908–99) termed *iatroversalia* – poetry inspired by, or related to, medical practice (Iniesta 2012). We enlarge Iniesta's meaning by adopting a bricolage method, where any poetry, and not just poetry about medical practice, can be employed to gain insight into the medical mind. *Iatroversalia* is a starting point but not an end point. Our focus again is medicine inspired by poetry. It naturally follows according to our belief that poetry is everywhere, then medicine can be sought everywhere.

The work of re-uniting poetry with medicine is set in a wider contemporary problem born of the gradual forcing apart and opposing of scientific and arts/humanities cultures primarily since the Second World War. In the late 16th and early 17th centuries, for example, there was not such a separation. John Donne, suffering from stomach cancer late in life, gave impetus to the modern genre of autopathography in writing about his own illnesses and symptom patterns ("Make me new" said Donne, and, famously, of the misery of isolation: "No man is an island". Writing about illness has a longer history – for example the Greek orator and rhetorician Publius Aelius Aristides, in the first century AD, gives an account of his hypochondria (Phillips 1952)). Donne had no medical training but was insatiably curious about medicine (Honigsbaum 2009).

John Keats – both doctor and poet – wrote about his time at Guy's Hospital, London from 1815–17 in an incomparable wedding of medicine and verse, packed with bodily metaphors. Keats attended the Physical Society at Guy's, a meeting of literary-minded doctors, surgeons and scientists as well as philosophers and poets, where papers would be read and discussed. The Society was founded in 1769 and moved to Guy's in 1783, attracting the leading radical thinkers of its age. In the 1790s Joseph Priestley, Thomas Beddoes, and Samuel Taylor Coleridge were regulars (Barnard, in Roe 2017). Here, science, politics, and poetics were inseparable. Indeed, it was unthinkable that the scientifico-medical and poetic imaginations would be split or opposed; rather they were inter-dependent.

As noted earlier, because of his work at Guy's Hospital, Keats made a transition from a poet of hollow-ringing metaphysics to one of muscular, embodied verse where his poetic imagination was thickened, enriched, and rendered sensual by the medical imagination:

> Before Keats went to Guy's, his poems had featured bland conventional figures of 'Pity', 'Despondence', 'Passions' and 'Hope'. After Guy's, he could imagine the throbbing life of nerves, muscles, arteries, bones and blood … where phrases such as 'nervous grasp' … 'laborious breath' … and 'horribly convuls'd' … give the fallen Titans a forceful physical presence.
>
> Roe (2017: 2)

Recall our earlier concerns about Narrative Medicine's use of strenuous, muscular metaphors, ones of rigour ("tough" rather than "tender"). Here, Keats is on another level. In narrative medicine workshops we want to see students not "failing to meet narrative competences at the required level", but rather have a "nervous grasp" on a complex idea that the educator can scaffold to help the student to progress: With a "laborious breath" the leap of understanding was made.

Despite the legacy of doctor-poets such as Keats, poetry and medicine drifted apart as separate continents, part of modernism's positioning the arts/humanities and the sciences as irreconcilable – the topic of C.P. Snow's notorious 1959 Rede Lectures on "The Two Cultures" (Snow 1959) referred to in previous chapters. Snow bemoaned this effect, suggesting "There is, of course, no complete solution …. But we can do something. The chief means open to us is education". But education, as Liam Hudson (1966) suggested a decade after Snow, continued to reinforce what Hudson called "contrary imaginations": the convergent thinker drawn to sciences and the divergent thinker drawn to arts and humanities. These types, suggested Hudson, describe natural inclinations reinforced by tight academic furrows at High School/Secondary level in either the sciences or the arts.

In such an oppositional mindset, whatever sits between convergence and divergence, as "bivergence", is seen as unusual and puzzling. This is clearly what Rita Charon and colleagues wish to encourage through the "stereoscopic" vision of evidence-based-narrative-medicine, effectively reinventing Hudson's model of bivergence. But Hudson's model itself is muddled where it comes to bivergent academic inter-disciplines such as Geography (part humanities, part sciences) and the social sciences (that typically draw on quantitative approaches and favour evidence over speculation), rather than the identities of the persons who study these subjects. In other words, if convergers are drawn to sciences and divergers to arts, who is typically drawn to inter-disciplines that are bivergent such as Geography or Economics?

Convergent thinking – characterising those who enter medicine (identifying as science-based) – typically represses affect, whereas divergent thinking encourages cathartic expression. In contemporary life, poetry and medicine can be seen to intersect (bivergently) as,

(i) *concretely*: doctors who are poets/poets who are doctors;
(ii) *cathartically*: poetry used therapeutically as a vehicle of expression; and
(iii) *pedagogically*: poetry as a vehicle for education.

In (i) above, poetry might be thought of as the backstage (and rebellious) to the frontstage (and conformist) of clinical practice, while in (ii) and (iii) poetry is a frontstage (conformist) prop. We consider this classification in more detail below.

There are, relatively, only a scattering of people who identify as both published and respected poets (knowing the craft of poetry) and experienced doctors (showing adaptive medical expertise). Their writing may or may not describe their medical encounters, but it is inevitable that, like Keats above, immersion in a medical world will have shaped and emboldened their poetic imaginations. Our question again is not what medicine can do for poetry, but what can poetry do for medicine? How do doctors *use* their poetic imaginations, rather than just write about their work? We happily embrace the paradox of admitting (and insisting on) uselessness while also being all for application: imaginatively, cognitively, emotionally and practically. One of the best-known examples is William Carlos Williams (1883–1963) (Williams 1967), deservedly now a regular figure in this book. Williams illustrates the striking marriage of a stripped-back Minimalism in diagnostic utterance – typical of medicine – and the style of imagistic poetics that sticks strictly with emergence of "field" as the whole poem placed on the page; and is defined by epiphany through economy of language, metaphoric precision, angular phrasing, intensely close description of phenomena, and avoidance of abstract generalities. The painter Agnes Martin said, "Art is the concrete representation of our most subtle feelings".

In "Arrival" (https://www.poemhunter.com/poem/arrival) Williams opens with a mystery, a common trope in his poetry: "And yet one arrives somehow". We imagine this emblazoned above the door of consulting rooms. But for Williams, in this poem, it is arrival perhaps in a motel or hotel. Where the protagonist of the poem "arrives" he is already "… loosening the hooks of / her dress / in a strange bedroom". But, as the dress drops this reveals "The tawdry veined body" that is "twisted upon itself / like a winter wind". Williams introduces the theme of ageing in a mysterious way via indefinite pronoun and nonspecific adverb use that suddenly switches into precise description: Just as "one" (author or reader) "arrives somehow" at the point of "loosening the hooks of / her dress" so one "feels the autumn / dropping its silk and linen leaves / about her ankles". Now we are nicely settled into the passing of the seasons; but then "the tawdry veined body emerges" "like a winter wind". The change in register mirrors the change in perception. We, too, are shaken by this change.

The woman seems to have passed from her autumnal years to winter. "Loosening the hooks" is literal, but it can also be taken as a metaphor of the creeping in of age as the body loses the firmness and uprightness of youth. The woman emerges "twisted" on herself, maybe slightly hunched. In ten short lines, Williams makes us ponder deeply on an interpersonal encounter that moves from productive superficialities to specific noticing. He focusses us on the meanings of often-encountered enjambments in relationships, the sudden falling away of expectation in the face of reality; how the tender might abruptly switch to the tawdry; the wished-for, or expectation, faced with the real encounter.

The man's affect switches from expectation to acceptance. Importantly for medicine, the affect is subterranean. Williams's emotionally quiet poem frontstage, in fact, hollers from its backstage and wings store of implications, hints and double meanings, centred on the loosening the hooks of the woman's dress in unfamiliar surroundings. The reader fills in the rest. The doctor fills in the rest of the consultation. The surplus rests with the unsaid.

Seasons pass (the spring and summer of expectation, the autumn of falling leaves mirrored by the falling silk and linen of the woman's clothes leading to the winter of the tawdry, veined body twisted on itself) as time compressed into place, again in just ten lines. Williams models compression as Minimalism with quality maintained. Can doctors compress with such poetic quality in the ever-decreasing time they have available for consultations, especially with swirling surplus to scoop up or sample from? Can frontstage (protocol, what is actually said and done) and backstage (the informal, the unspoken, what broods, and what is felt) be brought into conversation? What else (unknown, ambiguous) lurks in the wings? Minimalist moments can appear as exposed gems: stark observations, instant pattern recognition, rapid confirmations, polished surfaces, and condensed insights.

As doctors meet new patients, "professionalism" is supposed to maintain evenness of emotional interaction in the encounter, as detachment. But such ironing out of affect is once again a frontstage performance strategy. Backstage affect runs its course and must be accounted for, making the work of medicine equate to the work of poetry. The more specific the observation, the deeper the emotional response and this affect must go somewhere, to be expressed somehow. Meditation on Williams's poem here is potentially worth more than a host of "clinical communication" sessions under conditions of simulation.

We have taken Williams's poem as a metaphor for the compressed clinical encounter that has a narrative, of course, but here the narrative is squashed so hard under time pressures that it may just make gems in another node. The gems, of course, that appear are the nodal metaphors that afford diagnostic clues and facilitate communication. Such metaphors utilise well the promise that a lot can be achieved in a brief performative encounter. The metaphors are bridges that link backstage and frontstage issues ("metaphor" means "to transfer"). As Laurence Kirmayer (2000: 153) says, "Prior to narratization, salient illness experiences are apprehended and extended through metaphors". Medicine's job, in our idealised concept, might be summarised as the production of new metaphors under pressure prior to, or despite, narrative insistence. Do metaphors help medicine? Of course, "take 'puff, puff' breaths," says the midwife to stop the woman pushing too soon; "cut confidently and cleanly" says the surgeon (alliteratively) to the trainee (the cut itself is a precise and incisive metaphor); "it's like a buzzsaw deep in my ears, doctor, I just can't turn it off" (tinnitus sufferer to GP).

Williams called doctoring an essentially creative activity. Yet in the face of so much red-blooded passion in medical culture, a historically determined mix of arrogance and lust in the face of death, the day-to-day reality of medicine is actually closer to what the Canadian poet Dionne Brand (2018) describes as an oxymoronic "systolic blue". Systole describes the heart at its apex pumping red, oxygenated arterial blood around the body; also pumping deoxygenated blood to the lungs. But Brand's oxymoron serves to describe a medicine of truth – embodied in the tired venous "blue blood" that returns to the heart. Blood is literally always red, but appears blue in the veins close to the skin as an optical illusion. Red light penetrates further into tissue than blue light. You see more blue than red reflected light due to the blood's partial absorption of red wavelengths. Here's another frontstage/backstage phenomenon. The poem, of course, provides the optic and the metaphor does the work.

The late Welsh doctor and poet Dannie Abse (1923–2014) (https://www.poetryfoundation.org/poets/dannie-abse), met earlier, is another example of a deeply passionate and compassionate poet and doctor. Poetry frames and shapes the medicine. His collection (1989) *White Coat, Purple Coat* describes the purple coat trumping the white, where: "I like to think I'm a poet and Medicine my serious hobby". Abse's poems about medicine are often sardonic. He gently mocks, rather than admires, "physicians who'd arrive / fast and first on any sour death-bed scene", where, "There are men who would open anything. // … Men who'd open men" while "others, mother, with diseases / like great streets named after them: Addison / Parkinson, Hodgkin" (https://www.poetryfoundation.org/poetrymagazine/poems/34137/x-ray-56d21793976b8). The reader is left thinking that Abse, while annoyed by the heroic in surgery and medicine, is also irritated by the need for recognition among doctors. How will history remember me? Anyone familiar with medical schools and their dark wood halls, reception rooms and lecture theatres will have noted the dour, formal portraits of the famous male deans (rarely a woman) punctuating the walls as monumental frontstage drama.

Abse recapitulates the tensions of frontstage/backstage conversations and how these can be facilitated. If backstage is poetry, then we see medicine in the same role as King or Queen Narrative Medicine who will forever subjugate poetry. We think medicine can accommodate poetry rather than assimilate it, and we show how. We do not think that poetry used therapeutically, or in the service of medicine in its typical role in the medical/health humanities to offer a "voice for expression" (personal confessional quasi-therapy via catharsis), allows poetry to shine. Rather, it is what psychotherapists call an act of "smiling demolition" – we love you as we smother you.

We will leave poet-doctors at this point because we provide so many more examples throughout this book, particularly in chapter 14.

ii   *Poetry used therapeutically as a vehicle of expression*

The Guardian newspaper for March 8, 2021 carries an article about hospital-based healthcare workers being helped through the Covid-19 pandemic in times of extraordinary stress, where "The arts are helping some staff decompress" (Campbell 2021). At Imperial College Healthcare NHS Trust in London "the poet in residence … is helping staff to write their own poems in writing workshops" (ibid.). Writing poetry is widely drawn on as a therapeutic tool, for example in community mental health (Baker and Bartel 2020).

Marilyn McEntyre (2012) shows in detail how writing poems about their illnesses affords patients a therapeutic opportunity, and also creates insights for doctors and healthcare professionals beyond the initial diagnosis. Poetry acts as cradle and comfort, but also a means for insight. The emphasis, however, is not necessarily on the quality of the poetry (again, vitally important to craft-sensitive doctor-poets – after all "poetry" is derived from an ancient Greek word meaning to "make", or "craft") but simply the act of writing, so that the medium becomes the message and "craft" is left on the backburner. Poetry here is rather a vehicle of expression, enabling catharsis, without the residue or legacy that can be passed on to others as a lasting work of art. Hence, while catharsis is the main aim, the medium for its mobilisation is secondary – it could be drumming, chanting, singing, visual art, or drama. We detect a problem here.

As an illustrative example, we return to the inciting stimulus of our introduction and offer a couple of stanzas of a poem from 2008 published in Johanna Shapiro's (2009) *The Inner World of Medical Students: Listening to Their Voices in Poetry.* Shapiro is a well-known figure in the medical humanities and narrative medicine, and was the first to systematically look at the roles of students' poetry as an element in medical education. As you will recall, her focus is largely on the therapeutic function of poetry. Her approach in this book sets out to satisfy both narrativists and scientists. First, she scoops up narrative and poetry together treating them as one body. Her critical apparatus is a combination of literary studies and qualitative inquiry.

As Howard Stein (in ibid.: x) says in his Foreword, Shapiro treats the poetry as "data" to illustrate her argument that medical education (of the time) is fundamentally dehumanising. Stein notes how Shapiro offers "a typology of narrative themes into which her students' poems can be classified – chaos, restitution, quest, witnessing, journey, and transcendent". Thus, we see again poetry disappearing into the maw of narrative and being digested, to reappear as stories-as-data open to classification. This is repeated in Shapiro's (ibid.: 2) introductory section where she frames students' poetry as "data" ("n = 589" poems), asking, "What narrative forms do these poems take?" But aren't poems themselves? Should we trust any biomedicalist applying scales and measuring sticks in the search to quantify love? The idea is ridiculous, but the prospect of reading poetry, and using it, for what it isn't happens over and over again.

Shapiro analyses a poem by a medical student "Reflections of a Pruned Medical Student", in which the poem compares a "sculpted" tree to a "socialised" medical student who "Has learned how to conform":

My sculptured shape is chiseled
By shears too sharp to see

> For pruning is the price I paid
> For this topiary me

"Here the author uses a classic rhyme scheme (abcb) and a traditional meter (a kind of modified iambic trimeter), as well as a consistent metaphor (a sculpted shrub) to describe her experience in medical school". We cheer this formal analysis, found rarely in academic writing by doctors. Shapiro makes a case that the form of the poem reflects the formal nature of her socialisation into medicine. It is this imaginative analysis that we find the most poetic thing about the matter, even though we dislike it when poetry is being shoehorned into pre-set categories, when it is being read to confirm expectations rather than being read as poetry; when it comes to the poem itself, we see a rather awkward piece of writing. First, there is no rationale for the rhyme scheme or meter, but this runs along fine until the last line itself chokes on "topiary", and we all fall down. The analogies are weird. That a "sculptured shape is chiseled" is ok, this is a tree; but it is shears that are doing the chiselling (wrong tool, wrong job, wrong metaphor), and what does she mean by "too sharp to see"? Does she mean the unseen forces of the medical school establishment? And why are the shears "too sharp to see"? Surely sharpness is felt? Wrong sense – nonsense. We'll grant this poem, though, some points for its concision and Dickinsonian imitation so far (see Emily Dickinson's "I taste a liquor never brewed": https://poemanalysis.com/emily-dickinson/i-taste-a-liquor-never-brewed/).

The medical student continues,

> Meandering through scented shops
> Lounging by the pool
> Watching goofy sitcoms
> And trying to look cool
>
> Crosswords and sudokus
> Magazines and jokes
> These were clipped and hauled away
> By the garden training folks.

Note the devolution. By moving from a more meta-reflective self, which was handled competently if rather confusedly, we come to a poem trying to define loss of self or individuated identity through the loss of detritus. The change in tone is severe, crashing into colloquialism ("trying to look cool" and the terminal "folks"). Medical education might be likened to gardening, perhaps; but isn't *tending* better? The parallel remains forced, in any case. If this is what the student really misses about life as she enters medical school, then our jaws drop. Perhaps on evidence of the lack of craft displayed in the poem, it is good that these trivial pursuits were "clipped away" we say. Time to buckle down and get a proper job!

The poetry is so light it floats out of consciousness immediately, making no impression. Where is the argument, the depth of feeling that comes in making the reader feel the conformity? Or if the poem intended to work in the zone of light verse, then where is the gnomic acerbicness of Ogden Nash? Or the devastating pith of Dorothy Parker? The poem strikes us as occasional verse lacking an occasion, a work that bids farewell to a juvenile self that could have succeeded in its attempted enumeration of grief if it had made something formally interesting of its trite thingy-ness rather than a few items used to fill out a deadening rhyme scheme. It seems to us that the poem itself reeks of conformity more than the medical school initiation and functions much as a virtual medical school graduation does: a frantic wave to uncommemorated transformation.

Hard-working anatomists, biomedical scientists, social scientists, clinicians, and so forth, buzzing away with their pedagogical fervour are reduced to "garden training folks"? Worse, the poem itself is subject to a couple of paragraphs of analysis sans close reading for aesthetics. It is again used as an instrument to make points about shortcomings of medical education, a means-end function: poetry as dishwasher. What's the point of dressing up bad poetry like this? If poetry is useless, then poetry oblivious to beauty is worthless. Although, everything is, indeed, information.

Patients/service users write (and sometimes read) poetry, with or without help from facilitators, as (a) a means of expression leading to catharsis or emotional release (untutored illness autoethnography); (b) a means of impression, as a way to gain insight or stabilise identity, or to gain a different orientation to others and to the world; and (c) a way of nurturing creativity in otherwise stagnant periods of life, for example during a depressive period. Again, the quality of the poetry is not at stake. Here, the medium is not the message – otherwise the point of poetry. The goal is "arts-based therapy", where the media for therapy are secondary to the goal. We do not denigrate the purpose of such therapeutic methods. We do, however, throughout this book point out some logical negative outcomes of such a relegation to instrumentalisation. We're not saying throw out the therapy, we're saying that's all it is. Poetry is more than that. And to really achieve what the therapy wants, maybe it has to be more too?

An extension of this lay use of poetry is to draw on published or well-known poetry as "prescription". This is again to use poetry therapeutically, not through an individual's own writing but rather by them receiving chosen poems matched to an individual's presenting symptoms. For example, William Sieghart (2017, 2019), discussed previously, has toured the UK presenting poetry "on prescription" at public venues such as libraries. In this framework, poetry not only diagnoses the symptoms of historical, cultural, and social ills but promises cures for such ills; pondering the cancerous mass is not just for the oncologist but also for the masses. The democratising impulse is to be celebrated, especially if this results in authentically patient-centred doctor-patient encounters and authentically inter-professional doctor-healthcare practitioner encounters. Ronna Bloom provides a similar service in Toronto (https://ronnabloom.com/events). But, again, the poetry is a medium and not necessarily the message. We say this even where the "on prescription" poetry is good, because the poem is used instrumentally and not necessarily aesthetically to improve "quality of life". Of course, we're skating on thin ice here because arts therapy enthusiasts tend to see such claims as elitist. But our point is, if drawing, pottery, singing or weaving can do the job of poetry, we say that we don't want poetry to act as stand-in, but as stand-alone.

iii   *Poetry as a vehicle for education*

Some medical/health humanities programmes and interventions for doctors and medical students involve writing poetry as a vehicle for "seeing otherwise", or re-imagining medicine (Bleakley 2015). This is a re-education. Our example above from Johanna Shapiro's book does not raise confidence about medical students' poetry as vehicles for therapy or education. Granted, the writing of poetry may map out new ways of understanding relationships with patients or give fresh insights into medical conditions; it may also have a therapeutic function as in (ii) above – for example as a means for catharsis in times of stress, or for insight in times of moral dilemmas. Yet again, the quality of the poetry is not necessarily at stake – it is used as a medium for release, insight or change, or reframing practice. But the message of poetry – primarily to create beauty, sometimes dark, is missed.

Our book is not an apologia for poetry. We don't want to convert doctors to poets or artists in general. We want to introduce a poetic imagination into medical work. We return to Aristotle's point that "poetics" included literary and drama theory, and set out *an aesthetics of engagement with the natural and social worlds.* Importantly, Aristotle (*Poetics*: 6) suggested that poetry should not be concerned primarily with human qualities but rather with activities (thinking with things) – their motives and consequences. While history describes the activities of persons in the past: "the thing that has been", poetry, said Aristotle, describes the "thing that might be" (ibid.: 9). While it may reflect on the consequences of history, poetry trumps history by reinventing humans, describing what humans could become. But again, while we have time and time again illustrated our arguments with poems and cherish poetry, we are not saying that doctors should sign up to poetry workshops or writing classes (although we are happy if they do), as Narrative Medicine enthusiasts may insist for their discipline. Rather, we are saying that by hook or by crook, we want to encourage Aristotle's plea for – again – an aesthetics of engagement with the natural and social worlds with beauty at its centre.

We have said a lot about what poetry does not do, or how it is instrumentalised, potentially abused as therapeutic medium rather than art form, occluded or buried. What then, in a nutshell, does poetry do? We think that art is not to be harnessed *only*; it is philistine to think so. Art is to transform one's perception, such that one is utterly changed. We have noted that Narrative

Medicine, of course, sets out to do this, but we have enumerated a variety of reasons of why its aims can be undermined: such as over-reach, distraction by business interests, overuse of a muscular metaphor frame, educational laziness concerning reductive "training" terms, and so forth.

Some art is much more humble than this lofty goal, but all art is conducted in the shadow of a canon of eternity, what we look at when we are sad, or before we knew what true beauty was; and, knocked back a hundred feet, we no longer are so sure of where we are, or why. In one of his best-known poems, "Thunder-and-Lightning Polka" (see in Collected Poems: https://b-ok.cc/book/4624031/683584?id=4624031&secret=683584), Peter Redgrove (1987) sets out a manifesto for clinical practice: tune your body like an instrument and play it well, to join "the hypersensitive cabaret"; educate the senses so that you have "staring ears"; and build institutions of learning that have "halls stuffed with thunderwork".

Kindling the poetic imaginations of medical students

We think that doctors can diagnose with Redgrove's "staring ears" (multisensory immersion, close noticing) without necessarily having to put on the cloak of Sherlock Holmes and narrativise patients' accounts as a form of sleuthing. We also think that every wood-panelled hall of every medical school could have a large sign at the doorway saying "halls stuffed with thunderwork". (This would offer a "sly civility" dig at those ever-present pompous portraits of – predominantly male – ex-deans, reminding us that Narcissists love an Echo). This multimetaphorical weather itself might echo around the place and produce epiphanies. Or at least raise questions, inquiring minds, and not just obsequious nods to the white forefathers who are the foreground to our suggested irritant background. Within these hallowed chambers of the medical school (not all schools, of course, are so stuffy or dark-wood-panelled in their architecture or their ways) how then shall we kindle the poetic imaginations of medical students? Let's just imagine two possibilities: poetically infecting sterile "clinical skills training", and re-visioning science education (these two topics are books in their own right, so we apologise in advance for our turning the key in the lock without showing the room. Space is short).

Clinically, medical students, as doctors-in-waiting, could be encouraged to see their patients' "histories" through the lens of poetry as Bahar Orang (2020) again models in *Where Things Touch: A Meditation on Beauty*, developing Redgrove's "staring ears". Orang (2020: 72) talks of "how to skin / an essay and pare it down in spite of your attachments" as if she were describing at once dissection, autopsy, diagnosis – or "taking" a history (why do we not describe this as "receiving" a history?). Through "staring ears" we listen into the history and see the patient for what she is. This means that we take the history both literally and metaphorically. Orang (ibid.) notes that a "dry" history does not capture the liquid complexity of patients' needs, where,

nearly every body is
moist; nearly every body oozes. And what a relief it
might be, what a possible pleasure, to hear a patient's
unadulterated version of events, to allow the story to
seep through its own cracks.

On the doctor's part, as poet, Orang (ibid.) demands close noticing and witnessing, as an act of beauty:

a beauty concerned
with thick sentences, detailed ekphrasis, descriptions as
analysis, abundance as the most interesting aesthetics.

We are interested in not just what the patient presents but what may become of the patient as potential. "Taking a history" (again, we prefer "receiving a history" to avoid the imperialistic taxis) relies on concrete and factual description, while poetry enhances such description through use of metaphor as a vehicle of possibility, both springboard and lens for deeper appreciation and understanding. Thus, Aristotle says that the work of the poet is to convince us not of what we are (plain diagnostic description), but of how we can be or what we can become (prognostic possibility). Paraphrasing Aristotle (ibid.: 25), poetry describes a convincing improbability as preferable to an unconvincing probability, the latter accepted by a tamer imagination.

The diagnostic arc must operate at first sight of the patient, at first meeting. Again, this need not be framed as an unfolding narrative, but rather as an unpacking of instants in space that contain a myriad of clues about prognosis. As Marilyn McEntyre (2012) suggests, with poetry: "You have to let go of the expectations that you bring to story", where "Poems set their own terms". In particular, this means accepting and dwelling in ambiguities that may never be resolved through plot; and managing multiple possible meanings simultaneously. Our following three chapters pick up this theme of ambiguity – central to both medicine and poetry.

References

Abse D. 1989. *White Coat, Purple Coat: Collected Poems 1948–88*. London: Hutchinson.
Alduy C. (Undated). Against Narratives III. Or a Certain Kind of Narrative. Blog. Arcade: Literature, the Humanities & the World. Retrieved from https://arcade.stanford.edu/blogs/against-narratives-iii-or-certain-kind-narrative
Aristotle. 2013. *Poetics*. Oxford: OUP.
Baker C, Bartel H. 2020. Poetry and Male Eating Disorders. In: P Crawford, B Brown, A Charise (eds.) *The Routledge Companion to Health Humanities*. London: Routledge, 248–54.
Barnard J. 2017. John Keats in the Context of the Physical Society, Guy's Hospital, 1815–1816. In: N Roe (ed.) *John Keats and the Medical Imagination*. London: Palgrave Macmillan, 73–90.

Bleakley A. 2015. *Medical Humanities and Medical Education: How the Medical Humanities Can Shape Better Doctors.* Abingdon: Routledge.

Brand D. 2018. *The Blue Clerk: Ars Poetica in 59 Versos.* Durham, NC: Duke University Press.

Campbell D. Health Service: Hospital Workers Rewarded with Holidays and Hot Food. The Guardian. Monday March 8, 2021. Retrieved from https://www.theguardian.com/society/2021/mar/07/hospitals-offer-holiday-bonuses-covid-weary-staff-england-nhs

Charon R. 2006. *Narrative Medicine: Honoring the Stories of Illness.* Oxford: Oxford University Press.

Charon R, DasGupta S, Hermann N, et al. 2016. *The Principles and Practices of Narrative Medicine.* Oxford: Oxford University Press.

Encke J. Taking Its Pulse: Poetry in the Context of Narrative Medicine. EOAGH. Undated. Retrieved from https://eoagh.com/taking-its-pulse-poetry-in-the-context-of-narrative-medicine/

Foucault M. 1976. *The Birth of the Clinic: An Archaeology of Medical Perception.* London: Routledge.

Goffman E. 1959. *The Presentation of Self in Everyday Life.* New York: Anchor Books.

Honigsbaum M. The Patient's View: John Donne and Katharine Anne Porter. *The Lancet.* 2009; 374: 194–95.

Hudson L. 1966. *Contrary Imaginations: A Study of the English Schoolboy.* Harmondsworth: Penguin Books.

Iniesta I. The Iatroversalia (Doctor Poems) of William Carlos Williams. *Clinical Medicine* (London). 2012; 12: 92–93.

Kirmayer LJ. 2000. Broken Narratives: Clinical Encounters and the Poetics of Illness Experience. In: C Mattingly, LC Garro (eds.) *Narrative and the Cultural Construction of Illness and Healing.* Berkeley: University of California Press, 153–80.

Kneebone R. 2020. *Expert: Understanding the Path to Mastery.* London: Penguin.

McEntyre M. 2012. *Patient Poets: Illness from Inside out.* San Francisco: University of California Medical Humanities Press.

Nowottny W. 1965. *The Language Poets Use.* London: The Athlone Press.

Orang B. 2020. *Where Things Touch: A Meditation on Beauty.* Toronto: Book*Hug.

Phillips ED. A Hypochondriac and His God. *Greece & Rome.* January 1952; 21(61): 23–36 (14 pp).

Raj D, Williamson RM, Young D, and Russell D. A Simple Epidural Simulator: A Blinded Study Assessing the 'Feel' of Loss of Resistance in Four Fruits. *European Journal of Anaesthesiology.* 2013; 30: 405–8.

Rancière J. 2013. *The Politics of Aesthetics.* London: Bloomsbury Academic.

Redgrove P. 1987. Collected Poems.

Ricoeur P. 2008/1970. *Freud and Philosophy. An Essay on Interpretation.* Denis Savage (transl.). New Haven, CT: Yale University Press.

Roe N (ed.) 2017. *John Keats and the Medical Imagination.* London: Palgrave Macmillan.

Sartre J-P. 1956. *Being and Nothingness.* New York, NY: Washington Square Press.

Shapiro J. 2009. *The Inner World of Medical Students: Listening to Their Voices in Poetry.* Oxford: Radcliffe Publishing.

Sieghart W. 2017. *The Poetry Pharmacy: Tried-and-True Prescriptions for the Heart, Mind and Soul.* London: Particular Books.

Sieghart W. 2019. *The Poetry Pharmacy Returns: More Prescriptions for Courage, Healing and Hope.* London: Particular Books.

Snow CP. 1959. *The Two Cultures and the Scientific Revolution*. Cambridge: Cambridge University Press.

Theune M. Against Narrative. Structure & Surprise: Engaging Poetic Turns. Blog. Retrieved from https://structureandsurprise.com/theory-criticism/against-narrative/

Vaihinger H. 2000/1924. *The Philosophy of "As If"*. London: Routledge Classics.

Williams WC. 1967. *The Autobiography of William Carlos Williams*. San Francisco, CA: New Directions Books.

11 Kinds of ambiguity in clinical work

How to resist cutting the Gordian Knot

In this chapter we resist cutting the Gordian Knot, embrace the *pharmakon* or healing poison, and view contradiction as a resource. We lift off the beat to create space, open the brackets, and strike through the word to put it under erasure or in suspension. All of these are well-established techniques in writing, criticism and thinking (and in the musicality that shapes these activities). We see their value in medicine too. In a previous chapter we recounted the impatient and impetuous surgeon's satirical words on seeing a doctor deliberating by a patient's bedside: "Don't just do something, stand there!" (The surgeon, of course, may be right). We are going to stand there on and off during this chapter, deliberating issues that centre on ambiguity and uncertainty (we will differentiate between these below, although they are often conflated; the dictionary will give them as synonymous). We frame ambiguity in medicine as a resource and not a hindrance, and we note that it is central to practice, where tolerance of ambiguity marks the reflective practitioner. Ambiguity is central to poetry. What might medicine learn from study of ambiguity in poetry? This and the following two chapters address this question.

Professions such as law and medicine might be seen as ambiguity specialists. In both the law and medicine's cases, ambiguity is formally a suspended term, or bracketed out. While both professions recognise everyday ambiguity in their work, they also see their work as one of clarification or reduction of ambiguity. This creates an ambiguity in its own right, of course. Contemporary legal and medical education however have brought the ambiguity skeleton out of the closet and now nakedly admit that ambiguity should not be treated as a problem or constraint but as a resource. This and the following two chapters explore the meanings of ambiguity as a resource in medicine illustrated through borrowing poetry's view that ambiguity is central to the quality of writing, whereas once it was seen as a hindrance to style. For example, Yelland, Jones, and Easton (1950: 199), in a handbook of literary terms, and under the heading "Style", write, "Young writers are often told that they must avoid certain so-called style faults" such as "AMBIGUITY" (*capitalisation in the original*), but rather "cultivate the virtues of accuracy, simplicity, economy

DOI: 10.4324/9781003194408-13

and clarity". This would mirror the tenor of advice given to medical students and young doctors of the time.

Clinical reasoning is social and efflorescent (bursting forth and flowering)

Returning home from a late night of animated discussion with friends after a Christmas pantomime in 1817, the poet and surgeon John Keats discussed the conversation with his two brothers, bringing fresh insights. He later wrote that "several things dovetailed in my mind" about what constitutes the poetic imagination and creative mind. He noted that Shakespeare above all possessed a certain quality that he termed "Negative Capability" defined by Keats as, "when a man is capable of being in uncertainties, Mysteries, doubts, without any irritable reaching after fact & reason". This, he argued, was a keystone of the poetic imagination (Roe 2017).

In 1949, the psychologist Elke Frenkel-Brunswik, while researching the phenomenon of ethnocentrism, coined the term "ambiguity tolerance-intolerance" to describe a character trait she observed in children. Intolerance of ambiguity became associated with racism and what we now call "unconscious bias" typical of separatism. After the atrocities of the Holocaust, Frenkel-Brunswik and other psychologists such as Theodor Adorno (Adorno et al. 1950) – who was also philosopher, sociologist, musicologist, and composer – coined the term "the authoritarian personality" to describe the Fascist type. At the cold heart of this personality type is intolerance of ambiguity. Peter Merrotsy (2013) calls tolerance of ambiguity "a trait of the creative personality", where Gail Geller (2013) among others has, significantly, called for high tolerance of ambiguity as a "criterion for medical student selection". Of the many characteristics that one might look for to mark a "successful" physician, and one who is less likely to burn out under pressure, tolerance of ambiguity is high up the list (Peterkin 2018).

Keats had earlier, in November of 1817, written to a friend, "O for a life of Sensations rather than Thoughts!" As noted previously, Keats's work at St Guy's hospital in London as a surgeon from 1810 to 1817 had brought embodiment to his language, entangling poetry and medicine in sensate rather than abstract descriptions. But herein lay a trap: the shelving of rationality for the passions. Embrace of affect should not involve exclusions and divisions, but inclusions and tolerance. Thus, Keats laid the groundwork for the marriage of the poetic imagination and medical mind under two principles: first sensate focus, and second tolerance of ambiguity, or actively resisting "irritable reaching after fact & reason". Living with, and in, "uncertainties, Mysteries, doubts" describes the doctor as expert differential diagnostician. Describing the use of metaphors in palliative care medicine, Vyjeyanthi Periyakoil (2008: 843) notes: "ambiguity is not always bad and that skillful use of ambiguity (by doctors) can help to transmit meaning (to patients) in indirect and nonthreatening ways". In a broad-brush way, authoritarian medicine (hierarchical, pushy, and suffocatingly self-assured) is at core intolerant of ambiguity.

The poetic imagination and the medical mind seem at first sight to be at loggerheads in one fundamental values area: where poetry educates for tolerance of ambiguity through its employment of metaphor, reliance on epiphany, and use of slippage (enjambment) and slantwise technique, medicine seems to seek certainty or to reduce ambiguity, distrusting sudden insight in preference for dogged accumulation. However, doctors know all too well that much of their work is carried out under conditions of uncertainty, uniqueness and values conflict (Schön 1983), and medical educators have sought ways in which to educate for tolerance of ambiguity. Doctors say that they have a duty to reduce ambiguity for concerned patients, but research shows that patients are less concerned about being presented with ambiguities where they trust their doctor (Bleakley 2014).

Doctors educated as scientists and tending to a biomedical reading are generally Aristotelian in their logic – there is true and false and no in-between. Yet science as a valorised way of elucidating truth through objectivity is a shortsighted view of science whose methods are subject to historical circumstance. For example, Lorraine Daston and Peter Galison (2007) trace how notions of "objectivity" in science have changed historically according to the development of means of gaining evidence through, for example, use of observational and measurement artefacts (such as anatomy atlases, telescopes, and microscopes) and rules of representation (such as standardised anatomical drawings) to study natural phenomena. For example, anatomy atlases relying on drawing have typically idealised bodies and standardised the anatomy. Ambiguity is inherent to "objectivity" as read historically.

Also, as noted in earlier chapters, expert and adaptive doctors tend to use abductive reasoning through pattern recognition or clinical Gestalt, even where they are aware of potential diagnostic error, rather than resorting wholly to evidence-based approaches. This has been called the use of "mindlines" rather than clinical guidelines, where, when faced with ambiguity or novelty or ethical conundrums, doctors will habitually confer with colleagues and draw on their experience rather than deliberately checking on formal clinical guidelines (Gabbay and Le May 2010). The objectivity of clinical guidelines is then stained with the reality of messier mindlines. This won't be news to clinicians. Doctors do not act as pure scientists in their clinical work, where their approach has often been described as a form of *phronesis* or applied "wisdom" gained from experience (Hunter 1991, 2005).

Medicine then has an ambiguous relationship with ambiguity – just, as will be seen, did William Empson (1930/1991) in his masterwork of literary criticism *Seven Types of Ambiguity*. (There is nothing more ambiguous than what we "somewhat mean", or "possibly suggest".) The voice of science- and evidence-based approaches calls for the rational (and radical) reduction of ambiguity, but this is a voice in a practice vacuum, an idealisation. In practice, ambiguity is rampant and is dealt with through several tactics: from rational, decompression approaches that are driven by intolerance of ambiguity and fear of emotional contamination, to embrace of maximum complexity at the edge of chaos encouraging affect flow.

How then does poetry see ambiguity and can this transmit to and infect medicine? Isn't poetry's field – even in Minimalism – at the edge of chaos, feeding on maximum complexity, with its thunderheads of metaphors? Ian Hamilton Finlay's work advertises this. The poem entitled "1794 A ONE-WORD POEM FOR THE LADIES OF ART PRESS, PARIS", is just one word: "knitting". The implications are helped by context. One of Finlay's "plaque poems" runs, "Knitting was a reserved occupation" (it refers first to the "reign of terror" during the French Revolution, where women would supposedly sit by the guillotines as the heads rolled, and knit; and in the Second World War conscientious objectors being given "reserved occupation" jobs, where knitting was a sleight for the men as a stereotypically woman's occupation). In short, Finlay's one word poem "knitting" (both verb and noun) has a complex root and is held in a complex web of associations and yet can be no more minimalist in its bare fact of the single word. The word itself, of course, denotes pulling two separate strands together. We thus knit metaphors.

The jarring harmony of things

The Roman lyrical poet Horace (*Epistulae* 1.12.19) described an oxymoronic "jarring harmony of things". Shakespeare (*Romeo and Juliet* 1.1.178–80) plays in both mischievous and heavy-handed ways with oxymorons to make a point about ambiguity in character, advertising Horace's oxymoron:

> O heavy lightness! serious vanity!
> Mis-shapen chaos of well-meaning forms!
> Feather of lead, bright smoke, cold fire, sick health!

At the opening of the play, Romeo professes his heavy heart to Benvolio, Romeo's cousin and friend. He is in love, but the feelings are not reciprocated. Romeo sees bloodstains, the residue from a fight, and this triggers an association with the bloody struggle he is having for his own unreciprocated feelings of love:

> (seeing blood) Oh my! What fight happened here? No, don't tell me—I know all about it. This fight has a lot to do with hatred, but it has more to do with love. O brawling love! O loving hate! Love that comes from nothing! Sad happiness! Serious foolishness! Beautiful things muddled together into an ugly mess! Love is heavy and light, bright and dark, hot and cold, sick and healthy, asleep and awake—it's everything except what it is! This is the love I feel, though no one loves me back. Are you laughing?

Uncertainty, suggests Helga Nowotny (2015), has a level of "cunning". The poet Adrienne Rich (1969) agrees, in "Tear Gas" (https://nepantler-ablog.files.wordpress.com/2016/02/the-dream-of-a-common-language-adrienne-rich.pdf):

> I need a language to hear myself with
> to see myself in
> a language like pigment released on the board
> blood-black, sexual green, reds
> veined with contradictions.

Oxymoron (two contrasting words clumped together: "blood-black", "jumbo shrimp", "cold fire in his eyes", Rich's "reds / veined" – where veins are blue, an optical effect as blood is always red) is a significant literary device as it allows the author to use contradictory or contrasting concepts placed together in a manner that actually ends up making sense. Rich also sets a steep step, an enjambment, for the reader to negotiate from "reds" to "veined". (For an innovative reading of Rich's "Tear Gas" through the lens of Julia Kristeva's work, see https://www.slideshare.net/audenhugh/richs-tear-gas). "Reds / veined": this rhetorical device produces a sudden gasp, a sense of stepping sideways into the blue, or stepping down perhaps too far and losing balance, as if hit by tear gas. The red are veined with contradictions, says Rich, so it is not really colour at all that matters, but infiltration of pattern.

The physician is lumbered in some ways with ambiguities – it is bad enough having to do the work, but "medicine watchers" like non-clinical medical educationalists are obsessed with instrumentalising contrast devices: paradox, oxymoron, antithesis, and irony. They want to turn these complex literary devices into linear competencies. For example, Kassab and colleagues (Kassab et al. 2019: 155) reduce "interpersonal, cognitive and professional behavior", necessarily complex and best described through contrast devices, to a 10-item instrument with a 5-point Likert scale rating to be used by observers. There is a lovely line in the authors' article Abstract under "Methods", where, "Reliability of professional competencies scores was calculated using G-theory with raters nested in occasions". The first half of the sentence advertises instrumentalising of the otherwise complex issue of "professional behaviour", while the second half ("with raters nested in occasions") offers a literary flourish where the authors could have simply said that raters observed activities. Instead we get a kind of ornate ornithological metaphor fit for a 19th-century natural historian.

Ollie ten Cate (2013) describes an "entrustable professional activity (EPA) concept" that has become one of medical education's newer "god terms" and core curriculum practice. This activity-centred, "can-do/ will show" instrumental approach irons out both complexity (aiming for closed, linear and looped input and output) and ambiguity where it, allows faculty to make competency-based decisions on the level of supervision required by trainees. Competency-based education targets standardized levels of proficiency to guarantee that all learners have a sufficient level of proficiency at the completion of training.

The language could not be more expressive of distilling down to dry essences in medical education: "competence", "training", "targets", "standardized", "proficiency", "guarantee", "sufficient", and "completion". It is an engineering approach embracing minimalism but without the aesthetic. It is indeed artless and heartless. Doctors must now master these "entrustable" essences to become trustworthy practitioners. In "Burnt Norton" from *Four Quartets*, T.S. Eliot warns,

> Words strain,
> Crack and sometimes break, under the burden,
> Under the tension, slip, slide, perish,
> Decay with imprecision, will not stay in place,
> Will not stay still.

The frozen words above from ten Cate advertise competencies acting as disguises for taming ambiguity where, say the medicine watchers, is potential for medical error. We salute pedagogy around formal elements any day of the week. Except, of course, in the absence of the recognition of ambiguity, for as any master knows, the mystery of wisdom only deepens with knowledge. The more one knows, the more one realises there is more to know. This is wisdom. To embrace ambiguity in our way is to accept the fact of error.

Such frozen descriptors freeze out doctors as caring persons, where we recognise an obvious (and welcome) source of ambiguity, because emotions (hurray!) are conjured, warming the frozen phrases of competency, allowing them to liquefy as life. No wonder that, as far back as 1998, a family doctor Alistair Short (1998: 866) complained: "the caring doctor is an oxymoron". Short sees as oppressively demanding expectation that doctors be "caring" under all circumstances. Rather, doctors can be "professional" says Short, without being impersonal. His rationale is that all doctors now work within systems, including teams. These are supportive by definition, but for Short "caring" is a kind of syrupy therapy-speak, the obverse of ten Cate's frozen competencies (where "care" is chiselled out of the granite block of learning outcomes as a stony stare). Such therapy-speak and competence-fixation can infantilise.

As medical educators squeeze out the irritant complexities and contradictions (in language, again, the contrast devices such as paradox) for uniform competences and outcomes either cold-pressed or constituted as syrup, "care" really loses all of its meaning as antiphrasic, paradoxical, oxymoronic, antithetical, or ironic. The poet John Ashberry, discussed later, sums this up as "the division of grace". The first step is to bring back the rich language and metaphors of care, its imaginative frame, its emotional underpinnings, as these can be found first in life experience; and then transfer to the "professional" in medicine.

This move does not have to be flowery or excessive. Poets are experts in compression of language to create emotional and descriptive intensity, with a view to production of ambiguity. "Collapse" is a good method in poetry. We see this particularly in haiku and in William Carlos Williams's work that we draw on throughout. A disciple of Basho, Katsushika Hokusai (1665–1718), writes,

> I write, erase, rewrite
> Erase again, and then
> A poppy blooms.

It would be hard to find a better nutshell description of the process of differential diagnosis. Riches are collapsed into tight forms and the Big Bang happens in the poem's reception: in the bodily sensations, emotions, minds and imaginations of readers. Intrinsic ambiguity is left at the reader's doorstep where she may resolve, deepen, or despair over it, and where the primary purpose is to create a sense of inquiry, a thinking otherwise or a critique, as it creates beauty – sometimes exuding light, sometimes dark and chilling.

Bahar Orang (2020) notes in her meditation on beauty,

> If you pick a poppy, it withers
> within the hour. How simple a practice, then, to let flower, let flower,
> smelling its
> own
> earth.

The enjambment at "own" to "earth" is appropriate and lovely – we don't own flowers, picking them guarantees as death, so let's return to earth. The parallel with diagnostic work is clear: don't jump to conclusions and pick the poppy (symptom) but look first at the earth that nourishes the flower (context for symptom). This is a productive ambiguity. Koans often provide dwellings for meditation on knotty problems, multiple options, or ambiguities.

Pinning ambiguity down as it slips away – a lost cause?

Having circled around the campfire that is ambiguity, let us now attempt to pin it down, or warm oneself at its definition's dying embers, as that definition dies before our eyes! "Ambiguity", says William Empson (1930/1991: 1), "gives room for alternative reactions to the same piece of language". The parallel with medical diagnostic work is straightforward: there are often alternative reactions to the same symptom presentation. But while the poet (and her audience) may be happy to leave the linguistic ambiguity to simmer, the doctor may seek a definitive meaning or closure on behalf of the patient. Often, such closure is not possible or must await further investigations, so that tolerance of (or for) ambiguity is central to the diagnostic process. Irritability, a scratch, and not patience, often occupies the space between certainty and uncertainty.

"Ambiguity" is defined as "inexactness". Synonyms include ambivalence and uncertainty, while its opposite is "clarity" or "exactness". This suggests a potentially negative state of equivocation, obscurity, vagueness, or abstruseness – synonyms for ambiguity. Ambiguity might be thought of as what disturbs order, system and predictability. But there is a more generous definition, as: "the quality of being open to more than one interpretation". This suggests a measure of tolerance and is an apt definition for how ambiguity can be mobilised as a productive presence in clinical reasoning. Ambiguity invites a juggling act rather than logical, cold-blooded culling.

One of us (SN) recalls a favourite poet who shall remain anonymous, a mentally ill and addicted Canadian Maritimer, who was famous for shouting: "Life is contradiction!" We love the image of this guy shouting loud from the stage to people who prefer he, and most likely that very idea, would just go away. Antonin Artaud, of course, famously developed a "Theatre of Cruelty" by shouting at and insulting his audience to provoke them into response and engagement. This would produce unexpected couplings of mock pulpit bullying (poet as Groucho Marx playing Banana Republic dictator of Freedonia in "Duck Soup") and spontaneous audience interactions.

The French mathematician and polymath Henri Poincaré (1854–1912) talked of the progress of science as dependent on "unexpected couplings", and this surely offers a description of the work of both the diagnostic and the poetic imaginations. Coleridge said that the imagination: "dissolves, diffuses, dissipates, in order to re-create". Once the language of medieval and Renaissance alchemy, these words came to describe the operations of the new experimental science in the Enlightenment, particularly the language of chemistry. That the imagination might dissolve, diffuse and dissipate in order to re-create offers, simultaneously, a set of metaphors and literal reactions. Where alchemy, pre-dating chemistry, was chemistry prefigured as fantasy, medicine is material chemistry expressed semiotically as signs and symbols addressing symptoms.

Symptoms are chemistry in the sense in which we talk of "chemistry" in relationships, or what Goethe called "elective affinities". These are the lines of flight (necessarily unpredictable in trajectory) of symptoms from person to context. The doctor meets the person but is actually dealing with the line of flight of the symptom in developing a diagnosis, prognosis, treatment, and care plan. Doctors' medical minds must be stained by psychology and sociology to appreciate this – the logos or reason of both the embodied mind and its extensions that appreciate the power of context. But their minds too must be linguistically tuned – or take on a literary bent – to deal with metaphors such as "jangled nerves", "tired muscles", or "brain fog". The line of flight of the symptom requires the doctor to engage with predictive processing cognitively as diagnosis morphs into prognosis and treatment plan. While this line of flight thinking on the part of the doctor may be unsullied and engages a narrative arc, it simultaneously entangles with the abject matter that is the patient's troubling illness and this is the weighty anchor to whose grappling points the doctor must dive and then inspect.

The psychoanalyst Julia Kristeva (1982), in an account of the abject (that which is unacceptable, at the limits, or cast off as a terror or horror – such as serious symptom) notes that creative insights come not from noting patterns in everyday well-oiled communication (narrative order), but from what dislocates communication (nonlinear poetry). This is often as an emergence of irrational unconscious images and related feelings or emotions – the fermenting unconscious Well as opposed to the ordering conscious Will. Language and meaning are both formed and deformed by the irruptions of symbols and signs that emerge from below consciousness. These are driven and shaped by imaginative and emotional preverbal impulses and bodily forces rather than logic. Such a force of ambiguity, says Kristeva (1982: x): "provides the creative and innovative impulse of modern poetic structure".

Doctor and patient alike engage with this "innovative impulse" as the consultation unfolds. Even poets as outwardly rational as T.S. Eliot recognise the relationship between Will and Well, consciousness and the tacit dimension, or frontstage and backstage/wings. While reviewing a biography of another poet, Seamus Perry (2021) notes that

> a book called *The New Poetic* (1964) by the New Zealand poet C. K. Stead … portrayed an Eliot very different from the forbiddingly cerebral writer of popular reputation. Stead's Eliot spoke of the origins of poetry in the unconscious and the irrational, its material breaking through 'from a deeper level' of the poet's mind.

Eliot called this tacit source "that dark embryo … which gradually takes on the form and speech of a poem". Further, he even located the *rules* of transformation of such dark embryonic material, as "the feeling for syllable and rhythm, penetrating far below the conscious level of thought and feeling, invigorating every word; sinking to the most primitive and forgotten, returning to the origin and bringing something back". As the "animal snout" of the expert physician recognises a pattern for instant diagnosis, so the animal snout of the poet is grounded in sound and rhythm. A reminder too of the key line of Charles Olson's *Projective Verse* manifesto: "the HEAD, by way of the EAR, to the SYLLABLE" (https://writing.upenn.edu/~taransky/Projective_Verse.pdf).

Eliot's description separates even the actual forming of a poem ("syllable and rhythm" for example) from a prior "feeling for" that is cast as primitive and original. Here, Eliot slips from the Freudian personal unconscious to the Jungian collective unconscious as source of poetic inspiration. This primary or primal soil – Olson's "field" that we keep turning over and re-soiling, Williams' "festering pulp", Artaud's animal grunts, Kristeva's preverbal,

Peter Redgrove's literal mudbaths under a "thunder and lightning polka", Orang's "earth" for the vibrant, unplucked poppy – is surely our ground of metaphor. The more we sift this soil the closer we come to the claim that metaphor ("running on empty", "a riveting stare", "creeping flesh") is always embodied, as Lakoff and Johnson (1980, 1999) have said, as credo. Then, as a body symptomises, we can surely appreciate and then understand this metaphorically? This is primarily where medicine and poetry are hinged.

Certainly every object can become a metaphor and cannot be taken literally, as the new Object-Oriented Ontology (as a phenomenology) claims (see Chapter 7); and all objects are potentially abject in Kristeva's scheme of the preverbal as ground for metaphor. We return to Geoffrey Hill's Offa's scabrous earth and twisted roots as equivalent to bodily psychic scars. These can be limned through a perverse perception equivalent to the medical gaze (repeat mantra: "the undercut edges give an apple core appearance … this is a colonic carcinoma").

Everyday words can present as symptom expressions: "tired all the time". But we are more likely to be impressed by bigger knocks: bruising, burning, bleeding, festering, aching, irritation, inflammation, locking in, pulsing, engorging, prickling, rasping, blocked, dazed and confused, falling, swamped, depressed, hallucinating, outbursts, a deep sense of shame, and so forth. This is an embodied vocabulary for symptom that, as metaphor, mixes the literal with a deliteralising (metaphoric) impulse. Biomedicine reads literally where the imaginative consultation exercises de-literalisation. Both are necessary and feed each other.

Where psychoanalysts such as Kristeva suggest that a rational biomedical imagination cannot fully comprehend symptom, they are stating the obvious. It is not the work of biomedicine to make the psychoanalytic dive to inspect the tangling around the anchor. The quantitative and the qualitative must live side by side. Our argument again is that both can be poorly handled or done well. Biomedicine restricts access to qualitative inquiry. Overly territorial qualitative methods (narrative inquiry or otherwise) can snip out necessary numbers. But living side by side does not mean awkward fusions into one body such as "narrative as data".

The poem by Mary Cornish "Numbers" (https://www.poetryfoundation. org/poetrymagazine/poems/40877/numbers-56d21ecff2141) saves quantities from imperialistic trashing by the qualitative mob. Of course, numbers can act as qualities: "I like the generosity of numbers" says Cornish (addition, multiplication); "two pickles, one door to the room". But "Even subtraction is never loss",

> And I never fail to be surprised
> by the gift of an odd remainder

and, of course, "one sock that isn't anywhere you look". A good reminder for the operating theatre team as they chant the mantra of the instrument count to ensure that nothing is lingering in the patient's cavity.

Friendly fire and black suns

Uncertainty and ambiguity can present as "contradiction", that is, an incongruity or logical incompatibility between two or more propositions or states of being. "Face value" contradictions ("soft shell", "cold fire", "impulse control", "hard-wired") work as metaphors – they make sense in complex and strange ways through bypassing rational inquisition, appealing to affective and intuitive sensibilities. Such irrational pairings are "oxymorons" or contradictions in terms – rhetorical devices that light up the imagination, such as "friendly fire", "same difference", "ice burn", "virtual reality", and "only choice". The "making sense" is the same whether the example is grounded in poetry or science: for example, Milton's "darkness visible" taken up by the writer William Styron as a metaphor for chronic depression, echoed by Julia Kristeva (1987) as the "Black Sun" of melancholia.

John Ashbery writes of "Paradoxes and Oxymorons" (https://www.poetryfoundation.org/poems/50986/paradoxes-and-oxymorons) with an opening line that is oxymoronic and ambiguous: "This poem is concerned with language on a very plain level". Of course, it isn't. This is a nice introduction, entirely free of metaphor or imagery, unless you want to read "plain level" as a geographical metaphor returning to the equality Ashbery conjures: we're all in it together. But it is more complex than that.

The language offers a series of games. Ashbery is playing with you, while he puts "language" as the main protagonist: "Look at it talking to you". Ashbery has the reader turning her back on language, pretending it isn't there, prompting, provoking, but "You miss it, it misses you. You miss each other". "Miss" has a triple meaning – a loss (emotional, bereavement), a shot gone wide (practical, poor understanding, misappropriation), and a feminising or a turning of absence into tenderness (at the risk of employing feminine stereotypes). Cleverly, and with increasing complexity, Ashbery puts all feeling not in you the reader but in the poem itself as a living being: "The poem is sad because it wants to be yours, and cannot". The poem is actually out of your reach at this point as plays on words that conjure nothing but a "plain level". But these plays on words, says the poet, are, in fact, the poem's desire to play with you the reader, as "A deeper outside thing, a dreamed role-pattern" that is,

> the division of grace these long August days
> Without proof. Open-ended.

Ashberry toys with us here again, implying that engaging with the poem is filling in the time, coming to no conclusion; indeed the words (as poem) that held so much promise as potential friend "gets lost in the steam and chatter of typewriters". This is a sudden animation in a flat "very plain level" poem. He then says to the reader, "I think you exist only / To tease me into doing it" (writing poetry) "on your level"; "and then you aren't there / Or have adopted a different attitude". Ashbery seems to be saying: how do we poets keep our readers' attentions? The final lines resolve the dilemma:

> the poem
> Has set me softly down beside you. The poem is you.

The gnomic quality of the poem gives it the structure of a Gordian Knot, and the poet cuts the knot to release the tension. There is no mystery after all – the poem is your friend and your mental nourishment. It is a mild epiphany, a puppy (mind, one that thinks and bites). There is no story with resolution, because Ashbery is telling us what we knew from the opening lines: "This poem is concerned with language on a very plain level. / Look at it talking to you". The plain level is that the poem sees eye to eye with you. You are both its subject and objective. Ashbery is notorious for writing like a mind wandering, unchecked, but actually it is a mind rehearsing angles around a theme. It is a perspectival or diagnostic mind at work. But it is also a model of how to "lean in" to a patient, creating an atmosphere of trust: "sit beside me, talk". "My words are yours". "The diagnosis is yours".

We have analysed Ashbery's poem as we might a transcript from a clinical consultation, but actually we ask you to feel or experience these words, and not to see them as disinfecting infectious affect. Ashbery is a master of dressing up currents of feeling in seemingly affectless tone. You have to see through it and sit next to the poem that is ready for embrace or "play" in the poem above.

Ambiguity is not an absolute good: unproductive vs productive ambiguity

Dangerous ambiguity is of Orwell's "double-think" kind, used to frustrate and stun productive thinking by consciously dealing in unproductive contradictions such as double binds. Orwell may actually be describing a deliberately cynical way to think. The point is not that one truly believes both things are possible at the same time when it is plain that they cannot be. The point is that one publicly displays such a belief and is in possession of an ideological apparatus that can resolve the contradictions in a nonsensical, but consistently cynical, manner, for example, war is peace, or freedom is slavery. There is the bluntness of the surface interpretation, and then, peering deeper, one sees the profundity inherent in all abstract three-word-phrases. But the bluntness forces one to rub up against the contradiction and get carpet burn. It is a mark of our current "alternative facts" age where a cynical ambiguity is a functional one. The purpose is to serve power which thrives on all possible interpretations being possible all of the time, especially the allowed ones, which change arbitrarily, and often require the most outrageous contradictions to be accepted in order to reflect the totality of control.

Double binding is a classic technique of authoritarians, who gain control through offering contradictory messages, or making statements that appear to be important but carry no substantial message or conclusion. The medium itself becomes the message – the fate of 20th-century mass communications, as Marshall McLuhan famously predicted. The classic double bind used by authoritarians is, "you are either with me or against me" that some would take as a good example of non-Derridean aporia. Set as an apparently simple binary choice, the injunction immediately stuns and bruises any thinking person because relationships are more nuanced than that.

In contrast to unproductive contradiction is productive ambiguity, advertised in William Empson's seven kinds, detailed below and addressed critically in the following chapter, where we challenge our own schema below as "too neat for ambiguity's tastes". Empson shows how ambiguity – again, "any verbal nuance, however slight, which gives room to alternative reactions to the same piece of language" – is central to the poetic imagination, and can be readily anatomised. His scheme is undeniably brilliant in scope, but horribly shaky as a classification device. Nevertheless, doctors listening to their patients could gain inspiration from Empson's scheme as we look for productive overlaps between the poetic imagination and diagnostic clinical reasoning. A word of warning however – Empson does not make clear that language carries moral obligations as well as technical ones, where it can take by surprise and deceive. Ambiguities – that doctors grapple with in diagnostic work, and poets employ in writing – must be worked on and employed ethically. They cannot simply be admired. Again, it must be stressed that where poets produce and study ambiguity, a doctor's task is to tolerate ambiguity but as an engine of change. Doctors can learn from poetry *about* this.

Seven levels to chaos

When William Empson, only 24 years old, published *Seven Types of Ambiguity* in 1930, it was part of a closely clustered grouping of works that ushered in a new form of literary criticism reliant on "close reading" of texts. We have illustrated this throughout. I.A. Richards had tutored Empson in close reading, but if not its true origin, a pre-occurring method (by about five years or so, though defining the start of movements is not exact) can be found in the Russian Formalist movement that began in the late 1910s, as explored in Chapters 3 and 5. Empson's book can be counted among the most influential literary criticism texts of the 20th century. Such "New Criticism" focussed on productive conflicts not only in the author but also the reader, as the text takes on autonomy (its capital open for sharing). Further, as Empson notes, his scheme considers unproductive outcomes "due to weakness or thinness of thought" on the part of the writer that include intentional obscurity, opportunism, and incoherence. It has long been essential reading for English literature students, but we recommend it for medical students and doctors, for reasons that unfold in this and the following chapter.

Ambiguity, for which "uncertainty" can be taken as a synonym and "contradiction" a close relative, was considered to be a double-edged sword for Empson in the exercise of the poetic imagination. While ambiguity could be used productively, it could also act as a blunt instrument or spiral out of control, producing poor poetry and illuminating confused states of mind in the writer, and then confusing the reader. Empson's book provides a road map for how ambiguities and contradictions can be drawn on as resources not only in creative writing and reading but also in thinking in general. Here, we generalise to the medical mind. As noted, medicine is infamously caught in a double bind and contradiction: patients' symptom presentations, especially in psychiatry, are ambiguous, yet doctors are socialised into a culture in which certainty and surety are embraced as virtues. Education for tolerance of ambiguity should be at the core of the medicine undergraduate curriculum to mitigate against the poor outcomes militated by the cultural preference.

Empson's book, articulating seven types of ambiguity as both intended and unintended poetic devices, was revised in 1947 and again in 1953, ironically to address its ambiguities. It can be read as an account of tonal registers in poetry – created by ambiguities – that can in turn be compared to dissonances and rhythmic experimentation in music. These registers are often created by ideas presented simultaneously that may at first sight appear to be unconnected and even contradictory, but offer creative tensions or invite unusual resolutions. There is always an unknown quality, a surprise around the corner. Again, Helga Nowotny (2015), in the context of ambiguity in literary texts, calls this the "cunning of uncertainty".

Empson's seven types of ambiguity constitute not just a list of devices or means to create poetic effect such as tension. It is a schema of a gradual descent into the loss of mind through what might be seen as increasing doses of the Circe effect, the gradual loosening of grip on a poem by its author as the poem breaks free and becomes an object of the attention of readers and critics. Ambiguity becomes untethered from its role as authorial technique to occupy a space between the poem and its audience reception. Patients' symptoms as poems and the doctor as reader mirror this. Empson's entropic scheme unfolds as a series of appearances of symptom in the body of language.

The first type of ambiguity is mild – merely the use of metaphor: meat and potatoes to the poet and doctor alike, where metaphors often appear as resemblances ("raspberry tongue") or fancies ("kissing tonsils").

A second and unstable notion is the use of two metaphors at once. These may be resolved in one common meaning. Differential diagnoses are common in medicine and may embrace two or more metaphors: Covid-19 is characterised by a continuous "hacking" cough, feeling "feverish", and "bland taste" (anosmia). Or, two resemblances may describe the same condition. We think here of "plaques and tangles" when it comes to Alzheimer's disease. Both point to the same disease, yet one is an intracellular feature on histographic analysis (plaques) and the other extracellular (tangles). This is fascinating in terms of what plaques and tangles are (Wippold et al. 2008). For example, "plaques" are small spheric structures within the cerebral cortex and tangles are "flame-shaped fiberlike bundles" – a Russian doll of metaphor.

A third level of ambiguity is that two ideas are given simultaneously that can be connected by context and resolved into one descriptor. Again, in medicine this can be a differential diagnosis. As Kenan Malik (2020) has written in a review of Matthew Cobb's *The Idea of the Brain*, "The coronavirus is both a physical threat and a metaphor for everything from the failures of globalisation to the menace of foreigners".

So far so stable; but the fourth level of ambiguity begins to introduce a level of instability, even a touch of madness: two or more meanings do not agree, but combine to make clear a complicated state of mind in the author. The reader is left with a lot of work to do here, perhaps to guess precisely what that state of mind might be. In medicine, we might be entering the territory of "disputed diseases" or high levels of complexity, such as chronic fatigue syndrome, irritable bowel syndrome, or long covid – diagnoses embracing both physical and psychological interventions, or crossover treatments such as anti-depressants.

By level five, the author is shooting in the dark. The ambiguity appears as the discovery of an idea through the act of writing itself, not through pre-planning. Serendipity in medicine is not uncommon – after searching and searching, the doctor almost gives up hope and then a crack appears and the light floods in. This is illustrated in Jerome Groopman's (2007) *How Doctors Think*. Groopman, a doctor himself, developed pain and swelling in his right hand, visiting six prominent hand surgeons and getting four different opinions, none of which he felt comfortable with in terms of treatment options. Eventually, he saw a surgeon who, by examining his left hand, came up with a correct diagnosis. A defamiliarisation was needed.

By level six, the writer has lost control of the process where her words are so ambiguous that the reader must invent a meaning of her own, and this may conflict with that of the author. (Perhaps you feel this way now, reading our medical-themed version of Empson's already ambiguous version of ambiguity). Multiple readings gain legitimacy. Here, the doctor has run out of ideas or the limits to competence. The doctor hands over control to other specialists and to the expert patient, the latter informed by her online support group of lay experts.

And, finally, at level seven, the words on the page reveal a clear and troubling conflict in the author's mind – "due to weakness or thinness of thought" as Empson puts it – a misunderstanding or a fundamental division or conflict of ideas. The reader is left to abandon the poem or make meanings through her own critical responses. The doctor can no longer treat the patient due to failings perhaps on both sides.

These seven levels offer increasing levels of poetic experimentation. We can readily form an analogy bridging these seven types of ambiguity with the clinical diagnostic process to amplify the examples above:

Level one is the everyday use of likeness or resemblance as adaptive expertise: for example, a basket full of fruit metaphors such as "strawberry tongue" of scarlet fever, or "peau d'orange" of breast cancer.

Level two is a resolved differential diagnosis: symptoms suggest two causes but one is rejected after physical examination, second opinion, and/ or test results.

Level three mirrors level two where the focus switches from symptom presentation and tests to context for appearance of the symptom. Once we know that the patient was recently bereaved, symptoms of depression are explicable.

Level four is where a differential diagnosis will not resolve due to conflicting evidence. The doctor is unable to offer a clear route for treatment to the patient.

At level five, ambiguity is omnipresent. There are several possible diagnoses and the doctor is unable to offer any certainty. Chronic high levels of fatigue in the patient cannot be pinned down to a specific cause such as vitamin or iron deficiency.

At level six, the ambiguity has been taken on fully by the patient. Suffering from a rare illness of which her GP has little knowledge and her specialist can find no further route for treatment, the patient joins an online support group formed around fellow-sufferers and they become experts in their own conditions.

At level seven, ferment is so high that the doctor is unable to offer further help and disengages from the patient. Perhaps the patient is an addict, of drugs, drink or sex, and keeps relapsing; or is on the streets where the primary cause of symptom is social and all the doctor can do is provide temporary alleviation or comfort. Perhaps the doctor has reached the limit of her competence. What more can I do for this chronic pain or fatigue, these migraines, this irritable bowel, loss of libido, or persistent anxiety? How can I go on treating symptoms where the cause of inequity and social injustice remains untouched?

A riposte to Empson's scheme

Empson's scheme, brilliant in many respects, frankly unravels as an architectural plan, inviting a formal critique. We base this on the work of the literary critic Winifred Nowottny, who does not specifically critique Empson, but whose work can be mobilised as a riposte to Empson's scheme. Nowottny (1965: 150) argues that, in principle, ambiguity is resistant to classification through typology, as detailed by Empson above, where, "The temptation to set about constructing a typology of ambiguity and a terminology for the different types is strong. The deterrents, however, are stronger still". Where Empson sees types, Nowottny sees scales: at one end are explicit and intended devices such as use of metaphors and explicit contradictions (of the sort that Empson turns into types), and common public ambiguities such as double-entendre jokes. At the other end are unintended ambiguities such as muddled syntax or weak argument. She notes that terms such as "ambivalence" and "dilemma" can be readily substituted for ambiguity.

Nowottny persistently attempts to democratise the text to allow for reader response. In contrast, while Empson's literary-critical eye is motivated to help readers to make sense of texts, it can also be suffocating such that the reader is hampered rather than helped in navigating poems through Empson's typology. Where Empson (1930/1991: viii) can sound quasi-dictatorial (if admittedly a little tongue-in-cheek): "I claimed at the start that I would use the term "ambiguity" to mean anything I liked", so Nowottny (1965: 151) democratises texts by turning statements (this is what is happening in the text) as sureties into a web of questions, to open debate. She makes this point in particular by an appeal to a "common-sense view that one knows what meaning is, sufficiently to be able to survive without defining it", where meanings rest not in the ambiguity or otherwise of what is spoken or written, but rather the *context* in which it is spoken, heard, and discussed or given meaning.

Here "More often than not we remain unaware of the extent to which the meaning we ascribe to remarks depends upon what Gombrich calls our application of situational clues to "make sense" of what is being said" (ibid.: 152). Everyday empathy or identification allows us to tolerate high levels of ambiguity in making meanings of speech (and therefore of poems and of doctors' diction as patients). Thus, while "inserting a central line" for a clinical context is unambiguous, in a lay setting the phrase is initially meaningless, puzzling, or ambiguous, but readily clarified. However, its surplus is also readily carried over as material for punning or introducing metaphorical worth into conversation.

Where Emspon finds ambiguities of discrete types in the texts of poems, Nowottny suggests that ambiguity is diffusely spread across contexts for poems, scooping up writer, reader and critic in interplay. Here, ambiguity is not an object to be discovered or revealed, but a complex, liquid system whose affordances may include ambiguities with inconsistent sources, appearances and meanings (according to context). Again, there is a democratic intent at play: "If we have no objection to having two (or more) meanings, we may be struck chiefly by the presence in the context of equipollent sets of relationships. A tolerable term for these cases might be the term 'extraloquial', if one might suppose that it would suggest *having extra meaning* or *leaving extra meaning in*" (ibid.: 155–56). Nowottny suggests that such "extralocution" is another way of conceiving "ambiguity" where "People could please themselves whether they approved or disapproved of the extra load" (that Derrida calls "surplus"). Parataxis (Caesar's "I came, I saw, I conquered") offers a democratic ambiguity, for each clause, without the illumination of conjunctions, is of equal status. This also represents an archetypal teasing anti-narrative, a story without story.

Nowottny's "extraloquial" is an important notion in the context of ambiguity. Poetry (with the exception of some contemporary verse and performance poetry) brackets out foibles of everyday speech such as non-sequiturs, but primarily paralanguage such as hesitations, filler words, and slang. Yet simultaneously poetry creates an inbreeding of ambiguity through craft (and sometimes as a consequence of accident and sloppy writing). Medicine too, if one looks at transcripts of consultations, as in Chapter 5, is shot through with the ambiguities provided by paralanguage slippage in everyday speech. Sometimes this creates high levels of ambiguity and potential for misunderstandings, while at other times, the ambiguity provides a springboard for negotiation and dialogue (including tics such as "do you know what I mean?"). Sometimes too, the ambiguity is surplus or dross and fails to attract meanings. Ambivalences too may be read as a character trait and tolerated as such.

Thus, Nowottny alerts us to differences between "ambiguity" as everyday speech (perlocutionary and negotiated) and "Ambiguity" as technical use of language in poetry for example (elocutionary, drawing on locution and illocution). This warns us against a too-literal application of a typology such as Empson's. We carry this advice through to our Chapters 12 and 13.

Such schemes as Empson's typology cannot in any way represent ambiguity, but rather (oxymoronically) rationalise ambiguity – holding its presentations at arm's length, refusing the body odour of another. These models are like carnivorous plants that attract you with their outward display – colour and smell – their outrageous efflorescence. As you seek to inspect in the guise of curious insect, they snap and devour you, and their acids dissolve you (see Tolu Oloruntoba's poem "My Therapist Assesses Suicidal Ideation" in Chapter 12). In the next chapter, we throw you a curveball as a close reading of Empson's *Seven Types of Ambiguity* that dissolves the logic of our "seven levels" analysis above in a sap drawn from a crooked tree. We pulped the tree and manufactured the paper for a limited edition of The Poetry Uselessness Red Book.

References

Adorno TW, Frenkel-Brunswik E, Levinson DJ, Sanford RN. 1950. *The Authoritarian Personality.* New York: Harper & Row.

Bleakley A. 2014. *Patient-Centred Medicine in Transition: The Heart of the Matter.* Dordrecht: Springer.

Daston L, Galison P. 2007. *Objectivity.* New York: Zone Books.

Empson W. 1991/1930. *Seven Types of Ambiguity,* 3rd ed. London: The Hogarth Press.

Gabbay J, Le May A. 2010. *Practice-Based Evidence for Healthcare: Clinical Mindlines.* Abingdon: Routledge.

Geller G. Tolerance for Ambiguity: An Ethics–Based Criterion for Medical Student Selection. *Academic Medicine.* 2013; 88: 581–84.

Groopman J. 2007. *How Doctors Think.* New York: Houghton Mifflin.

Hunter K. 2005. *How Doctors Think: Clinical Judgment and the Practice of Medicine.* New York: Oxford University Press.

Hunter KM. 1991. *Doctors' Stories: The Narrative Structure of Medical Knowledge.* Princeton, NJ: Princeton University Press.

Kassab SE, Du X, Toft E, et al. Measuring Medical Students' Professional Competencies in a Problem-Based Curriculum: A Reliability Study. *BMC Medical Education*. 2019; 155. Retrieved from https://doi.org/10.1186/s12909-019-1594-y

Kristeva J. 1982. *Powers of Horror: An Essay on Abjection.* New York: Columbia University Press.

Kristeva J. 1987. *Black Sun: Depression and Melancholia.* New York: Columbia University Press.

Lakoff G, Johnson M. 1980. *Metaphors We Live By.* Chicago, IL: University of Chicago Press.

Lakoff G, Johnson M. 1999. *Philosophy in the Flesh.* New York: Basic Books.

Malik K. Like a Moth to a Flame, We're Drawn to Metaphors to Explain Ourselves. The Guardian. March 15, 2020. Retrieved from https://www.theguardian.com/commentisfree/2020/mar/15/like-a-moth-to-a-flame-we-are-drawn-to-metaphors-to-explain-our-world

Merrotsy P. Tolerance of Ambiguity: A Trait of the Creative Personality? *Creativity Research Journal.* 2013; 25: 232–37.

Nowotny H. 2015. *The Cunning of Uncertainty.* Cambridge: Polity Press.

Nowottny W. 1965. *The Language Poets Use.* London: The Athlone Press.

Orang B. 2020. *Where Things Touch: A Meditation on Beauty.* Toronto: Book★Hug.

Periyakoil VS. Using Metaphors in Medicine. *Journal of Palliative Medicine.* 2008; 11: 842–44.

Perry S. We Did and We Didn't: Are Yez Civilised? *World Catholic News.* April 28, 2021 (on Seamus Heaney). Retrieved from https://www.worldcatholicnews.com/seamus-perry-%C2%B7-we-did-and-we-didnt-are-yez-civilised-%C2%B7-lrb-6-may-2021-london-review-of-books/

Peterkin A. 2018. A Brief Guide to Close Reading. In: B Sibbald (ed.) *Encounters: Selected CMAJ Narratives.* Ottawa: Joule Inc., 4–5.

Roe N (ed.) 2017. *John Keats and the Medical Imagination.* London: Palgrave Macmillan.

Schön DA. 1983. *Educating the Reflective Practitioner: Toward a New Design for Teaching and Learning in the Professions.* San Francisco, CA: Jossey-Bass Inc.

Short AD. The Caring Doctor is an Oxymoron. *British Medical Journal.* 1998; 316: 866.

Stead CK. 1964. *The New Poetic: Yeats to Eliot.* Harmondsworth: Penguin.

ten Cate O. Nuts and Bolts of Entrustable Professional Activities. *Journal of Graduate Medical Education.* 2013; 5: 157–58.

Wippold FJ, Cairns N, Vo K, et al. Neuropathology for the Neuroradiologist: Plaques and Tangles. *American Journal of Neuroradiology.* 2008; 29: 18–22.

Yelland HL, Jones SC, Easton KSW. 1950. *A Handbook of Literary Terms.* Urbana-Champaign: University of Illinois Press.

12 General change and the poetry uselessness red book

More or less useless?

Neil Pickering's (2000) wonderfully blunt article "The use of poetry in health care ethics education" argues that "since reading poetry is of no use, it can be of no use in health care ethics education". Pickering softens this rhetorical wrecking ball by engaging with poetry as poetry — as itself — and concludes that the benefits of reading poetry are those attendant to reading poetry, which is an incredibly obvious point, but one that emphatically needs repeating, year after biomedical year. And yet, isn't this a point that can, possibly, be operationalised? Can there be a use for uselessness?

Our party line for poetry in the discipline of medicine has been that it need not "do" anything, and in its glorious refusal, or laziness, or declination of applied science status, it can yet be the thing that makes all the difference (Neilson 2019). The essentialised core of this larger party platform — let's call it the Poetry Uselessness Red Book — is simple: by virtue of its neglect and the disrespect afforded it, poetry has a subterranean power. Denials, refutations, and simple ignorance of poetry's power are very much beside the point because poetry is not meant for specific application as much as general application; poetry is not about a specific outcome, it is about general outcomes. Who knew it was Evidence-Based Medicine in disguise?

If poetry were appreciated and understood *as* poetry by medical practitioners, then we would be referring to a group of practitioners quite different than the majority of those working now. Think of it, though: health care practitioners who think in terms of quality of relation, who appreciate beauty as a foregrounded (and not sublimated) property, whose lives revolve around aesthetic as well as functional principles. This circumstance is not impossible, for we know physicians like this, doctors able to straddle arts and humanities despite the prevailing biomedical gravity. Such a wish involving poetry-conversant practitioners would require a wholesale transformation of care. Into exactly what we wouldn't know, but we've made careers out of guessing (Bleakley 2020).

Up until recently, our resolute party line has been: poetry because it's useless (and in the uselessness, somehow be of use by resisting an instrumental culture); poetry because the act itself has meaning; poetry because it creates

DOI: 10.4324/9781003194408-14

its own good which need not be measured, but which is felt and experienced as true; poetry because, in the emancipatory uselessness of writing it, one transforms the self over time into ... a different kind of practitioner. A doctor in conversation with beauty as much as pharmacology, physiology, neuro-anatomy, and so forth. Though we've itemised some specific beneficial items that poetry can provide in medical encounters during the previous chapters, all of these stemmed simply from thinking like a poet. Poetry because ... by engaging with the subject *generally*, one experiences a *general* change.

This is something to do with climate rather than culture. Practical applications of poetry within the realms of medical pedagogy and medical research might be abhorred because such a desire contravenes poetry's spirit itself. We certainly recognise the danger, as reflected in our engagement with Johanna Shapiro's book. But this may not necessarily be the case. A slippery, beautiful thing, people can be warned off poetry forever by bad teaching; this is a Huge Truth in Our Culture. True in the general classroom, it has to be doubly true in the biomedical one. One might wonder: what kind of universe wants to corrupt poetry, to spawn a hybrid monster that is a biomedicalised poetry oriented to direct improvements in patient care? Indeed, SN in particular has actively spread the Poetry Uselessness Red Book doctrine in Canadian territory, giving gleeful seminar after seminar plying poetry on physicians who attend narrative medicine conferences, opening with an attack on the instrumentalisation of poetry. But, again, that question creeps up: "can there be a use for uselessness?"

> Yes yes yes
> Help me me me

There it is – an echo from the biomedical battlefield and its war zone filled with the dead husks of martial and machine metaphors. "All Day Permanent Red" says the poet Christopher Logue (2003) in his loose "translation" of Homer's *Iliad* where battle rages (https://poetryarchive.org/poem/all-day-permanent-red-extract/). All day permanently unread we say of poetry in medical circles. And in the rare instance when read, poetry's either misunderstood or appropriated for the wrong reasons.

We hear, through the battle's din, the voice of General Change atop his steed. General Change is hirsute William Empson, and he's yelling at us from back in 1930, when the biomedical initiative was in full swing, but nowhere near as entrenched as it is in 2021. Empson certainly knew something about science – he was a promising mathematician, gaining a first degree in the subject before the English Literature bug infected him and the mechanics of ambiguity changed, cleared and scrambled his mind simultaneously.

Poetry-thought for the medical masses

The issue limiting our progress on the road to poetry pedagogy in medicine has been what William Empson – General Change – might call habitual, a literary tic. Empson (1930/1991: 4) explains how "poetry has powerful means of imposing its own assumptions, and is very independent of the mental habits of the reader". What exactly does he mean by "habit?" Where Empson (ibid.) writes on the difference between a poetic line versus a prosaic one, he says that poetry largely requires one to "assume a habit" rather than read the line as prose, as "a piece of information". We have already spent a good deal of this book distinguishing between the work of prose and poetry, and between the informational, the knowing and the wise. A monkish adoption of poetry-thought – and attendant lifelong commitment to continue to try to bend a life towards poetry-ness – can result in an equivalent of poetic navel-gazing. However,

> Poetry need not be reduced to meaning but rather experienced as an experience!
> Poetry need not be reduced to meaning but rather experienced as an experience!
> Poetry need not be reduced to meaning but rather experienced as an experience!

Prosaic minds of the world, unite! Be one with unity of effect! Throw off your chains!

Our belief in the Poetry Uselessness Red Book waned over the years in part because of a dimly perceived, possible utility that came to full fruition in this book as a book; but more so because we became increasingly aware of the epistemology-fusing ambiguities inherent to what goes by the name the "general case". Allow us to explain. By referring to the "general case" – not to be confused with General Change, our valiant hero – we impishly rejoice in language which sounds not only biomedical in vocabulary ("case"!) but also in terms of epistemology. The supreme irony inherent in a latter-day awakening to the instrumental use of poetry in medical education is that poetry, too, has a homology with biomedicine. SURPRISE. But here is the case.

If poetry is to have a general *usefulness* to any individual practitioner by virtue of its *uselessness* at the level of specific outcome or application (as already argued), meaning that it informs practitioners' sensibilities as something they do in their lives and thereby this personal reading practice affects their public professional practice rather than existing as a ghastly, actionable "competence", well, this "general case" gist is at least sister to the biomedical epistemology, is it not? For the biomedical epistemology also seeks to gather together specific knowledge in order to create generalisable, generic principles. This is its essence and power, and we are all better off for it in many senses. For example, we have vaccines for Covid-19 at breath-taking speed and efficiency.

Poetry is hardly a purely aesthetic discipline without analytic tools. Indeed, there is a tool kit as old as language itself, and these tools are consistently being renovated and improved. Centuries of this productive work inform new kinds of analysis constantly being generated. MFAs in poetry feed off this stuff. Biomedicine too is being added to by its monks, just as poetry is being added to by its Empson acolytes or naysayers. Notice that we are proceeding *generally*. Specifics are on hold. It is our simultaneously ironic and sincere method in this chapter. More specifically as Empson (ibid.: xv), our leader for this skirmish, has written:

> there is always in great poetry a feeling of generalisation from a case which has been presented definitely; there is always an appeal to a background of human experience which is all the more present when it cannot be named.

Do you see how General Change has led us to the general case? Follow us in our reasoning through example. Specific case: this man's angina episodes are exacerbated by the microaggressions of his boss in the workplace; general case: angina is linked to anxiety.

To go too deeply into the full implications of the irony of the partially shared epistemologies of biomedicine and poetry is beyond the scope of this chapter, which is not housed in the disciplinary home of the philosophy of medicine but rather in the more general and rapscallionish domain of literary criticism meeting medical practice. No, what we want to do is valorise the general case, to make it communicable, to bring you the reader into that condition – via the spirit of sheer appreciation. To be very ambiguous in a mischievous way, but then again in a very practical and concrete one, we aim to generalise poetry's applicability to your, the reader's, practice, but only in the general sense.

Let us bring back Neil Pickering (2000) in order to crystallise the idea:

> Any usefulness which poetry may have in health care ethics education must be as a by-product of a quite different educational activity. That educational activity is directed towards the poem in its own right, and it guarantees no predictable outcome.

This "different educational activity" *is exactly the point* – the reading and discussing of poetry, maybe even writing it. Intellectual apparatuses have been constructed to encourage this heretical idea because the idea is not as heretical as you might think. Strangely, but felicitously, biomedicine and poetry are both generalisable categories (of course) that, as traditions of knowledge, are not so incompatible as previously understood.

What's missing to connect them and make them more permeable to one another is a means of appreciating the dialogue always already happening in doctor-poets' heads with medicine. This book is an attempt to consolidate what's known as well as make a long-overdue attempt to push past impediments to the general poetrification (as opposed to the long-established narrativisation) of medicine. It's our goal to have (albeit for a largely clinical or clinical education audience) the effect of Empson himself, one that John Gross (https://www.poetryfoundation.org/poets/william-empson) summarised as a "gift" in which Empson was "able to show you qualities in a work you would never have seen without him, and the even more important gift of enlarging your imagination, encouraging you to go on looking for yourself".

A manual for poetry-thought in medicine?
Why, yes. Our general case for this

We say hallelujah to the spectacular lack of applied functions for poetry in the medical realm. In honour of ambiguity (or at least one kind) we will illustrate the applicable non-applicability of poetry to medicine. If we were to choose a text for all physicians to read as an introduction to how form is important to poetry it would be Lucy Alford's (2020) magnificent *Forms of Poetic Attention*. We are aware that physicians are among the world's worst when it comes to looking after their own health, but we would expect them to respect the health of poetry by paying attention to its forms. After all, they don't just freestyle their medicine. One mode, commonly used rather than accidently incurred, in poetry is ambiguity. Doctors know that ambiguity is central to their work too, ever-present. But they resist ambiguity, making for an ambiguity in its own right in medical practice – doctors want to reduce ambiguity just as they must suffer it on a daily basis. It is well established that tolerance of such ambiguity is a mark of a good practitioner, now a mantra in this book.

How then to best engage ambiguity as a shared issue of poetry and medicine? We introduced this in the previous chapter. We will continue to make a sustained engagement with a seminal practical text in literary criticism. That the text was originally published in 1930 only shows that there is a lot of catching up to do in the field. We chose William Empson's *Seven Types of Ambiguity* as our starter-kit applied text for a number of reasons. The first is that the book is a signal instance of the New Criticism that developed in the 1930s in the UK and flourished until the end of the 1950s. This form of criticism was especially interested in understanding the formal properties of literature – such as use of metaphor, tension, irony and paradox – so as to comprehend the piece of literature on its own terms without reference to context (such as the writer's biography, the historical setting of the work, or its political implications).

If we go back to our gloss on Sylvia Plath's poem "Tale of a Tub", New Critics would be interested in the whole notion that the objects in the bathroom have "voices" in the poem that create tensions, ironies, and ambiguities. But they would not be interested in our extension to psychoanalysis, Plath's mental state or her unresolved relationship with her father. The poem floats free from the poet as a work of art in its own right deserving scrutiny for its formal structure and voice. The poem opens up, again, like the bonnet (hood) of the car and underneath is the engine ripe for engineering.

The manual for "fixing" the car is the poem itself, word by word, image by image, atmosphere by atmosphere. Entering the poem this way becomes habitual. But – and this is obviously critical – engaging with the poem and its parts in a meticulous manner (close reading) affords defamiliarisation. Your habitual ways of looking and engaging will be undone for another kind of habit in another kind of habitat. This habitat, as we have shown, is the poetic *umwelt*, rich in affordances; not a culture but a climate.

We might have chosen I.A. Richard's *Practical Criticism* or *The Meaning of Meaning*, since these titles are also inherently manual-istic, but the special element of Empson's manual is that it is concerned with ambiguity, a quality we have taken book-length pains to establish as something to cultivate a tolerance for in medicine. Furthermore, a delicious irony is that Empson's book is written in a deceptively systematic way, seeking to taxonomise what had not been generally understood (that poetry has many meanings) in an implicit, but not explicit, fashion. We say "deceptively" because, as Jon Cook (https://www.worldofbooks.com/en-gb/books/jon-cook/poetry-in-theory/9780631225546) points out, Empson offers "not a theory of literature or a single method of analysis but a model of how to read with pleasure and knowledge". There is of course much here for doctors to savour as they read their patients as texts (Bleakley, Bligh and Browne 2011), trying to stick with what the body says in a formal sense and not get too wound up in biography or context.

The necessary use of an ambiguous concept like "ambiguity" frustrates any attempt to contain its definitional ambiguities, a point we will return to later. As seems obvious, the appeal of such a model to the lay practitioner is high. Perhaps the chief temptation for us to use Empson's book is that our act of usage is, at root and ironically, a misapplication of Empson's book. Rightly thought of as a work of literature in its own right, and suggested by many as the unfortunate victim of those who would dully try to use the book as a taxonomy or typology rather than as a means to establish a cosmology of interpretation, to shove *Seven Types of Ambiguity* at medicine as we do is to instrumentalise that which is beautiful exegesis in instantiation.

In other words, we enthusiastically make the same kind of error that biomedicine does with narrative, or vice versa. After all, isn't Narrative Medicine the beautiful imperfection we needed to make a small stand against the cultural dominance of chilly biomedicine, itself a much larger mistake made centuries ago when art was discarded on the road to science? We proceed to make familiar, avoidable mistakes as proof that we are ridiculous creatures. Such is the beautiful foolishness that poetry sometimes goes by on the way to abstracting to the general case.

Let us quickly sketch Empson's (1930/1991) methodology so that a general frame of interpretation can be set. We'll start slow, by way of analogy. Consider a medical student or an experienced clinician interviewing a perplexing patient. They are halfway through and are baffled but fascinated. They think they know what the condition or conditions might be, or they think they partially apprehend a small portion of the totality of the person before them, but they aren't sure. Now pull them from the interview room and have them write out their impressions. You might get something like this, if you changed the literary terms below to medical ones:

> It seemed to me that I was able in some cases to partly explain my feelings to myself by teasing out the meanings in the text. Yet these meanings when teased out ... were too complicated to be remembered together as if in one glance of the eye; they had to be followed each in turn, as possible alternative reactions [...] and indeed there is no doubt that some readers sometimes do only get part of the full intention. In this way such a passage has to be treated as if it were ambiguous[.]

The hermeneutical method described here strikes us as one that recommends itself to us by virtue of its curiosity, provisionality, and humility. At bottom, Empson tries to crack open poetry's gestalt appreciation for subsidiary elemental contributions to the whole understanding in an encompassing "glance", reminding us of Foucault's (1976) description of the embracing glance as opposed to the penetrating medical gaze. He examines poetry's excess of meaning – what he calls "ambiguity" – by trying to identify manifestations of that ambiguity in canonical poetry, not to develop some kind of overarching theory of poetics but rather to honour and celebrate poetry itself, developing an expertise and learning that recommends itself much like poetry-thought recommends itself to the medical practitioner.

There is another recommendation to discuss. Empson (1930/1991: 15) writes,

> It is true that no explanation [of a poem] can be adequate, but, on the other hand, any one valid reason that can be found is worth giving; the more one understands one's own reactions the less one is at their mercy.

That Empson ultimately subscribes to a relational model to gainsay his critical efforts is eminently applicable in our view to the plight of the medical practitioner awash in data about a patient, anxious to analyse. Obtaining data is more obviously a relational process, yet considering the data as non-informational, *as poetry*, is a relational one too. A doctor under orders from General Change might ask herself questions like: *What is it about this data that is somehow affecting me? What interpretative capacities am I bringing to the data?*

Beginning the ambiguine

To begin with, there is a glorious hole at the heart of Empson's critical enterprise and, thereby, our own. We enjoy this fact because it is an enactment of our goal, which is to embrace ambiguity. The hole is simple: any definition of ambiguity worth the name must be ambiguous. The poet Peter Redgrove called this a "hole-in-the-day" – a pun on "holiday" – as an opportunity to take a break from conventions by riding the ambiguity train into ambiguity territory, rather than repairing the hole and returning to the mundane, or attempting to rationalise the irrational.

Empson's (ibid.: 1) definition, met in the previous chapter, meets this challenge: "any verbal nuance, however slight, which gives room for alternative reactions to the same piece of language". In the second edition of the book, due presumably to the "infamous" reception of the original definition (Ossa-Richardson 2019: 1), Empson (1930/1991: 1) adds a footnote in which he says the definition is not exactly a definition at all, that it's "not meant to be decisive" and that what "the best definition of 'ambiguity'" is "crops up all through" the book. The contingent nature of Empson's analysis – which, it must be admitted, creates "types" that blend into one another the longer one looks at them – delights, rather than vexes, us. Rather than the separation out of types, we get fermentation and dissolution of category boundaries: A de-territorialising within a mock territorialising text, a delicious irony and a meta-ambiguity.

Indeed, the truly compromised nature of the analysis is the exact quality we find irresistible. For Empson (ibid.: 9) was forthright that the occasion of the book was simple: as a critic, he finds that "unexplained beauty arouses an irritation in me, a sense that this would be a good place to scratch" and that the book is the result of his trying to "reason" about the "roots of beauty". The book is a symptom of a deeper condition, that of the expectation at all that literary texts would be stable or clear, like engineering manuals, train timetables, or chemical formulae.

As Ossa-Richardson (2019: 3) explains: "The book's method, despite its title, turns out to be tactical rather than strategic, arriving at insight not by systematic theorisation but hap-hazard, as if on the way to something else, in the course of a chat over sherry in the combination room". If there is systematicity inherent to *Seven Types of Ambiguity*, it can be found in the relief of prurience when apprehended – but not fully understood – beauty comes calling. To put things another way, the systematic (rather than formulaic) approach rests in asking, "Why do I love this thing, this line, this poem, this image?" The question is asked in order to honour the beloved more deeply, and not as an occasional practice, but as a routinised one, much like the way a doctor interrogates pieces of information and tries to synthesise them into a whole or wholes, consultation upon consultation. That a line or two does not fit or contribute to a synthesised whole only makes for a more complicated beauty, an ambiguity that defies integration into summative simplicities known as diagnostic categories; the line or two of history that doesn't fit can become rebellious personhood itself, a non-functional beauty that adds to the richness of life.

To return to Ossa-Richardson once more, the reading of poetry can hardly be called strategic unless one already understands its spiritual necessity; yet it is gloriously tactical in thought, a constant remonstrance with meaning, sound, form and experience in order to generate relational properties. Empson's strategic brilliance in wringing interpretations out of works is a wonderfully useful model. We recognise the strategic lack in such an argument, since his book is almost a hundred years old and has already infiltrated the mechanics of close reading on a molecular level; we celebrate the tactical use of the text for our own purposes in this moment. Following the orders of General Change, in the next chapter we move on to tactical deployment!

References

Alford L. 2020. *Forms of Poetic Attention*. New York: Columbia University Press.

Bleakley A. (ed.) 2020. *The Routledge Handbook of the Medical Humanities*. Abingdon: Routledge.

Bleakley A, Bligh J, Browne J. 2011. *Medical Education for the Future: Identity, Power and Location*. Dordrecht: Springer.

Empson W. 1991/1930. *Seven Types of Ambiguity*, 3rd ed. London: The Hogarth Press.

Empson W. The Poetry Foundation. Retrieved from https://www.poetryfoundation.org/poets/william-empson

Foucault M. 1976. *The Birth of the Clinic: An Archaeology of Medical Perception*. London: Routledge.

Logue C. 2003. *All Day Permanent Red*. New York: Farrar, Strauss & Giroux.

Neilson S. Poetry Will Save Your Life. *Canadian Family Physician*. 2019; 65: 820–22.

Orr D. 2011. *Beautiful and Pointless*. New York: HarperCollins.

Ossa-Richardson, A. 2019. *A History of Ambiguity*. Princeton, NJ: Princeton University Press.

Pickering N. The Use of Poetry in Health Care Ethics Education. *Medical Humanities*. 2000; 26: 31–36.

13 Tactical ambiguity spelunking amidst Canadian physician-poets

Informed consent for poets

Consider this chapter the equivalent of obtaining informed consent from a patient. The coordinates of the analysis are close to what academics call their "archive", but the method here is one of setting such terms as evincing "place-thought", what the Indigenous Scholar Vanessa Watts (2013) (Mohawk and Anishinaabe Bear Clan, Six Nations) explain as a means whereby our personal relations to materials can be understood. This echoes our insistence throughout the book on the importance of place and of object relations. SN did the fieldwork here to gather the evidence – as a poet who is also a physician, he felt it a righteous thing to include work by other poets who are also physicians. More, as a Canadian who has long recognised the relative paucity of Canadians in international poetry venues, he insisted on Trojan Horse-ing some contemporary Canadian work into what has admittedly been largely a sampling of the European canon. In his *Lives of the Poets,* Michael Schmidt (2000) infamously referred to the work of Canadians as a "short street", but, due to a recent renaissance of poetry written by physicians in Canada, this dated view can be ditched. Where Schmidt saw a short street we see an expanding field.

SN kept in view Canadian literature's relatively new, but permeating, emphasis on anti-oppressive practices and sensitivities towards representation. Thus the analysis in this chapter will consider work by racialised poets primarily, though this qualifier again is hardly an impediment since the newest wave of physician-poets in Canada is predominantly a racialised one. Missing in the analysis is the work of an Indigenous poet working within the settler-state designated as Canada. Identifying such a poet would have been quite productive, since it throws into question a series of assumptions that underwrite the entirety of the premises in this book. For example, should an Indigenous person who was trained in Western medicine be included? Why even think in such an exclusionary way? What about an Indigenous person who practiced "traditional" medicine, keeping in view the fact that the category "traditional" has been problematised by Indigenous scholars as itself a Western construct? Isn't the work of Indigenous poets in a more

DOI: 10.4324/9781003194408-15

general sense, in a place-thought sense, contributing to the cultural health of its community?

To illustrate the identified ambiguities in poems most productively, we have decided to fulsomely quote in the Canadian case and to more broadly survey in the non-Canadian one. We felt it important to provide, in a chapter that is essentially the culmination of what came before "on" poetry, entire poems in which to suss out different kinds of ambiguity. (In the introduction we gave an apology for not being able to reproduce entire poems due to copyright issues and associated permission costs). We also wanted a place for poetry to shine in its whole cloth in this book. We return to poems in order to demonstrate different manifestations of ambiguity in order to keep the references close and the meanings tight. We trust that this decision provides dividends to the reader unable or disinclined to seek out the original works. We also hope to give poetry-savvy readers a range of identified ambiguities in canonical poems as we range far and wide to prove the general case, necessarily quoting judiciously as we go. Thus, broadly speaking, there are two ways in which we demonstrate ambiguity.

Finally, we deliberately chose medical-themed poems not out of dogmatic themedness or limited imagination – all of the included poets write wonderfully about unlimited subjects – but because we feel that the clinicians reading this book will more readily relate to the material because of its clinical substance. We want there to be face validity, in other words, to the poems we close read for ambiguity. Since the ambiguities William Empson (1930/1991) discovers only loosely cohere as categories and unravel as a typology on close scrutiny as already noted, *we think that the demonstration of close reading these poems with ambiguity in mind is one that is itself a usefully ambiguous enactment of how readers might carry a close reading of ambiguity forward in their own practicing lives.*

Thus, we don't "discover" or disclose ambiguity but rather enact it. A close reading of a close reading of ambiguity in texts is a shift of emphasis from source (Empson) to target domains that itself carries ambiguity and is necessarily a metaphorical gesture. Let us descend, carefully spelunking, to those potholes and caves as the territories for re-imagining Empson's seven types of ambiguity. By the way, our spelunking is not a pastime, but a commitment to the life of poetry itself. Our work of exploration is to reveal what those caves have to offer, to articulate their beauties.

First-type ambiguities arise when a detail is effective in several ways at once

As can be seen, "first-type" ambiguities are, by Empson's stated summary – the heading above is a quote of his own chapter heading from the table of contents – broad, and they are, at bottom, metaphor. The commonality between them is that each complicates, somehow, a fixed meaning. The most notorious example of Empson's (ibid.) of the type – "that choirboy controversy" – came as follows when quoting Shakespeare:

To take a famous example, there is no pun, double syntax, or dubiety of feeling, in ["]Bare ruined choirs, where late the sweet birds sang["]. But the comparison holds for many reasons; because ruined monastery choirs are places in which to sing, because they involve sitting in a row, because they are made of wood, are carved into knots and so forth;, because they used to be surrounded by a sheltering building crystallized out of the likeness of a forest, and coloured with stained glass and painting like flowers and leaves, because they are now abandoned by all but the grey walls coloured like the skies of winter, because the cold and Narcissistic charm suggested by the choir-boys suits well with Shakespeare's feeling for the object in the Sonnets, and for various sociological and historical reasons (the protestant destruction of monasteries; fear of puritanism), which it would be hard now to trace out in their proportions; these reasons, and many more relating the simile to its place in the Sonnet, must all combine to give the line its beauty, and there is a sort of ambiguity in not knowing which of them to hold most clearly in mind.

The point of including this example at such length is to show just how close one can close read, how the technique can become a form of scrying; that this example was, in time, massively contested by Shakespearean scholars is an occurrence we celebrate for its irrelevance. For what matters here is a virtuoso interpretation. Correctness or truth is not at issue here. We celebrate the sheer power to see this far, rightly or wrongly, and encourage more seeing like it amongst physicians. It is close noticing deluxe. We point to it as a mighty example of how much can be made of a line and how much a line can demand of its reader. Empson followed up on the quote above with the comment that "the machinations of ambiguity are among the very roots of poetry". His close readings of lines seem like the products of a relational meaning-making machine cued by a curiosity itself pricked by beauty. His process is to take a line and to make something of it – an inherently practical attitude for what is otherwise a pointless purpose save to derive further enjoyment.

Let us emulate Empson's process when demonstrating ambiguity of the first type which, again, is inherently about metaphor, but which in our hands is about the inherently metaphorical properties contained in every word in the English language. Rather than consider a choir in Shakespeare, we take on the associational like-properties of a whole line in Tolu Oloruntoba's (2021) poem "Medicine":

MEDICINE

It was only ever about my own patient
excision, incision, tunnels as train
religion, hugging the walls in oncoming
shake, flattening in the perpendicular
congress of tracks, the points of spaced

insults, at speed, coalescing
into the becoming: man of faith,
here's a man of doubt.

Opening crawl:

lightning chalks a descending cumulonimbus.
Dramatis persona: we know the prime
as he enters the frame, his foreshadow
a skin of death, a long hood. But if the canary-
down torch lights in this funk,
he'll be golden. Drained in hot morgues,
the substance of mind is harder still

than the soft sheath of belief, scarified
with a swaddling of inky inoculation:
hamsa, haibun, halter hitch, ampersand, hymn.
Febrile, I leach sweat into the mattress,
takeoff maimed. But, doubtful apostle,
there is some breath left to me. And if anyone
could find me in a valley of ribcages,

you could.

Strap me to your cart.
Run me, if you can, from the city.

Let us close read the lines:

But if the canary-
down torch lights in this funk,
he'll be golden

in relative isolation, not plugging the lines too much into an awareness of the
rest of the poem, of which much more sense could be made – there will be
time enough for that – all the while recognising that it is the process which
matters, not so much the individual insights.

The first item that makes us scratch a little at beauty is the appearance of
"canary-down." Just what is that? The senses that seem most appropriate in
context – meaning that we're already in the land of first-type ambiguity – are
'down' used as a noun in terms of "An elevated stretch of open, uncultivated
land with gently rolling hills" as well as "The fine soft feathers forming the
inner layer of a bird's plumage, often used for stuffing beds, pillows, etc."
Also: the similar soft covering of a young bird before it is fledged (OED).
If the intention is the former, then land – probably Oloruntoba's Nigerian

countryside – is connected to colour, but also, quite interestingly, to a bird – to flight itself. The association with flight is not unintentional, for the poem is about fleeing *something*.

The canary has further connotations in English as a bird of warning (the proverbial "canary in a coal mine") and that sense is perfect, of course, in the context of the poem also (which can be interpreted to be partially symbolic of lynching). "Canary-down" is then ambiguous – the canary has downy feathers and goes down when dead. There is much in the poem about the body and skin tied to death. The Grim Reaper is invoked ("his foreshadow / a skin of death, a long hood"). Yet the canary-down is a compound adjective in the use of the poem that offers an instrumental, similitative function (such compounds bring two things into a fused relation), and it further modifies "torch", investing into an object which provides illumination a pre-existing colour and texture that is, in the context of the larger sentence in which these lines occur, a conditionality. We are not sure if the torch will light. It is part of the drama of "but" and a further fraught condition of "if".

The "funk" is the condition itself that seems to be threatening the torch's ability to catch fire, and "funk" is defined as "a powerful, unpleasant smell, or musky odour of sweat or other bodily excretions; a stink" (OED). The connotation of moistness makes sense, although the surrounding lynch-like conditions certainly strike us as miasmatic and materially wet; then again, "funk" also refers to a "state of panic, extreme nervousness, agitation, etc.; utter fear or terror" which fits for the same reason. In black culture, "funk" (as in funk music since the 1960s, such as James Brown) means "getting down", or, as the OED puts it, a form of music "characterized by a prominent, repetitive bass line and a propulsive, heavily syncopated rhythm that typically accentuates the first beat in the bar, with other instruments such as guitar, keyboards, and brass used primarily to provide a rhythmic counterpoint". We like the idea that below or within the funk that the poet implies as the musky stink is heavy bass, rhythm, a formulation of song. Finally, there is an obsolete use of "funk" that demonstrates the richness of the language: funk is also "a spark." Wet, yet also combustible? Inherent in the word is a singularity of ambiguity. All of which is to say that, in the same case as "down", we are in the presence of a productive ambiguity.

"Flattening", "crawl", "descending", "down", and "maimed" culminates in "a valley of ribcages" – but there is some breath left in the protagonist who stands up to the oppressor: "Run me, if you can, from the city". This is a delicious turnaround – somebody is being run down, is rundown, but turns on the pursuer to say I dare you to run me down.

But we are not done looking through the grasses of these ambiguities. The end of the line, "he'll be golden", might strike one as a mere cliché, an ossified piece of language marring the line. Look closer. The "he" pronoun is the first appearance of the second person in a poem that switches speaker points of view throughout. More can be made of this switch, and we will do this in a moment. Suffice to say, this creates another form of ambiguity, i.e., who is spoken of? Who is speaking? Another facet is the homology to "hell" that "he'll" has, albeit for an errant, impositional apostrophe to make the contraction. He, in other words, is contracted into hell. And the poem's terrain is, at least to one reading, a hellscape. Finally, the "he'll be golden" is a kind of conditional promise made to connect to the opening "canary-down." The torch is yellow; the torch will make yellow light; the man will reflect yellow when illuminated. The colour-sense intrinsic to these lines is continuous. Yellow signifies cowardice, but the man responds with courage and challenges back.

There may be a bit of virtuosity here,

> the substance of mind is harder still
> than the soft sheath of belief, scarified
> with a swaddling of inky inoculation:
> hamsa, haibun, halter hitch, ampersand, hymn

where Oloruntoba takes amulet, literary form, glyph, and knotty poem itself as emblems for praising and raising life, just as they scarify, making incisions in our beings, the alliterative "h" acting as tattoo, or a surgical trace. We take this to mean that we are marked from birth to death, while we can also read these marks as imbrications, scaly overlappings of cultures with their differing emblems. The language is tactile, scratchy.

Do you see the ghosts, too? Although perhaps the most ubiquitous and general form of ambiguity possible – that meaning can be bent and warped and pushed based on the richness of language itself, its vault of definitional and associative extensions – one can see that a line or two of good work can be wrung out so that a poem can seem better known and yet no less beautiful for the speculative knowledge.

In second type ambiguities two or more alternative meanings are fully resolved into one

It is now time to return to Oloruntoba's pronomial use to see how alternative meanings arrive at a final unity. A complete unpacking is impossible, but enough can be done in a short space to demonstrate the point. Consider, first, the "it". We start with the singular, neuter, third-person pronoun that in this case kicks off a line that refer to the speaker's patient, were the first line to be considered in isolation, but which also refers to surgical procedure on the speaker's body (among other things) – the nest of additional experiences is irrelevant to our purpose here. Note, though, that the "It" that refers to a general situation is qualified later in the same line with "my" designating the first-person possessive determiner of the situation. There is no ambiguity, really, in this line at the level of pronomial use though the stage is deliberately set from the outset for ambiguity later on.

Near the end of the first stanza, we actually seem to be in a dramatic narration, an unveiling, as if the self is recognising it is taking a kind of stage or making an address to another: "man of faith, / here's a man of doubt." Things become stranger: the "dramatis persona" is singular. "Dramatis personae" – literally "masks of the drama" – refers to frontstage characters – yet it is collapsed to the singular. This is the backstage observer who becomes the single frontstage performer. And he "enters the frame, his foreshadow / a skin of death, a long hood". Is this Death, straight out of Ingmar Bergman's 1957 film "The Seventh Seal"?

The pronomial use changes radically at this point, becoming a "we know the prime as he enters the frame", and this change can be understood as being embedded in a new stanza, set apart from the first, which had "it" and "my". The new stanza is deliberately ostentatious, scored with an introductory stage direction ("opening crawl"). The implication might be that the "we" is now a crowd of onlookers who are both the collective speaker of the poem now, but also a performative "we" in a newly performative space with, in actuality, the same original speaker as the speaker who is wearing a plural mask. There is no certainty in this interpretation, only ambiguity. Moving forward in the same stanza, there is the additional third person "he'll" glossed in the first-type ambiguity section.

In the next stanza, we move to an outright "I" and "me" first-person use, which resolves us back to the original speaker idea that began this analysis. And yet the final lines of the poem obliterate this resolution as they are, themselves, a resolution. The second person singular appears, and it reads as ominously as when the earlier observer, the plural "we", appeared. In this appearance, it is a "you" that can find the speaker in an ominous environment ("valley of ribcages"). Indeed, it is the closing imperative that amplifies the poem's prevailing atmosphere of menace. "Strap me to your cart" it commands, "Run me, if you can, from the city".

In other words, this poem creates in the reader an awareness that, as readers, we are the audience, that we must act to remove the speaker from danger. As if by magic, the speaker was always first-person singular and the audience was always the reader, but careful play with pronouns resulted in an ambiguous fusing of identities that are, ironically enough, resolved at the conclusion via direct, clear imperative.

An ambiguity of the third type, considered as a verbal matter, occurs when two ideas, which are connected only by being both relevant in the context, can be given in one word simultaneously

As one can see as we progress, focussing on particular kinds of ambiguities leads to different readings of a poem, some of which are at a variance to one another and which can't be resolved into one, as per the second ambiguity; rather, these readings sit alongside one another, informing each other. In this reading for ambiguities of the third type, we make the most "medical" interpretation so far.

The title of "Medicine" signals the surface importance of the subject. But it is also medicine that is intended in the poem when the world "religion" or its synonyms/accoutrements appear. Medicine might refer to any healing tradition, substance or balm. The same is true for the word "poetry". In the poem, the shifting speaker mentions the following items that stand in place of one another:

- "train religion" – what is medicine if not a secular, rite-and-rote-filled practice? "(T)rain / religion" might refer to acolytes, where medicine is a self-perpetuating community of practice, a procession (train referring to trail, like the trail of a dress; or what is behind and pulled by the front men).
- "man of faith" and "man of doubt" – we have here a contrast between confident biomedicine and a sceptic; but also, as the singular is used, the contrast may be between life and death, the man of doubt being the Grim Reaper: "his foreshadow / a skin of death, a long hood".
- "soft sheath of belief" – even if represented as somehow soft, medicine is somehow the sheath for something hard. Where "the substance of mind is harder still // than the soft sheath of belief" the poet may be referring to "hard" science set against "soft" faith.
- "inky inoculation:" – this is not just vaccination but getting a metaphorical jab of poetry, faith, and medicine as revealed by the next line, explained below. While the "soft sheath of belief" is "scarified / with a swaddling of inky inoculation" – the ambiguity being that to scarify is to cut the skin, either in surgical incision or tattooing, yet this is described as a "swaddling", a way of settling through soft wrapping.

Then: "hamsa, haibun, halter hitch, ampersand, hymn" – a complicated line in which the hamsa, a protective talisman that brings good fortune, health, and happiness is included in a list that mentions a poetic form (haibun), a kind of knot typically used to connect a rope to an animal (halter hitch), the lopogram (&) representing the conjunction "and", which originated as a ligature of the letters *et* in Latin; and the final container of "hymn" which denotes the poem entire but also is the container largely for poetry and medicine together. The poet seems to say that a connection has been made. Here, two ideas (piercing/cutting the skin and swaddling) are connected by one symbol, repeated (knots, talisman, common artefact, common ritual).

"Doubtful apostle" – the paradox, an obvious ambiguity of faith and doubt again; but it is made more ambiguous by the nature of what kind of apostle is intended here. Based on the poem, it is an apostle of poetry and medicine with faith possessing a double meaning. Yet the linkages of these disparate words occur in the context of the verbal device of the poem.

An ambiguity of the fourth type occurs when two or more meanings of a statement do not agree among themselves, but combine to make clear a more complicated state of mind in the author

As Empson himself wrote, "Evidently this is a vague enough definition which would cover much of the third type" but he insists that the distinction setting the type apart from the third is that it more overtly reflects a conflict in the poet or speaker's mind. One can easily see a differential weighting of medicine and religion and poetry in Oloruntoba's "Medicine", suggesting a conflict in the author's mind denoted by the equivalence of concepts as if they were nested within one another like Russian dolls; yet Empson wishes to signal in the fourth type a greater psychic split, a more intense tension. Let us turn to "My Therapist Assesses Suicidal Ideation," another of Oloruntoba's poems:

MY THERAPIST ASSESSES SUICIDAL IDEATION

My own stigmata are different:
I never return calls, another way of cutting
myself from the mind of the world.

I go to my
carnivorous plants out back:
trigger plants, with velcro pantsuits of death, clutch stomachs;
powdery strap airplants and guiding pilot lights,
to sticky strips for the unknowing;
pitcher plants and pitcher-trap ambushes awaiting the totter,
the topple, the drown in digestive drums;
twining bladderworts and purple, delicious, dervish skirts;
venus flytraps belching beyond tripwires and the clap of cymbal doors;
waterwheel plants, whorls of snap-traps sieving, wading the water,
washing me down;
Sundews, anyone, anemone home for a warm shower?
Here, midges around a touchscreen moon, I can slurp
the capsized roof
of the pond.

My mind has bent the facts, I know.
The facts have bent my mind.

In this poem, the equivalence of mental distress and gardening terminology is foregrounded in much the same way the poet signalled that faith, medicine, and poetry were important variables in the previous poem. Yet there is a curious effect in a poem that, at first glance, seems to make a simpler mix of a more obvious split or duality. To pick things up after the (un)clear orientation of the title – we are never definitely shown a therapist, office or screen, suggesting that we might actually be appreciating the speaker-as-his-own-therapist – we encounter the speaker demonstrating that rather than bear marks of self-harm on limbs, his telltale indicators of injury are, instead, those of invisible retreat from labour ("I never return calls, another way of cutting / myself from the mind of the world").

The rest of the poem is a verbal feast of plant types that have alternatingly lush, tantalising, and ominous descriptors that seem to develop a phantasmagoric other life as the speaker's extended self; penultimately, we linger at obliterated labour again mixed with garden "midges around a touchscreen moon, I can slurp" but with a lineation that seems to arrest with two short capping lines ("the capsized roof / of the pond") perhaps enacting the "capsizing" action. Yet the mental strife that is occurring is sublimated in the garden imagery and is best reflected in its blend and embodiment there – the action is almost calm, an embedding or banishment of the problem into the external world that, paradoxically, the poet is cut off from in other ways; there is a dissociational quality amidst plant life of great fierceness – until we return again to the business end of the poem, the conclusion, which, like the title, is up front about its subject. The speaker is in distress.

Even so, the matter is spoken in a restrained way, as if the verbal excess permitted to flourish in the garden must coalesce in plain speech here, yet for that fact, it is all the more affecting. Compared to the third kind, this ambiguity is less intended to indicate a multiplicity of meaning when a word appears but is more so an orchestrated, poem-wide attempt to demonstrate its overarching concept of mental difficulty, and it accomplishes it as a verbal phenomenon (the means that Empson prefers), yet it also does so at a formal level as well. Note the field's shape: the line lengths of the poem, printed just as they appear in Oloruntoba's (2021) *The Junta of Happenstance*. Many overspill the margin and are orphaned on the next line. Reality, as the final couplet puts it, is being distorted by its facticity.

If we return to Empson's definition: "An ambiguity of the fourth type occurs when two or more meanings of a statement do not agree among themselves, but combine to make clear a more complicated state of mind in the author", we can see in this poem that suicidal ideation – the complicated state of mind in the author – is illuminated by the marriage between martial and pacific nature. Martial nature is the carnivorous plants, made more so by the acidic and snapping alliterations: "drown in digestive drums", "snap-traps sieving", and more. Pacific nature is the balm of the gnat swarm around the light of the touchscreen, and the promised nourishing slurp of the upturned pond. As these forces (of snapping and acid-bath plants) and presences (of benign gnat clouds and pondwater) meet, so the state of mind of the poet is complicated and framed as an enantiodromia. In the final stanza: "My mind has bent the facts, I know. / The facts have bent my mind". Surely this type of ambiguity – to entertain enantiodromias as calling and lifestyle – is the mark of the poet.

An ambiguity of the fifth type occurs when the author is discovering his idea in the act of writing, or not holding it all in his mind at once

Of all the ambiguities Empson suggests, this one brings forth vividly to mind the "read my mind" questions that medical students come in for so often with a certain kind of preceptor who has a very particular and uncurious manner of teaching, in which the things that are known (well, that they know, the two or three things, tops) could be easily discerned and packaged in the form of a question that required divine inspiration to answer, unless one had happened to overhear the antique bonesetter do their impression of sphinxitude the day prior at the nurses' station when some other student had fallen victim. "Read My Mind" questions are unfair and infuriating. They can be differentiated from the "Socratic Method" questions, which students seem to dislike nowadays, derogatorily referring to them as attempts to "Pimp Us Out" but which we quite like for their openness and sense of mutual discovery when done well.

But we digress, just like the bonesetter who knows two or three things and whom can really draw out that knowledge. The only quality recommending the sphinx-bonesetter's bloviations is the extreme ambiguity of his questions. Yet biomedical questions need not be ambiguous by their nature, correct? Being in the presence of ambiguous certainty in the bodily form of Royal College personhood makes the sphinx-bonesetting question experience bizarre. *What is the next thing to do in this general situation?* I think they were/are asking. *Well surely, the answer is clear!* was/is their demeanour. And the answers somehow *are*, when they triumphantly say them. But they weren't, until they did. Which is to say, ambiguity is bullshit if it shouldn't be ambiguous at all. Biomedicine, take your own inventory here.

We get to a dangerous juncture in our analogic thought experiment that is this wilfully idiosyncratic journey to fifth-type ambiguity: just when can we presume to know a poet – who otherwise writes beautifully, whom is worth reading – is stumbling towards ecstasy by dim half-awareness? How could we possibly know that, if they didn't tell us themselves?

Yes, we rebel a little against Empson here. It is routine for a writer to discover in the process of writing; in particular, poetry can be partially defined as an attempt to uncover or reveal what one already knows, or rather what is already there in the world, when one lacks the clear prose logic to articulate the facts of the case. This porous body lives and breathes fifth type ambiguity. Empson's position here is one fraught with … ambiguity?

This said, we would like to think that the final couplet of "My Therapist Assesses Suicidal Ideation" is the idea Oloruntoba suddenly discovered after writing out the verbal feast of the middle section where he blended self with what is typically a healing space (the garden) but which in his case seemed rather more violent and disturbing. He had to sit with the enantiodromia that we discussed in the last section. The ouroboric worm eats itself from the tail only to appear whole, refreshed. What the poet refers to as "stigmata" in the opening stanza – "I never return calls" – is deliciously ambiguous, made more so by (our) addition of a pause: 'I never return, calls'.

The calling of "never returning" is vocation, a way of life, a professional commitment. In opposition, infantile regression, retrieval, habit become tic (obsession, compulsion) are "never return(s)". The poet, like Empson, moves on through the levels. Doctors move on from apprenticeship to moderate competence, to full competence, to capability, expertise and then adaptive expertise or labile authority (expertise + high tolerance of ambiguity + innovation + democratic collaboration). Activity theory activists call this "expansive learning", a process of negotiations and border-crossings as learning is widely networked with no end in sight, just a receding horizon.

We'd like to presume that the poet realised that his life was being deformed and the deformation was his life, that he just half-knew it in the middle section and then the point suddenly rose up from the "capsized roof / of the pond." But we wouldn't know for sure. And we don't want to know, making this thought experiment more so our own half-realised discovery of an idea we couldn't hold together all in the head at once, until we had written it out ourselves. We notice that the writing has a habit of changing its mind, trajectory and identity mid-stream.

An ambiguity of the sixth type occurs when a statement says nothing, by tautology, by contradiction, or by irrelevant statements; so that the reader is forced to invent statements of his own and they are liable to conflict with one another

Empson's account here could describe the psychoanalytic encounter. By mirroring back to a person what she has just said, no "analysis" occurs at all. But, of course, the mirroring is deadpan, Beckettesque, and supremely ironic because the analyst knows a lot and has a lot to say. But interpretation is for later. For now, we say to the poet (as analysand in this example): "you say nothing, by tautology, by contradiction, or by irrelevant statements" (so now the analysand "is forced to invent statements of his own and they are liable to conflict with one another"). Poets, in conversation with themselves, like to play analyst and analysand simultaneously, of course.

We will now turn to the work of Tamar Rubin (2020), a paediatric immunologist currently practicing in Winnipeg, Manitoba. Rubin's debut, *Tablet Fragments*, is a thematic blend of medicine, motherhood, and biblical myth. The switch seems appropriate in terms of our analysis, for Rubin's book considers her Jewish heritage, and Empson's chapter on this type of ambiguity begins with a biblical example from Moses. Rather than recapitulate Empson's biblical exegesis (it turned out to be a rather ambiguous example of the sixth type, which Empson himself endearingly admits), we'll jump immediately to Rubin's "I" and hope we can explain the type ourselves:

I

written often,
say nothing

about myself.

Repeatedly.

This poem is about my mother.
This poem is about my father.
This poem is about

some trauma, having to wear my older brother's lime green sweatpants.

I have not undressed this. I'd rather wear something other than bareness.

I write in first person,
say nothing, often,

without interrogating

pronouns, really asking: Who
might I be?

The poem invites an analytic reading. Let's suspend for a moment, as the Russian Formalists would urge, the desire to contextualise the poem by analysing the poet's motives, but simply analyse the poem itself. Further, we use the technique above of suspending conventional analytic readings for a mirroring of what is said back to its source. In other words, the poem analyses itself (ouroborically, swallowing itself from the tail and re-appearing refreshed). The words of the poem must look at themselves for a slantwise refreshment. The subject of the poem is the pronoun ('she', 'he', 'it', 'them'). Pronouns stand in for nouns and names. The child wants to be known in the family by specific name and not referred to as a generic "she" or worse "it". Family dynamics squeeze the identity of the child into being through pronouns but coax the best out of the child through the beauty of names. Identity is in the naming. The analyst gives the words back to the poet as analysand so that she "is forced to invent (names of her) own and they are liable to conflict with one another" as Empson urges.

Our objective in selecting for this ambiguity was not to pick a poem that contained a single example of the type required – Empson tends to select a line or lines in isolation – but instead to pick a poem comprised of the essence of the sixth type. For the trick of Rubin's poem lies is in its suggestive concision, consistently refreshed with new tableaux on which to project the meanings suggested by the brevity of the phrases themselves. Consider the beginning: does "written often, / say nothing" mean that the speaker's "I" in poems is a repeated gesture, an empty signifier, hollowed out of meaning and selfhood? That the "I" says nothing? Yet the word used is not "says", it is "say." So the reflection pertains to the person itself, not a reflection on the act of saying. As you can see, we are already some distance into trying to make meaning of what is inherently ambiguous.

The next line throws meaning into further disarray. The "I" is not saying anything about the poet in poems but then reads also as an imperative, as if this "I" must not say anything about the poet and her life, as if it is an admonition.

The next line, a single word, reads as declarative – as if "Repeatedly" refers to the fact that the "I" is consistently deployed in a host of poems that somehow "say nothing". Yet one also wants to add to the single word, to resist the period, to fill it out. Repeatedly – what?

We then encounter simple statements that begin in relatively fulsome declaration – "This poem is about my mother. / This poem is about my father." – in which the poem is somehow shifted from the self, to another subject, yet is inescapably phrased in personal possessive terms ("my"). But then the poem begins to shave itself, or devour itself from the tail, becoming more gnomic in the next line ("This poem is about") and, quite purposely, unfinished. Further, the lines about mother and father attract full stops (periods), making for a severe separation of the lines, as if mother and father too are divided for separate treatment by the poet, but such treatment is not disclosed. Glaringly absent, the mother and father are not brought into connection by something warm or tender.

The next two lines are both precise and imprecise, deliberately mixing an abstract and imprecise ("some trauma") significance with a relatively specific insignificance ("older brother's lime green / sweatpants"). Is the trauma the embarrassing hand-me-down sweatpants-wearing? Or is it more significant, and unstated to gain power in contrast with the stated lesser? There is gravity in levity.

The poem continues in its strangeness. We're finally introduced to an "I" in the body of the poem proper, yet this "I" does not specifically refer to an action (again), but rather a nonspecific one. Does the speaker mean the "this" of the previous stanza's lime green pants? Or does the speaker mean the "this" of the not saying anything about the self from the first stanza? Or does the speaker mean the "this" of the possibly unstated "trauma"? As per the sixth type, we're forced as readers to speculate, to fill in, to meaning-make. The manner of close reading this poem is, as might be intuited from those already in clinical practice, a productive way of interpreting encounters with ill persons. The poet asks insistently: "Who / might I be?" as if the reader has answers. The patient asks: "what is wrong with me?" gnomically, but provides clues only slantwise (what is the "trauma" in wearing her brother's lime green sweatpants that remains "undressed" and not 'unaddressed'. What is the tantalising "bareness"?)

The poem is not yet done with its intentional confusions. It comments on preferring to wear something other than "bareness" – an intentional bareness, its intention signalled by the first appearance of the "I" pronoun in a poem of the same title. More analysis of this kind can be done, but we'll skip to the end that acts as a meta-commentary on all of the analysis just conducted by us: "Who might I be?" A poem sceptical about a self that says anything of worth or note, with a background drama of self-worth playing out, makes its scepticism the content of its utterance, all the while readers filling in its semantic gaps. Identity undressed and exposed seems to be an identity ad-dressed and re-dressed, the question: "who am I?" re-posed.

We leave it to you to consider the ambiguities between our two readings, one analytic and one synthetic. But we ask you to see which parts of the poem you particularly identify with and then dig where you stand.

An example of the seventh type of ambiguity ... occurs when the two meanings of the word, the two values of the ambiguity, are the two opposite meanings defined by the context, so that the total effect is to show a fundamental division in the writer's mind

Rubin's "I" conjures deep divisions between the moral responsibilities in-curred in adulthood as opposed to childhood. The naïve child endures the family context as subject and not agent. The adult takes on the mantle of moral agency. There is nothing more pressing than introjecting such agency so that moral dilemmas are constantly rehearsed (inter)subjectively. And yet the question remains "who might I be?" or "what might I become?" The poem dwells on the moral problem of shifting identities: an 'I' for an 'I'. The seventh kind of ambiguity in Empson's scheme is the poet's burden to mirror back to the world fundamental division's in the collective mind, as a "diagnostician of culture" to draw on Nietzsche's descriptor of the role of the artist.

The "I" in Rubin's poem could also be run through this seventh kind of ambiguity where the title of the poem (and its ostensible subject) is both the substance of the poem and also not; the "I" is intersubjective, becoming a more permeable I-with-others that can sometimes be, despite its yearning to be complete and contained, I-am-in-terms-of-others; it is this opposition that is the essence of Empson's seventh type, but because the opposites are more ideational as opposed to images or specific words, we've elected to in-clude a different poem to illustrate the concept alternatively.

Bahar Orang (2020) is a queer Persian-Canadian poet who published her debut collection, *Where Things Touch: A Meditation on Beauty,* in 2020. A fragment from the book reads in its entirety:

> I interview for residency programs, and they point out that I list "imaginative" as one of my strengths in my written application. Tell us more about that. I blank. I don't have a thing to say. We sit in a brief silence, and my mind, in a way that cannot be explained or accounted for, remembers the ocean. A sliver of sunlight escapes through the blinds behind my interviewers, and I wish I could free that light into the sea, where it would be free to play its games of reflection and refraction into oblivion.
>
> ibid. (88–89)

A striking ambiguity within this fragment is the phrase "I blank". We can read this as Orang intends, as she literally blanks out at that point, frozen. But we can also take this as a general dictum: "I blank": a comma helps "I, blank". Back to Samuel Beckett's 'Ping' where the 'I' disappears into background and is then reclaimed as essentially mysterious. The history of continental philosophy – following the deconstruction of Existentialism's search for 'authenticity' – is to blank the I. Certainly it can be multiplied up as numbers of identities, but in Beckett's world, the I-blank is Being. This is a Zen celebration of clearing. Orang sits in this clearing and silence, clearly moved by it as she is pinned. And then her I is named, pronoun to noun, in the best traditions of namings – she is absorbed by sunlight and sea, reflection and refraction. Oblivion means "to forget". And so we move on.

Clearly the "meditation" intended in the title holds true in this fragment of Orang's accretional book-length prose poem. There is no cataclysmic drama occurring here. Yet there is an opposition unfolding, in which a previously "imaginative" speaker is asked to comment on her status as imagineer, as, possibly, poet. In the moment, the poet is unimaginative, not able to provide a gloss or demonstrate her imaginative powers. Yet the lack doubles back into imaginative capacity, in which the imagination asserts itself as a godlike quality that can free light itself so that light can not just be ("let there be light") but instead so that light can be light ("free to play its games of reflection and refraction"); yet even this power becomes, somehow, terminal and approaches "oblivion" where, of course, the imagination cannot be.

We hope that our readings of these poems bring you closer to reading these poets yourself. We also hope that our readings prompt in you a close and critical reading of our words.

We also signal up again the exasperation we have with how poetry is often used instrumentally in medicine and healthcare, via the medical humanities, for therapeutic purposes in particular. Our close readings may be taken as mirroring the diagnostic arc, especially with complex symptom presentations, where Poetry=Medicine. It again puzzles us that poetry that would not pass muster in poetry circles is so readily acceptable in medical/health humanities circles (and not taken as seriously as medical work for its techniques). This is in no way a sleight against those who write the poetry, because we really do want to encourage people to do this. Rather, our concern is with the seeming inability across medical/ health humanities circles to set up cultures of informed tuition for aspiring poets based on close, critical reading. The first step in this is reading widely in poetry, and not imagining that you can just produce a poem out of nothing without immersing yourself in poetry itself. Our plea to members of the medical and healthcare professions is – don't believe what we say here about poetry's relationships to medicine without the acid test of immersing yourself in poetry and seeing what this does to your perceptions.

In the following chapter we evidence this with first-hand accounts of poet-physicians-academics, including Bahar Orang.

References

"down": OED Online, Oxford University Press, June 2021.
Empson W. 1991/1930. *Seven Types of Ambiguity*, 3rd ed. London: The Hogarth Press.
"funk": OED Online, Oxford University Press, June 2021.
Oloruntoba T. 2021. *The Junta of Happenstance*. Windsor, ON: Palimpsest Press.
Orang B. 2020. *Where Things Touch: A Meditation on Beauty*. Toronto: Book*Hug.
Rubin T. 2020. *Tablet Fragments*. Winnipeg, MB: Signature Editions.
Schmidt M. 2000. *Lives of the Poets*. New York: Vintage Books.
Watts V. Indigenous Place-Thought and Agency amongst Humans and Non Humans (First Woman and Sky Woman Go On a European World Tour!). *Decolonization: Indigeneity, Education & Society.* 2013; 2: 20–34.

14 Practitioner-poets do the footwork

We wrote to twenty doctor-poets and doctor-writers to invite them to contribute to this chapter. We wanted to hear from the horse's mouth how poetry and medicine engaged. We explained that we were particularly interested in the diagnostic thinking process in this respect. Eight persons responded with copy. Many others promised but were unable to deliver, mainly due to clinical pressures brought on by the Covid-19 pandemic crisis. We are grateful to those who have contributed, drawing our book to a close with some first-hand testament that provides a rich context for contemplating our previous chapters.

Bahar Orang

Bahar is a psychiatry resident in Toronto and a writer. A hybrid of lyric essay and prose poetry, her much acclaimed first collection *Where Things Touch: A Meditation on Beauty* was published in 2020 by Book★hug Press. She has a BASc from McMaster University and an MA in comparative literature from the University of Toronto. She completed her MD at McMaster University.

So you feel dangerous: poetry as method, abolition medicine, and Palestine solidarity

What is poetry to do? What is poetry to articulate in the present political moment? What can, what must, poetry articulate, or disarticulate, in the present political moment, in this time of breakage? I consider these questions, am perhaps perpetually considering them, but these days with a differently urgent orientation as I help to plan a teach-in for health workers about the meanings and practices of solidarity with the struggle for Palestinian liberation. One member of our planning group suggests to us all that yes, we can elucidate those links between medical violence and state violence, but how can we also suggest to health workers the possibility of working otherwise? How do we put forward that it is possible – *it* being something radically other than what is? How to corral that careful, difficult, nourishing analysis of the

DOI: 10.4324/9781003194408-16

world that in turn brings us to life and meanwhile redirects us towards the great risk of reimagination?

Poetry, as the poet Muriel Rukeyser (1996) suggests, stands only in "curious relationship" to our "*acceptance* of our way of living" (emphasis mine). I qualify Rukeyser's suggestion with the world *only* to signal that naming poetry's curiosity, while exciting, is, nonetheless, a restrained and a careful naming that does not (dangerously) over-suggest poetry's capacities for affecting life, or social and political life. If our ways of living are violent, as they tend to be, poetry is curious about our *acceptance* of such a violence. Poetry's curiosity does not necessarily imply a destabilisation of violent arrangements, nor does its curiosity always, or ever on its own, mobilise new orders of life. In fact, poetry's curiosities are sometimes satisfied towards reifying and beautifying tyrannical orders of the world and even obfuscating resistance and protest. However, to be curious could be to not take for granted, which could be to realise a new set of radical political demands.

To be specific and explicit, such a poetry would write somehow against modernity, which is to write against the co-constitutive and co-foundational organisations of settler-colonialism and apartheid, militarised police power and carceral violence, racial capitalism and white supremacy, and global and border imperialism. Which may seem a gargantuan and unruly task for poetry and I would think carefully about an excessively didactic or utilitarian writing or a writing that takes the place of political action. Poems that write somehow against modernity might be the poems that are held as banners at protests and chanted at marches. They might be poems that critique the technologies of power and domination under which we are continually crushed. Sometimes they are poems that want to rescue language from state-sponsored language. Other times, they escape politics entirely, and grapple with, or play with, or gesture after, the large and small details of a utopian otherwise vision, the strange, unpredictable, and improvisational dreams of alternate realities.

In the *Lancet* article "Abolition Medicine" (Iwai et al. 2020), the authors, writing amid the global Black-led uprising for police abolition that followed the public police murder of George Floyd, ask, "What might a public health approach to public safety look like? At this time, this question is an act of radical imagination". They go on to explain: "Abolition medicine is a practice of speculation, of dreaming of a more racially just future and acting to bring that vision to fruition". Narrative medicine, they argue, can bring abolition medicine into view as we "renarrate and re-envision justice, healing, activism, and collectivity". I want to think about poetry as a different but related method of activating the radical imagination for health workers. The poet Gwendolyn Brooks (1990) has said, "Remember that poetry is life distilled". Encountering a poem, then, is something quite different than thinking with and through narratives. The poet Dionne Brand (2018) has said, "The reader interrogates narrative. Poetry interrogates the reader". Narrative (medicine) usually keeps certain things intact; poetry (though not every poetry) invites us to give everything up (towards liberatory futures).

Like Brooks's poetry as distillation, Brand speaks of poetry as "pressure, pressure on verbal matter, on air, sustained pressure on space". Narrative tends to be less attentive to the truly elemental, tends to spend less time with elemental matters like the verbal or the spatial. Narrative tends to take such things for granted, where in the overwriting, in the renarration, the molecular matter of the story has remained the same, has something essentially in common with the originary narrative it has tried to reject. We can think, then, of narrative intervention as having a greater capacity for reformism, for little more than "renovation" of narratives of racism, colonialism, imperialism. But poetry can distil life, and in doing so, can bring us face-to-face with the most inherent and intrinsic terms of our collective demise. Poetry, to return to Rukeyser, is radically curious about those murderous terms, assumptions, sounds, resonances, tones, languages, and arrangements that we continuously employ (and all that they enact) and, as per Brand, applies a powerful pressure unto them, and unto us as poetry's readers. It is this kind of pressure, poetry's pressures, that one might hope to offer during a Palestine solidarity teach-in for health workers.

I want to suggest poetry as a method towards abolition medicine – a method that does not jump immediately to renarration, but that in its inevitable abstraction, its deep curiosity, can release us from those violent narratives that otherwise seem impossible to radically abandon, and compel us to excavate meanings and possibilities that exceed every assumption and give us new bearings for dreaming.

In the following sections, I will think, towards abolition medicine, with two poems – "Desired Appreciation" (Sharif 2016) and "The Workers Love Palestine" (Alsous 2021) – to consider first, the carceral health worker as the state's agent, and second, the abolitionist health worker's obligation to Palestinian liberation. I read Alsous's poems alongside the essay "Palestine and the case for abolition medicine" (Abo-Basha and Beltrán 2021), which helps to clarify the urgent realisation that a vision for abolition medicine must not only include the internationalist struggle for Palestinian liberation but can also learn from the political work of Palestinian health workers.

The poem "Desired Appreciation," by the poet Solmaz Sharif, which she wrote after the "Senate Intelligence Report On CIA Torture", enfolds doctors, psychologists, and psychiatrists into the nation-state's complex mechanisms of subjection. To start, the speaker talks of her own (American) docility, her well-behaviour, her graciousness: "A learned helplessness". The speaker then explains, "I've learned the doctors learned of learned helplessness / By shocking dogs. Eventually we things give up". And later: "Or the teeth of handcuffs closing to fix / The arms overhead. There must be a doctor on hand / To ensure the shoulders do not dislocate". Three scenes the poem collapses: the doctor's research on torture and its horrific utilities; the description of torture where the doctor is on hand; and the poem's speaker who is entrapped in a culture of discipline and punishment, where at the poem's end, the speaker tells her psychiatrist: "*I feel like I must muzzle myself*".

The doctor's role as an agent of the state is indispensable in each of these three scenes; indeed, it is perhaps the doctor on whom the entire apparatus hinges. It is the doctors who produce and then study tortured and traumatised psychological states in their potentially depoliticised spheres of laboratory research; it is the doctors who provide a kind of medical attention that is not care, but the permission for the perpetuation of state-sanctioned violence (they help to sanction it); and it is the doctor to whom the speaker expresses her feeling of muzzlement and who can respond by exerting many kinds of discretionary power and control.

The psychiatrist in the poem asks the speaker the following questions:

> "So you feel dangerous?" she said.
> Yes.
> "So you feel like a threat?"
> Yes.

Though the poem does not address this fact, as a psychiatry resident, I know that these are questions for a psychiatric risk assessment, the kind that could lead to the invocation of a Form 1, whereby once filled, the police would forcibly escort the speaker to the hospital for possible further and greater incarceration and subject her to so-called caring therapies that are frequently (though not by doctors) called torture.

The health workers of "Desired Appreciation" practise a carceral medicine that reproduces the carceral state. The poem weaves three seemingly disparate threads – the lab, the torture chamber, the clinic – to make an argument about carcerality and violence. The argument is not made axiomatically but aesthetically, following its own infra-logic, making sense from inside the terms of the poem itself, and not according to narrative logic. The poem is not a representation of violence, but a presentation of violence. The demands on us as readers are therefore understood differently; the demands are impressed on us, are felt by us, are differently urgent and experiential. The poem distils; the poem pressures. The possible demand then, for abolition medicine becomes harder to reject, harder to argue; the poem is therefore a mode of speaking that is particularly politically relevant to abolition, because abolition cannot be an argument. As the academic and activist Dylan Rodriguez (2017) has said, "It is not only a logical consequence to be an abolitionist, but it is an ethical and historical obligation." Abolition is not to be played with in the market of ideas; abolition is a must; abolition is an injunction.

Let us now return to the question raised by my colleague: how to suggest to health workers the possibility of working otherwise, of knowing health as a site of struggle?

"The Workers Love Palestine", by the poet Zaina Alsous, begins,

> The week before the SUN announced hospice
> my great-great-great-great-grandchild the harpist announced:
> WORKERS OF THE WORLD
>   JOIN THE STRIKE FOR GUARANTEED LIGHT

The florists union in Caracas and the Algerian weavers presented joint proposals:

TOWARD ILLUMINATION THAT MULTIPLIES

The word "hospice" in the first line alerts me to a scene of total illness and dying, where even the sun has fallen interminably sick. Where "light" has somehow reached its end, and the most supposedly intractable necessity for existence has, nonetheless, been extracted, depleted, snatched away. So the workers are invited to suspend working and demand a guaranteed light, and imagine, alongside the florists union of Caracas and the Algerian weavers, that it is an illumination that multiplies, that expands infinitely in every direction.

We have reached a liminal setting of the future-present-past where the choice between annihilation and protest, between death and liberation, is inescapable, is all that is left. Without light, what medical work is ostensibly possible? Health workers might think of themselves as implicated in the invitation to strike. I am thinking with the poem not just through its theoretical and aesthetic concerns but also in explicitly material terms, because it asks that of us. The poem locates itself in actual rebellion that explicitly addresses workers, calls for striking, invokes a transnational solidarity, and names (with clarity and with urgency) the worker's (inevitable) love for Palestine.

There is much for us, as health workers from the place now called Canada, to learn from Palestinian health workers past and present, whose history of organising imagined and practised a liberatory healthcare disentangled from imperialism and colonialism. In the essay "Palestine and the case for abolitionist medicine", the writers ask: "What would it look like for healthcare workers and patients around the world to not simply advocate for funnelling resources toward researching decontextualised "health risks" and humanitarian relief but to advocate for defunding the imperial systems of harm that produce them?" This question rearticulates, through a different specificity, the questions of "Abolition Medicine": *What might a public health approach to public safety look like? At this time, this question is an act of radical imagination.* Perhaps such a radical imagining could study transnationally, learning from Palestinian health workers, and could envision historically, learning from Palestine's history of health justice work.

On May 18, 2021, Palestinian healthcare workers with Israeli citizenship joined the Palestinian general strike (Abo-Basha and Beltrán 2021). Palestinian healthcare workers, through their protest and their theorising, demonstrate how colonial mechanisms aim to depoliticize health care as sites of neutrality both locally by disciplining a professional class of 'native clerks' with Israeli citizenship as well as transnationally through rending the political horizon of resistance to occupation into a humanitarian effort.

In Israel's "colonial health care industrial complex", Palestinian healthcare workers are needed both as "a source of medical labor and as eventual targets for the continued violent deprivation of the Palestinian population," and, into the historical present, Palestinian health workers are recruited as "brothers in arms" for the state's discourse of coexistence. By joining the general strike, Saleh Dabbah, a pharmacist and cultural writer who took part in the strike explains, health workers "burst through Israeli citizens' denial." *Burst through* – I think of Alsous's an *illumination that multiplies*, the *guaranteed light*.

Palestinian healthcare workers with Israeli citizenship call our attention to how the "violence that aims to discipline and depoliticize them through their professionalized labor also works to depoliticize global healthcare workers through humanitarianism". Such a humanitarianism is the purportedly apolitical medical work of attending to consequences of violence, rather than looking at what it is (colonialism and imperialism) that produces that violence. Ultimately, then, "the case of Palestinian healthcare workers shows us that 'health disparities' cannot be properly addressed without naming and challenging the structural harms that produce them" (ibid).

The doctors of Sharif's poem "Desired Appreciation" provide what could be considered a humanitarian care as described by "Palestine and the case for abolitionist medicine", which is a warped care that "ensure(s) the shoulders do not dislocate" and that "basic dietary needs" are met. But it is an ostensibly humanitarian care that advances a dispossessing politics. What if the torturer's doctor went on strike? Then the brutality of the state's subjection could no longer be tampered. The illusion of care would be lifted, and the health worker could no longer be narrativised into a somehow more palatable and somehow more tolerable imperialist violence. By striking, the terms of the struggle are distilled. The Palestinian healthcare workers, by joining the strike, reject and make explicit the colonial narratives of citizenship and border-making. Just as in "The Workers Love Palestine", the stakes of the struggle are a matter of life and death; as the Palestinian healthcare workers suspend their work and abstract themselves from the coloniser's narrative techniques, they too, in a manner, struggle for the sun. The sun is and is not a straightforward metaphor in the poem. The sun stands in for everything. The poem distils; the poem pressures.

"The Workers Love Palestine" – the title, and the proceeding poem, is, like the demand for abolition, an injunction. Though it is not in the scope of this essay to articulate the poem's Marxist politics, to see oneself as a worker, and not as a professional (a doctor, a member of the elite), and to realise one's alienated labour, is an important step in a political self-consciousness that is tied to abolition and to Palestinian liberation.

The last lines of "The Workers Love Palestine" read:

Language is merely the placeholder
for what the LAND has always known
Species being is an observation of MOM (preface)
Absent the wet painting of a razed village (sold)
This land is land
Land is land
    LAND LAND
I AM COMING
HOME

Inside the realisation that "language is merely the placeholder/for what the LAND has always known" is the reckoning that not every language is such a placeholder, and not every language holds the land's knowledge. Indeed, colonial languages intend to obscure what the land has always known and to work in tandem with the obliteration of that land. One work of the health worker is the discernment of such languages. We could call it a poetic attunement: to stay almost recklessly curious, to encounter with great intimacy where things are distilled (such as in poems), to be almost painfully open to the pressures of some languages (poetries). Attentiveness to this particular poem should necessitate an anti-colonial work, an anti-colonial health work that is interested in accessing and grasping something about care that has been forgotten or concealed by our present sequestrations of health and life. To be recruited by the poem and join the strike for light, rather than to be recruited by the nation-state as a state agent to incarcerate, torture, colonise, and advance imperial agendas, all the while ensuring "the arm does not dislocate" and maintaining a distinctly political apolitical position, also perhaps called a humanitarian position.

Importantly, even the placeholding language of Alsous's poem trembles, vibrates, and changes to the poem's own pressures. "This land is land" shifts to "Land is land" and then finally "LAND LAND" – the poem begins to forgo language, words are shed as land speaks of land. The poem performs its distillation of life as it leaps ahead and against how language, any language, binds. The poetry editor for *Jewish Currents*, Claire Shwartz introduces "The Workers Love Palestine" and writes of its last lines: "In the poem's final, struck-through line, even the language refuses, joins the strike". Whatever our poetic attunements, our narrative sensibilities, our radical curiosities, whatever our study of language, of the poem's distillation and the poem's pressures – we too, as health workers, must practise our own refusals, discursively and actually, and, sooner or later, join the strike.

Monica Kidd

Monica (https://www.monicakidd.ca/bio/) is a family physician working in Calgary, Canada. She is a mother, and runner. Originally educated as a biologist, she has worked in radio journalism and medical education, including the medical humanities. She has an extensive list of publications including poetry, and is an audiophile (https://www.curiaudio.com/monica-kidd/).

Monica writes: Well, hasn't this been an interesting thing to ponder? You asked me to consider the idea that "the medical mind (most clearly developed in diagnostic reasoning) and the poetic imagination (primarily in lyrical poetry) overlap – indeed, might be seen to be one and the same". You said, "If this is the case, then arguments for the value of the medical humanities in medicine are made redundant, as poetry is the same as medicine".

I initially recoiled at this. It sounded too much like poet-physicians using the (largely theoretical) pedagogical value of the medical humanities in fostering empathy, improving visual diagnosis, teambuilding, whatever, as a stalking horse behind which we would continue to happily scribble, justifying our own creative passions in the context of our medical professional lives. I often wonder why we try always to broadcast its worth to our more materialist, positivist colleagues? I think most people, when they lower the flags of their own knowledge traditions, recognise the worth of diverse epistemologies.

Ensconced in clinical practice and raising children and dealing with a pandemic and all its attendant uncertainties, I had begun to think of the perennial "Why does poetry matter in medicine" question as handwringing, mostly a matter of ego, à la Rodney Dangerfield ("I don't get no respect"); I wanted to move past it and just read, write and love the damned poetry.

But, of course, you know I can't quite.

In medicine, and medical education, the fundamental currency is the "case". A person has a troublesome symptom or sign and seeks medical assessment and resolution. The healthcare professional hears the person's story, seeks clarification through dialogue, examines the person's body and/or thoughts, triangulates all these data points with what she recalls from her recollection of pathophysiology, epidemiology, natural history, anatomy, pharmacology, the social determinants of health, local healthcare resources and health beliefs, and eventually comes up with a plan of investigation and care. She gathers empirical knowledge to which she applies schemata and arrives at a diagnosis through abductive reasoning.

Because there are a host of other "cases" in line behind this one, sometimes that process needs to happen in fifteen minutes or less. Also, healthcare professionals are increasingly evaluated according to how well they adhere to the latest clinical guidelines crafted by international panels of experts. Diagnosis gives way to pattern recognition, treatment to recipes. Little wonder then that medical pedagogy draws on machine learning, the study of how algorithms improve through repetition and revision. Or that artificial intelligence begins to make its way into the clinic.

But anyone who has sat in a room with another person and tried to figure out what they want and need, knows something premedical is also happening. Something largely social, maybe even moral. Something required in the listening and the synthesis that machines can't do yet. In the 1990s and early 2000s, literary criticism took a turn toward ethics, and, among other questions, whether reading makes us better people. This was already a central preoccupation of the medical humanities, as modern treatises on the importance of bridging the supposed art/science divide in medicine are more than a hundred years old. Foundational to this literature is the (contested) idea that an education in the humanities makes the student (doctor) more humane. Contained within literary ethics is the concept of a "readerly ethic", something discussed at length in a PhD dissertation entitled *Felt Thought: Neuroscience, Modernism and the Intelligence of Poetry* by Matt Langione (2016) at University of California, Berkeley.

Let's say that a patient can be considered a text, and the doctor a reader. This is not intended to dehumanise patients, but to suggest that in any diagnostic encounter, a physician will be presented rich complexity with which she will need to find a way to engage. She will always miss some things and overemphasise others, according to her own receptivity, experience, recall and computations, not to mention whether she is hungry, or was up all night with an elderly dog, or her pager is going off. The readerly imperative for a person reading a novel to be present with the text is largely internal; the readerly imperative for a physician sitting with a patient is internal as well, but also imposed externally by professional ethics and fiduciary responsibility.

As a poet, I'm probably biased in saying this, but I believe the effort, the readerly ethic, one brings to reading (and writing) poetry is parallel to the effort one brings to receiving and synthesising information in a clinical encounter. The twentieth century German philosopher Martin Heidegger described this as *Dasein* (Being, or presence) and defined it as an interpretive disposition. In other words: curiosity, patience, sitting in the discomfort of non-understanding. I guess in this way I am simply agreeing with Rita Charon when she says medicine practised with narrative competence requires "the ability to acknowledge, absorb, interpret, and act on the stories and plights of others".

But you are wondering if we should move on from that, as educators and professionals. When I came back to you for clarification on your proposal, you also asked me to consider whether poetry and medical diagnosis occupied the same epistemological space: that is, if they both relied on epiphany. Whether acknowledging this might open up new methods of teaching.

Back to Langione's PhD. He argues that poets were understood during the Romantic era in the first part of the 19th century as lone geniuses; the fact that a poet belonged to a culture, or occupied a social rank, or a moment in history, mattered little – his words came in a flash of brilliance based entirely on his *a priori* qualities. When along comes T. S. Eliot, who believed that the work of the poet, talent notwithstanding, was first to be as well versed as possible in tradition; i.e. the poet can display flashes of brilliance only to the extent that he is a beneficiary of the culture in which he is immersed. Langione compares Eliot's beliefs to those of the 19th century mathematician and philosopher Charles Peirce who argued that scientists rely on intuition primed by careful empirical study: "For while the poet or the scientist absents himself at the crucial moment—in the sense of an 'unconscious' cognitive absence—he is responsible for conditioning his mind to perform correctly in his "absence"" (ibid.: 144). Put another way: "poetry is not a turning loose of emotion, but an escape from emotion".

This is the closest I've come to offering a "proof" of your idea that medicine and poetry are both epiphanic, relying on cognitive spaces in a conditioned mind into which intuition steps. How to teach (or even model) that is another matter entirely. It may be that poetry's bigger contribution to medicine is through *ostrananie*, or defamiliarisation: making the familiar strange. Jolting us to attention, waking us up again to presence and the readerly ethic.

Caroline Wellbery

Caroline (https://sites.google.com/a/georgetown.edu/mdarts/) is a Professor in the Department of Family Medicine at Georgetown University Medical Center, Washington, DC. She has a wealth of experience in family medicine, medical education, and medical humanities. Caroline completed a PhD in Comparative Literature at Stanford University, California. Her burning passions are climate change education and social advocacy for health improvement. Oh, by the way, she speaks French, German and Spanish as well as her native tongue.

Once when I was a medical student, I approached a patient who was hospitalised for investigation of a mysterious diarrheal illness. I dutifully began my structured questioning, but instead of answering, the patient asked if he could recite some of his poetry. He stood behind the tray table as though speaking from a podium and began to declaim his verse.

While poetry rarely plays such a direct role in the clinical setting, there are, nevertheless, moments when some understanding of poetry illuminates what is happening in the patient encounter. One example that comes to mind is a conversation I had with a patient who had body contouring after significant weight loss following bypass surgery. I asked her for her back story, in which she described a drowning accident that killed her husband and daughter. She ate her way out of sorrow. A while into the narrative, she mentioned that she was "drowning in fat". I don't think she even realised the connection she'd made. Clearly similes and metaphors are a place to search for patients' explanatory models.

At a more complex level, one can explore an analogy between the poem and what is called the "clinical gestalt". This term is sometimes used for "overall impression" which can be broken into the network of different pieces of information that "seasoned" clinicians (re)assemble to make their diagnoses. It turns out, at least according to one study on the diagnosis of heart failure, that a physician's sense of "clinical gestalt" is an excellent diagnostic predictor exceeding the informative value of any concatenation of individual diagnostic components. It seems to me that the formation of clinical gestalt is similar to the kind of structural and metaphorical cross-referencing we do when we interpret a poem. This clinical intuition serves the experienced clinician not because of some vague aura, but rather is derived from the precise assemblage of closely observed clinical instances that together set a tone and form a coherent whole.

But maybe a more basic, layman's version of "clinical gestalt" is what truly brings together poetry and clinical medicine. Most of us clinicians know what it is like to step into a patient's room and, after just a few words, understand something about the emotional and psychological needs of this patient. Ronna Bloom, a psychotherapist and poet in residence at the University of Toronto, put this intuition to use when she experimented some years ago with a "spontaneous poetry booth" in public spaces, announcing her services by posting a sign that said "The Poet is In". Strangers would sit down with her, while Ms. Bloom offered to write them a poem and asked what they needed that poem to be about. Then, as she describes her process in a YouTube video, "I listen to them as widely as I can … to what's alive in the moment in the room, and I write whatever is coming" (https://www.youtube.com/watch?v=u9btLEBvaB8).

There is, she states, "a strange kind of chemistry that happens with the poem and the person". In other words, the poem becomes the locus of connection. Without this emotional resonance, the aforementioned role of metaphor and clinical gestalt alone do not fully account for the ways poetry informs the clinical encounter. The interactive, interpretive space created between the clinician and patient is where the poetry of healing occurs. If there is an actual poem to facilitate this outcome, so much the better.

Marta Arnaldi

Here is Marta's autobiographical summary:

> I grew up in Sanremo, in the Ligurian region of Italy, not far from the French border. After studying Medicine and Surgery at the University of Turin (2005–2007), I obtained a BA in Italian Literature from the same university (2010). My graduate education includes a MA in Modern Philology from the University of Pavia (2013), a MSt in Modern Languages from the University of Oxford (2014), and a DPhil in Medieval and Modern Languages, also from Oxford (2018). Since 2017, I have been a Stipendiary Lecturer in Italian at St Anne's College, Oxford, and I arrived at Queen's as a Laming Research Fellow in October 2019. In addition to my academic career, I am a writer and a ballet dancer (London RAD). My first collection of poems, *Itaca*, has won two international literary prizes.

Marta's contribution here is entitled "The Translational Imagination". She argues that this transcends our book's interest in the conversation between poetry and medicine, or offers the perspective through which both poetry and medicine can be re-visioned. Marta claims that patients are "foreign texts that call for translation".

The translational imagination

"The place of the other is the maybe."

I would like to evoke this sentence by Italian poet Chandra Livia Candiani (2018: 34) to introduce the idea of the translational imagination. The translational imagination is more than the sum of the lyrical and the medical imagination. It is the porous interzone between the two. At this point of intersection between the poetic and the clinical, diagnostic crossing, therapeutic meaning and perspectival changes are produced.

Diagnostic crossing

Illness is an encounter with alterity. Some patients become foreign speakers of their own mother tongues (Kristeva 1987), resisting standard language and resorting to figurative speech, as disease confronts the sufferer with the challenges of inexpressibility (Scarry 1985). This sense of estrangement becomes apparent during consultation, "because a [linguistic and] cultural gap always exists between the [doctor] and the patient" (Kortmann 2010). Patients are not just texts (Charon 2006); they are foreign texts that call for translation.

Therapeutic meaning

This translational act mobilises imagination. It is the way in which patients articulate their inner speech to give their body and mind a language (inward translation). It also represents patients' and doctors' interpretative efforts to step into each other's worlds (outward translation). This negotiation between the self and the other, the foreign and the familiar, loss and change is therapeutic. "New worlds are born between the lines" (Steiner 1998: 239).

Perspectival change

Illness asks us to think differently; it is a loss of the destination map that used to guide the ill person's life (Frank 2013: 1). It poses us before a prism of possibilities, not all of which are good. Medicine and poetry share with translation an ability to refract, reflect, and sometimes extend and/or improve life. They can be a promise of survival, one based on a paradoxical dosage of hospitality, uncertainty, aberrance, imperfection, error and trust. We need the doctors' as much as the poets' words to keep alive. The translational imagination carves out a space where we may be able to navigate between, and comprehend, our own as well as other peoples' speech.

The colours of translation

By nature, translation is the time-space of the other. Poets are doctors that treat our foreign condition, and vice versa. One has to turn the personal into the universal and the universal into the personal in order to heal and/or write. Translation is the postcolonial space where the poetic and the medical not only mirror one another but also coalesce and coexist.

The other place is the maybe.

Maybe the place is the other.

The other is the maybe-place.

Allan Peterkin

A veteran of the medical/health humanities movement in Canada, Allan is a professor of psychiatry at the University of Toronto. He is a founding editor of *Ars Medica: A Journal of Medicine, the Arts, and Humanities,* and has published poetry, fiction and critical essays on the arts in medicine, narrative-based medicine and the use of the humanities in medical education in Canadian and international journals. Allan has a first degree in English and French Literature and originally worked as a family physician before specialising in psychiatry. He is Program Head, Health, Arts and Humanities, University of Toronto.

To a young doctor

Make every diagnosis
a poem

The words you choose
will never matter more
(or be less forgotten)

Arrows and missiles to unseen targets
a reverberation of souls

For you
another organ or limb or brain
for them
the only one

Your words
do not just foretell
the odds of life or death
(or something in between)

They deliver hope
or render it stillborn
they make you a trusted ally
(or something else)

Choose them well
they are already
unforgettable

Make the words beautiful
a vessel to
carry whatever comes next

(Originally published in *CMAJ.* 2013; 185: 13)

Quentin Eichbaum

Quentin is professor of medical education and administration at Vanderbilt University School of Medicine (Nashville, Tennessee) where he developed and directs a programme in medical humanities. He is professor of pathology, microbiology, and immunology at Vanderbilt University Medical Center where he directs a clinical fellowship program, the pathology programme in global health, and the pathology education research programme. He was raised in Namibia and South Africa and attended Harvard Medical School and Harvard School of Public health in Boston. But this is just the foreground. The background is Renaissance man: writer, painter, humanities and arts devotee, medical humanities mover-and-shaker. He is a high-profile figure in global health and a passionate advocate for equity, equality and access to healthcare provision, particularly in African countries.

For Quentin, visual art, narrative and poetry intersect and feed the beating heart of medicine:

As a physician, poet and painter (watercolorist) working at a large academic medical center, there are a number of ways in which my poetic imagination and medical mind mirror each other. The first pertains to the nature of attention. Writing poetry keeps me paying attention to the world. While painting (as a visual art) compels me to pay attention to mostly the 'seen' world, poetry compels attention to both the seen and 'unseen' because language captures the full spectrum of our sensory input.

In practicing medicine, my poetic imagination compels me to pay close attention to the patient's words and use of language (sentences, phrasings, spaces between words, intonation, silences). Students and trainees sometimes appear perplexed at the time I take talking and listening to patients, and how I will follow a train of thought or a narrative thread that appears irrelevant to them. Even more frustrating to some students, I will sometimes start a discussion with a patient about the book(s) s/he is reading. The students may look bored and I read their minds as imploring me: "What does that have to do with the patient's care?" But I have been sufficiently surprised in my medical career to know how clinically relevant information can emerge from unlikely sources – just as unlikely sources feed into a poem. To these bored incurious students I suggest Faith Fitzgerald's (1999) essay "Curiosity" in which a "boring" patient with a broken arm is revealed, through the physician's curiosity, to be a survivor from the Titanic.

While talking to patients I may weave back and forth between the ambiguities and uncertainties of conversational narrative, and the specifics of the patient's diagnosis and care. Weaving back and forth between such domains of certainty and uncertainty has some similarity with writing a poem in which the imagination moves between clinching an exact word, phrase or line, and then re-entering domains of uncertainty and ambiguity.

In the US, senior physicians at academic teaching hospitals are called "attendings" (Epstein 2017). To my mind, the attending physician has to attend to three attentional domains at once. First, is the technical domain entailing the specifics of the diagnosis and treatment plan. Second, is the team of caregivers and trainees milling around and interacting with each other and the patient (are they functioning appropriately and professionally as they should, my attention asks). Third, and perhaps most demanding, is a domain of uncertainty and ambiguity of the dynamic and evolving clinical encounter with the patient and her family. This domain must also simultaneously take account of any uncertainties that emerge from the first two domains.

Developing the capacity to "attend" to all three domains at once takes years of experience – hence the term "attending". Trainees tend to focus mostly on the first technical domain (labs, numbers, data, radiology, EKGs, etc.) and often fail to understand that the attending has to move back and forth between all three attentional domains. In writing poetry there may be analogous levels of attention-shifting as the poet attends to: (1) the technicalities of language (words, avoidance of cliché, metaphorical consistency, etc.); (2) how the parts of the poem relate to and play off each other; and (3) the extent to which the technical aspects, the related parts of the poem, and its ambiguities and uncertainties contribute to the whole rather than unravelling the poem.

When I am with a patient, I will at some point casually ask: "So tell me your story" – by which I mean something less focussed than the "history of present illness" (HPI) which physicians generally tease from a patient at high velocity and with multiple interruptions. (Out the corner of my eye, I see the students cringe at my use of the word "story".) By story (versus HPI), I mean things like: how were you diagnosed, when did you first notice things were different, who was with you, where were you, how did you feel when you got your diagnosis, what was the context, what did you do next, how did your family and loved ones react? – and I let the patient speak uninterrupted.

True story usually starts with the question "What happened?" For the seriously ill patient that leads in quick succession to the next question "Why me?" I never cease to be surprised by the urge patients have to tell their stories naturally and uninterrupted rather than as part of a medical interrogation for the HPI. Stories want to come out into the world. As Arthur Frank (2013) writes: "Whether ill people want to tell stories or not, illness calls for stories". Stories want to come out from patients into the world the way a worthy poem wants to get out and breathe. Some of the best poems come out with least editing, and so it is with the patient's story – with least interruptions. Both have likely been incubating in silence for some time before being born. A patient's story that is forced out with multiple interruptions (as in the HPI) may miss critical elements and be susceptible to diagnostic biases such as premature closure and others (Croskerry 2009, 2013), just as a poem that is forced out and over-edited will lack capacity to breath and take flight in the world.

Finally, just as writing poetry (and painting) keep me paying attention to the world around me and sustain my wellbeing, so do paying attention and engaging in close noticing (Bleakley 2015) with patients in the clinical encounter, serving as mainstays against burnout in the demanding profession of medicine.

Megan EL Brown and Martina Kelly

Megan is a UK primary care doctor who has recently completed a PhD in medical education at Hull/York medical school UK. Martina is an Irish national family physician currently working in Calgary, Canada, and has recently completed her doctorate in medical education. She is Director of Family Medicine at the University of Calgary medical school.

Neither Megan nor Martina considers themselves to be poets, but they aspire to the role, as can be seen from their stirring contribution below.

Poetic diagnosis

Introduction

The controversial television character Gregory House, MD is renowned for his diagnostic acumen. Astute, witty, and insightful, he wowed public and physicians alike with his "eureka" problem-solving. Most diagnosis making is more painstaking, students learn predominantly by using hypothetico-deductive approaches to distil differentials into reasonable probabilities (Coderre et al. 2003). Diagnosis is approached as a logical progression, through which knowledge is synthesised, distilled and deduced. But is there more to diagnosis than the application of rational logic? Apollo, the ancient Greek god of healing, is also the god of music and poetry. How might poetic thinking inform diagnostic astuteness? Here, we explore the possibilities of poetry to pique, play, and provoke diagnostic thinking, inspired by a patient who presented coughing up "ropes of phlegm". Poetry too coughs up metaphors.

Our contribution opens with a poem, written together, in response to the patient's consultation. Reflecting poetically on our experience allowed us to exercise our empathic imaginations to grasp more deeply the patient's perspective, and, in doing so, opened up a new horizon of diagnostic understanding. We hope the reader will be prompted to consider how the language and imagery used within the space of the medical consultation may deepen diagnostic thought. We follow this poem with the presentation of a clinical summary, as traditionally communicated in the clinical setting. We then ground our reflection in phenomenological ideas to offer thoughts as to how poetic techniques can expand traditional diagnostic thinking.

Ropes of phlegm

> I give to you this handkerchief,
> Doctor,
> Made by my wife's worn hands
> Our best
> Christening white, embroidered
> With love, won't you look?

> Sticky cotton gently parted
> And nestled within
> Ropes of phlegm
> Wrapped and offered to you,
> Doctor,
> Won't you look?

> Thick and tangled, a
> Fist of knotted green, a
> Creature from the shadowed spittoon,
> Alien to these aged eyes but not to you,
> Doctor,
> Won't you look?

> I'm sure it's clung within
> Three months now
> At night it seems to climb
> Twist until the void where breath once stretched
> Collapses

You can hold it
If you like
Rotten lung fruit
I won't mind
Not if you don't,
When you look

Doctor
Now I've coughed
My ropes of phlegm
Into your hands
Take the helm and
Unmoor me
Please
Unmoor me
From this breathless pit

Clinical summary

Mr Smith is a 74-year-old male non-smoker presenting with a three-month history of worsening nocturnal dyspnoea and dyspnoea on exertion. He reports a cough productive of thick, green sputum. His past medical history includes recurrent community acquired pneumonia and osteoarthritis. On examination, he has finger clubbing and crackles were auscultated at the bases of both lungs. On review, patient's sputum appears purulent and profuse.

Reflection

We would like you to take a moment to reflect on the poem we have presented above, and the thoughts you have in regard to this patient's diagnosis and future care. We would then like you to do the same with the clinical summary we have presented. Once you have reflected on both accounts of this patient's presentation, take a moment to consider the differences between the two accounts, and whether or not they affected you differently. Below, we present our own thoughts on this matter, as authors of both summaries. It may be interesting for you to know whether your perspective aligns or differs from ours.

Diagnosis

Though in some ways, the ultimate diagnosis of this patient does not matter, as it is the process of diagnostic reasoning we plan to focus on and discuss, rather than the outcome *per se*, in the interest of completeness we offer you the ultimate diagnosis of this patient: bronchiectasis.

How do poetry and diagnostic reasoning interact?

Phenomenology is an approach to exploring individuals' lived experiences of significant or day-to-day events – of phenomena (Neubauer, Witkop and Varpio 2019). Hermeneutic or interpretative phenomenology maintains that understanding is subjective, and approaches adopting this orientation move beyond description of phenomena to explore the meaning of individuals' experiences (Bynum and Varpio 2018). For phenomenologists subscribing to a more hermeneutic worldview, poetry plays a large role in thinking – Van Manen (2014) refers to phenomenology as a "poetising project", while poetry preoccupied Heidegger's (1971) later publications. Exploring patients' lived experiences of disease, illness and circumstances is part of one's role as an empathic and holistic clinician and contributes to practicing in a person-centred way (Dearing and Steadman 2009; Doherty and Thompson 2014). Poetry can help attune clinicians to the lived experiences of patients, and to their own perspectives, in ways that help open them up to the patient's experience beyond a traditional hypothetico-deductive model of clinical reasoning alone (Finn, Brown and Laughey 2020; Sgro 2021).

The phenomenologist Gadamer (1989) proposes that understanding and knowledge be conceptualised as a mode of being. For Gadamer, spending time to reflect on and consider the language another person uses and, within this the poetic conventions of that language, is the way in which understanding of that person's lived experience is constructed (Galvin and Todres 2009). Language opens up and extends our thinking – indeed, understanding itself is a "language event" focussed on a "silent agreement" between participants in a conversation (Gadamer 2006). This silent agreement, built up of conversational aspects held in common, is what makes social solidarity possible and shows that the traditional scientific approach to understanding is an inappropriate starting point for self-awareness.

Simply put, words get their meaning from the open space of living conversation. We can pay attention to this space, by thinking poetically about our experiences to sharpen our sensitivity to language, in reflecting on the language and imagery another uses (Rosenblatt 1978; Richardson 1992). Constructing the poetic summary of our patient's presentation attuned us to the remarkable and vivid phrases he used to describe his breathlessness and sputum: "ropes of phlegm" was a descriptor – a striking embodied metaphor – that particularly stood out to us, invoking imagery of thick, coarse ropes. It was a descriptor that did not only perfectly describe the sputum this patient had brought with him but offered us insight into his struggle with this sputum. Ropes are usually substantial, long and easily knotted, we could imagine and empathise with the way in which he had pictured them as dense, heavy and choking, as though the effort of coughing them up was like dragging wet, heavy ropes to moor a boat.

Gendlin (1981) employed the concept of "felt sense" that resonates in relation to poetic thinking within diagnosis. "Felt sense" is a sort of ongoing interaction we each have with the world. It involves an awareness that is embodied and helps us to make sense of the complex world before us in an intuitive way (Rappaport 2013). Felt sense and emotions are often conflated, though they do differ (Todres and Galvin 2008). Meeting a long-absent but close friend or relative may make you feel happy (an emotion), or it may engender a sweeping sense of warming glow that spreads through your body – this is a felt sense. Felt senses can be difficult to describe, but they help us make what Todres and Galvin (2008) term "embodied interpretations" of the world. In the context of the consultation room, paying attention to a patient involves simultaneous apprehension of their situation and the language they use, a meaning making.

Our recollections helped us to find "words which work" to put our shared felt sense within that consultation into words. In this case, as MB probed MK's recollections, each question enabled MK to recall her felt sense of this particular patient. She recalled in detail the elderly man and his wife sitting anxiously in her consulting room, fearful of a diagnosis of cancer. This was not stated but present, nonetheless, expressed through anxious eyes, hunched shoulder and the visit of husband and wife together. She recalled Mr Smith wearing a tweed suit jacket over his hand knit sweater. She recalled, later, after the poem was written that Mr Smith previously worked on the docks. In some manner, the poem seems to have captured that pre-reflective, or unconscious awareness, of Mr Smith's employment.

Considering our own reactions to the patient also facilitated reflexivity (Freeman 2001). We were able to consider the language the patient used, and how his actions made us feel, in particular the way in which the sputum was offered up in a delicate handkerchief. This led us to consider the vulnerability of patients in such situations and the shame and stigma often associated with bodily secretions. This further stimulated a discussion about the trust many patients place in clinicians. We also discussed our own preconceptions regarding the condition this patient was ultimately diagnosed with – bronchiectasis – that led us to considering the mystery of the term and how it must feel to receive a diagnosis using such an alien term. Stimulated by our attempts to poeticise our experience, this reflection offered us a chance to consider this patient's experience far more humanistically than we had previously in discussing the clinical features, signs and symptoms, of bronchiectasis. We had empathy for this patient, we felt connected to him, considering our own roles in a new and more deliberate light. Sgro (2021) recalls that, for the poet Edward Hirsch, poetry is "a way of connecting – through the medium of language – more deeply with yourself, even as you connect more deeply with others". This encapsulates our experiences of writing a poem about this patient encounter. Empathy and reflexivity are both critical to patient care (Hojat et al. 2001; Iedema 2011) including compassionate and person-centred diagnosis (Baarts, Tulinius and Reventlow 2000; Bellet and Maloney 1991). We then see a role for poetry in shaping and encouraging empathy and practitioner reflexivity.

We feel it is important to highlight that although our poem is written in the first-person, it is an interpretation of this patient's experience, akin to many forms of qualitative analysis within health professions education (Peshkin 2000). We do not assume we can speak on behalf of the patient we have represented here. We instead subscribe to Gadamer's (1989) conceptualisation of understanding as "a play between context and detail, the personal and the relational, the past and the future" and believe that constructing poetry to convey the experience of the medical consultation from the perspective of another communicates a shared understanding, or meaning created in the space between two people. In this way, we hope the poem that we have presented represents the voices and experiences both of us, as clinicians, but also of the patient, given the way we have paid close attention and made efforts to respect his voice through detailed reflection on his story and consideration of the ways in which he used language and imagery.

Summary

We believe that poetry has the power to expand diagnostic thinking. By engaging with poetry and poetic conventions, clinicians can integrate their experiential and embodied knowledge of a person to transform diagnosis from a cognitive dilemma of problem-solving into one of hermeneutic engagement.

Engaging with poetry and poetic conventions may take many forms – though we have written a poem with one another, we do not believe engagement with poetry needs to be formal. Discussing and reflecting on the language a patient uses, what this may mean for you and them, and considering how their words and actions imbue you with certain felt senses can also be done relatively informally, in personal or collaborative reflective spaces.

We envision that reading and discussing poetry individually or in groups concerning patients with similar conditions or experiences may also help attune clinicians to their own perspectives, fostering a humanistic connection with themselves, as well as encouraging connection with the lived experiences of patients. We speculate that our reflection about the need for humility within medical practice was, at least in part, stimulated by our own vulnerability, as we ventured into a relatively unfamiliar, shared creative space, exercising our imaginations to engage with language and our own artistic thoughts within a conversational space (both with one another, and with the patient we pictured). Before we felt connected to the patient's experience, we first felt we had to connect more humanely and honestly with ourselves, granting ourselves the dispensation to dwell among language, to express our "felt senses", be they emotional, joyous, or more negative and perhaps stigmatised felt senses, such as disgust.

In addition to attuning clinicians to their inner selves and outward to patients' meanings, we also speculate that considering and writing about diagnosis, or one's interpretations, poetically may open a portal of understanding to limited models of clinical reasoning. The traditional hypothetico-deductive model of diagnosis, prioritising scientific knowledge over the patient perspective, needs to be expanded. Contemporary diagnostic strategies within medicine represent a form of "epistemic injustice" that silences human expressions, replacing them instead with reductive biotechnical language. Fricker (2007) writes at length about epistemic injustice, noting that it is related to the silencing of some forms of knowledge, and can occur when others' experiences are not well understood.

Within medicine, the technical language used to describe disease, diagnosis and management is a form of epistemic injustice against patients whose experiences do not fit the concepts known to the technical lexicon of biomedicine. Physicians' lived experiences, too, are silenced through the way in which the hypothetico-deductive model prioritises scientific knowledge. We propose that engagement with poetry can acclimatise those seeped in the technical lexicon of biomedicine to other language codes and experiences. Poetic diagnostic thinking creates opportunities to affirm the testimonial value of patient narratives, and highlights the significance of hermeneutic engagement with patients. Where the hypothetico-deductive model advertises scientific fact, poetic approaches to diagnosis remind us of our constitutive engagement with the world – where meaning rests with involvement, one with another.

References

Abo-Basha A, Beltrán S. 2021, June 5. Palestine and the Case for Abolition Medicine. Retrieved from https://www.madamasr.com/en/2021/06/05/opinion/u/palestine-and-the-case-for-abolitionist-medicine/

Alsous P. 2021, April 16. The Workers Love Palestine. Retrieved from https://jewishcurrents.org/the-workers-love-palestine/

Baarts C, Tulinius C, Reventlow S. Reflexivity – A Strategy for a Patient-Centred Approach in General Practice. *Family Practice*. 2000; 17: 430–34.

Bellet P, Maloney M. The Importance of Empathy as an Interviewing Skill in Medicine. *Journal of American Medical Association*. 1991; 266: 1831–32.

Bleakley A. 2015. *Medical Humanities and Medical Education: How the Medical Humanities Can Shape Better Doctors*: Abingdon: Routledge.

Brand D. 2018. *The Shape of Language*. London: Poetry Foundation.

Brooks G. 1990. *Poetry Lectures*. London: Poetry Foundation.

Bynum W, Varpio L. When I Say… Hermeneutic Phenomenology. *Medical Education*. 2018; 52: 252–53.

Candiani CL. 2018. *Il Silenzio È Cosa Viva: L'Arte della Meditazione*. Turin: Einaudi.

Charon R. 2006. *Narrative Medicine: Honoring the Stories of Illness*. Oxford: Oxford University Press.

Coderre S, Mandin H, Harasym P, Fick G. Diagnostic Reasoning Strategies and Diagnostic Success. *Medical Education*. 2003; 37: 695–703.

Croskerry P. Clinical Cognition and Diagnostic Error: Applications of a Dual Process Model of Reasoning. *Advances in Health Sciences Education*. 2009; 14: 27–35.

Croskerry, P. From Mindless to Mindful Practice – Cognitive Bias and Clinical Decision Making. *New England Journal of Medicine*. 2013; 368: 2445–48.

Dearing K, Steadman S. Enhancing Intellectual Empathy: The Lived Experience of Voice Simulation. *Perspectives in Psychiatric Care*. 2009; 45: 173–82.

Doherty M, Thompson H. Enhancing Person-Centred Care through the Development of a Therapeutic Relationship. *British Journal of Community Nursing*. 2014; 19: 502–7.

Epstein R. 2017. *Attending: Medicine, Mindfulness, and Humanity*. New York: Simon and Schuster.

Finn G, Brown M, Laughey W. Holding a Mirror up to Nature: The Role of Medical Humanities in Postgraduate Primary Care Training. *Education for Primary Care*. 2021; 32: 73–77.

Fitzgerald FT. Curiosity. *Annals of Internal Medicine*. 1999; 130: 70–72.

Frank A. 1995/2013. *The Wounded Storyteller: Body, Illness, and Ethics*. Chicago, IL: University of Chicago Press.

Freeman M. Between Eye and Eye Stretches an Interminable Landscape: The Challenge of Philosophical Hermeneutics. *Qualitative Inquiry*. 2001; 7: 646–58.

Fricker M. 2007. *Epistemic Injustice: Power and the Ethics of Knowing*. Oxford: Oxford University Press.

Gadamer H. 1989. *Truth and Method*. London: Sheed & Ward.

Gadamer H. Language and Understanding. *Theory, Culture & Society*. 2006; 23: 13–27.

Galvin K, Todres L. Poetic Inquiry & Phenomenological Research: The Practice of 'Embodied Interpretation'. *Poetic Inquiry*. 2009; January 1: 307–16.

Gendlin E. 1981. *Focusing*. New York: Bantam Books.

Heidegger M. 1971. *On the Way to Language*. New York: Harper & Row.

Hojat M, Mangione S, Gonnella J, et al. Empathy in Medical Education and Patient Care. *Academic Medicine*. 2001; 76: 669.

Iedema R. Creating Safety by Strengthening Clinicians' Capacity for Reflexivity. *BMJ Quality & Safety*. 2011; 20: i183–6.

Iwai Y, Khan ZH, DasGupta S. Abolition Medicine. *Lancet*. 2020; 396: 158–59.

Kortmann F. Transcultural Psychiatry: From Practice to Theory. *Transcultural Psychiatry*. 2010; 47: 203–23.

Kristeva J. 1987. *Black Sun: Depression and Melancholia*. New York: Columbia University Press.

Langione MP. 2016. Felt Thought: Neuroscience, Modernism and the Intelligence of Poetry. PhD thesis. University of California, Berkeley.

Neubauer B, Witkop C, Varpio L. How Phenomenology Can Help us Learn from the Experiences of Others. *Perspectives on Medical Education*. 2019; 8: 90–97.

Peshkin A. The Nature of Interpretation in Qualitative Research. *Educational Researcher*. 2000; 29: 5–9.

Rappaport L. Trusting the Felt Sense in Art-Based Research. *Journal of Applied Arts & Health*. 2013; 4: 97–104.

Richardson L. 1992. The Consequences of Poetic Representation: Writing the Other Rewriting the Self. In: C Ellis, M Flaherty (eds.) *Investigating Subjectivity*. London: Sage.

Rodriguez D (undated). *Abolition Is Our Obligation*. Lecture.

Rosenblatt L. 1978. *The Reader, the Text, the Poem: The Transactional Theory of the Literary Work*. Carbondale: Southern Illinois University Press.

Rukeyser M. 1996. *The Life of Poetry*. Middletown, CT: Paris Press.

Scarry E. 1985. *The Body in Pain: The Making and Unmaking of the World.* New York: Oxford University Press.

Sgro G. Earthed Lightning: A Prescription for Poetry in Practice and Teaching. *Academic Medicine.* 2021; 96: 1105–7.

Sharif S. 2016. *Look: Poems.* Minneapolis, MN: Graywolf Press.

Steiner G. 1998. *After Babel: Aspects of Language & Translation.* Oxford: Oxford University Press.

Todres L, Galvin K. Embodied Interpretation: A Novel Way of Evocatively Re-Presenting Meanings in Phenomenological Research. *Qualitative Research.* 2008; 8: 568–83.

Van Manen M. 2014. *Phenomenology of Practice: Meaning-Giving Methods in Phenomenological Research and Writing.* London: Routledge.

Appendix 1

Links to poems

Due to copyright restrictions on how much of a poem can be reproduced in a critical work such as this book (known as "Fair Use"), poem extracts are short. The reader is encouraged to use the online links provided in the book to read poems in full.

Abse, Dannie: White Coat, Purple Coat (collection) https://www.poetry-foundation.org/poets/dannie-abse

Abse, Dannie: "Anniversary" https://www.poetryfoundation.org/poetrymagazine/browse?contentId=26744

Ashbery, John: "Paradoxes and Oxymorons" https://www.poetryfounda-tion.org/poems/50986/paradoxes-and-oxymorons

Beckett, Samuel: "Ping" https://astrofella.wordpress.com/2020/12/30/ping-samuel-beckett/

Cornish, Mary: "Numbers" https://www.poetryfoundation.org/poetrymagazine/poems/40877/numbers-56d21ecff2141

Coulehan, Jack: "I'm Gonna Slap Those Doctors" https://utmedhumanities.wordpress.com/2014/10/13/im-gonna-slap-those-doctors-jack-coulehan/

Dickinson, Emily: "Tell all the truth, but tell it slant -1263" https://www.poetryfoundation.org/poems/56824/tell-all-the-truth-but-tell-it-slant-1263

Dickinson, Emily: "I heard a Fly buzz – when I died" https://www.poetryfoundation.org/poems/45703/i-heard-a-fly-buzz-when-i-died-591

Ferry, David: "Soul" https://www.pbs.org/newshour/arts/weekly-poem-soul

Hecht, Anthony: "More Light! More Light!" https://allpoetry.com/More-Light!-More-Light!

Keats, John: "This Living Hand" https://www.poetryfoundation.org/poems/50375/this-living-hand-now-warm-and-capable

Khalvati, Mimi: "Afterwardness" https://www.theguardian.com/books/booksblog/2020/nov/30/poem-of-the-week-afterwardness-by-mimi-khalvati

Kinnell, Galway: "Wait" https://poets.org/poem/wait

Logue, Christopher: "All Day Permanent Red" https://poetryarchive.org/poem/all-day-permanent-red-extract/

Long, Rachel: "Hotel Art, Barcelona" https://www.panmacmillan.com/blogs/literary/inspiring-poems-by-female-poets

Milosz, Czeslaw: "Ars Poetica" https://www.poetryfoundation.org/poems/49455/ars-poetica-56d22b8f31558

Orang, Bahar: "Where Things Touch: A Meditation on Beauty" http://open-book.ca/News/Read-an-Excerpt-from-Bahar-Orang-s-Where-Things-Touch-A-Meditation-on-Beauty

Partridge, Elise: "Domestic Interior: Child Watching Mother" https://howapoemmoves.wordpress.com/2016/10/27/domestic-interior-child-watching-mother-by-elise-partridge/

Plath, Sylvia: "Tale of a Tub" https://plathpoetry.livejournal.com/

Plath, Sylvia: "Daddy" https://www.poetryfoundation.org/poems/48999/daddy-56d22aafa45b2

Redgrove, Peter: "Thunder-and-Lightning Polka" (see in Collected Poems: https://b-ok.cc/book/4624031/683584?id=4624031&secret=683584)

Rich, Adrienne: "Tear Gas" https://nepantlerablog.files.wordpress.com/2016/02/the-dream-of-a-common-language-adrienne-rich.pdf

Richter, Jennifer: "My Daughter Brings Home Bones" https://www.poetryfoundation.org/poems/90104/my-daughter-brings-home-bones

Sexton, Anne: "The Ballad of the Lonely Masturbator" https://www.poetryfoundation.org/poems/42574/the-ballad-of-the-lonely-masturbator

Sexton, Anne: "In Celebration of My Uterus" https://www.poetryfoundation.org/poems/42573/in-celebration-of-my-uterus

Stevens, Wallace: "Certain Phenomena of Sound" https://www.books-cool.com/en/The-Collected-Poems-of-Wallace-Stevens-738769/19

Stevens, Wallace: "Sunday Morning" https://www.poetryfoundation.org/poetrymagazine/poems/13261/sunday-morning

Stevens, Wallace: "The Man Whose Pharynx Was Bad" http://bactra.org/Poetry/Stevens/The_Man_Whose_Pharynx_Was_Bad.html

Whitman, Walt: "I Sing the Body Electric" https://www.poetryfoundation.org/poems/45472/i-sing-the-body-electric

Williams, William Carlos: "A Cold Front" https://www.poetryfoundation.org/poetrymagazine/browse?contentId=22429

Williams, William Carlos: "Asphodel, That Greeny Flower" https://poets.org/poem/asphodel-greeny-flower-excerpt

Williams, William Carlos: "Arrival" https://www.poemhunter.com/poem/arrival/

Young, George: "Tell Me" https://www.acpjournals.org/doi/10.7326/0003-4819-137-5_Part_1-200209030-00016

Zambrano, Maria: "Lengua" (language, tongue, lingo) https://www.wordswithoutborders.org/article/lengua-mara-zambrano

Index

Note: *Italic* page numbers refer to figures.

orientation to here-and-now space and place 163–164; subjectivity and confession 155–159; tolerance of ambiguity embracing empathy 159; *see also* poetry

Macbeth (Shakespeare) 182–183
Making Stories (Bruner) 35
"Making Strange: A Role for the Humanities in Medical Education" 87
Malik, Kenan 229
Marcus, Eric 80
Marsh, Alec 8
Marx, Karl 197
Matsuo Basho 147
McCrum, Robert 184
McEntyre, Marilyn 109, 207, 212
McLuhan, Marshall 227
McNamara, Patrick 34–35
medical gaze 139–142
medical imagination 167–187
medical interview 85–86; meticulously writing out the interview 89–92; poetry alone (text only transcript) 92–95; slow jamming 86–95
medical masses, poetry-thought for 235–238
medical moods 155–159
medical students: kindling poetic imaginations of 211–212; poetry of 4–5, 26, 38, 121
medical work 15–16
medicine: contemporary 124; manual for poetry-thought in 238–240; and memory 112–113; and poetry 7–10, 115, 130–131, 189–191; tacit rules of 111–112
memory and medicine 112–113
Mercian Hymns (Hill) 103, 109
metaphor count *see* metaphors
metaphors 8, 12, 116, 124, 126; engineering 52–53, 58; generating new 174–176; and imagination 71; "maximum pain" 131; and Narrative Medicine 44–45, 47; and poetry 13; as vehicles of expression 153–155; Well and Will 120
metaphor types *see* metaphors
method, poetry as 260–266
Meza, James 45, 48
Michaels, Anne 180
Milosz, Czeslaw 38–39
Minimalism 199, 201, 204
mnemonics 18

Montello, Martha 26
Montgomery Hunter, Kathryn 17, 24–25, 44, 50
mood 155–159
Mulemi, B.A. 177
My Own Country: A Doctor's Story (Verghese) 81

narrative: *vs.* discursive argument 12; illness 4; patients' as reconstructions and translations 72–75; as Procrustes's bed 62–72; and story 30–34
narrative-based medicine 26; *see also* Narrative Medicine
narrative competence 25, 31, 39–40, 44–45
Narrative Ethics: The Role of Stories in Bioethics 26
narrative imperialism 23–40; critiques of 34–37; false identification 37–40; generic narrative medicine 24–30; story and narrative 30–34
Narrative Medicine 3, 12, 81, 198–200, 203; absence of lyric poetry in 64–67; commodification of 32; defined 30; false identification 37–40; handmaiden to biomedicine 43–51; history of generic 24–30; interpretive tool 51–57; lack of self-critique within 32; patient's story *vs.* doctor's narrative 31, 37–40; problems of definition 62–72; reach 95–96; use of psychoanalysis 78–81
Narrative Medicine: Honoring the Stories of Illness (Charon) 32
narrative reciprocity 30
Narrativism 23–24
"negative capability" 159, 216
Nemeth-Loomis, Tisha 133
New Criticism 56, 78, 227, 238
Nguyen V-K. 58
Nietzsche, Friedrich 197, 257
non-narrative poetry 13, 15–16, 23–24, 29, 39, 57, 109
Nowotny, Helga 219, 228
Nowottny, Winifred 230, 231–232
Nussbaum, Martha 157

Oates, Joyce Carole 50
"objectification" of patients 131
Object-Oriented Ontology (OOO) 52, 104, 127–128, 168, 176, 224; Sylvia Plath's 129–134
objects 130; etymology of 130; fixation 133; orientation 131

For Product Safety Concerns and Information please contact our EU
representative GPSR@taylorandfrancis.com
Taylor & Francis Verlag GmbH, Kaufingerstraße 24, 80331 München, Germany